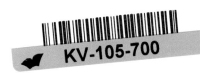

Health, medicine, and the sea

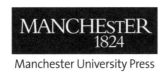

MANCHESTER
1824

Manchester University Press

Health, medicine, and the sea

Australian Voyages, c.1815–1860

Katherine Foxhall

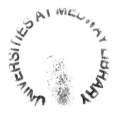

Manchester University Press
Manchester and New York

*distributed in the United States exclusively
by Palgrave Macmillan*

Published by Manchester University Press
Oxford Road, Manchester M13 9NR, UK
and Room 400, 175 Fifth Avenue, New York, NY 10010, USA
www.manchesteruniversitypress.co.uk

Distributed in the United States exclusively by
Palgrave Macmillan, 175 Fifth Avenue, New York,
NY 10010, USA

Distributed in Canada exclusively by
UBC Press, University of British Columbia, 2029 West Mall,
Vancouver, BC, Canada V6T 1Z2

British Library Cataloguing-in-Publication Data
A catalogue record for this book is available from the British Library

Library of Congress Cataloging-in-Publication Data applied for

ISBN   978 0 7190 8571 0 paperback

First published 2012

Typeset
by Carnegie Book Production, Lancaster
Printed in Great Britain
by TJ International Ltd, Padstow

Contents

Maps and figures

Maps

Figures

Acknowledgements

I spent seven great years in the History Department at the University of Warwick, where my doctoral supervisors, Margot Finn, Sarah Hodges, and Catherine Cox motivated and helped to shape my ideas for this project from the start. They turned me into a historian years after Andy Speake first engaged my interest. Hilary Marland, Colin Jones, Mathew Thomson, and Claudia Stein were also always generous with time and knowledge. Sarah-Easterby Smith, Lisa Grant, Debbie Toner, Lydia Plath, Kate Smith, Lucy Allwright, Philippa Hubbard, Jonathan Willis, Helen Cowie, Laura Sangha, and Tracy Horton made postgraduate work a distinctly sociable business.

Mark Harrison and David Arnold examined my PhD thesis, and I am grateful for their engagement, criticism, and ongoing support.

From 2008 to 2010 the staff, postdocs and students at the Centre for the History of Science, Technology and Medicine in Manchester gave me a whole new set of ways to think about disease, health, and medicine. Mick Worboys' practical advice and support was invaluable. Vlad Jankovic, Ian Burney, John Pickstone, Flurin Condrau, and Carsten Timmerman were generous with knowledge, Lyn Schumaker was an inspiration besides that. Rob Kirk, Elizabeth Toon, Duncan Wilson, Vicky Long, Emma Jones, Neil Pemberton, Mike Brown, and Leucha Veneer were great company, moral support, and astute readers in the 'West Wing'.

Molly Rogers read through this entire manuscript, some of it more than once, and provided a reassuring voice of experience just as it seemed impossible. I am glad to say that she has turned from colleague to friend. Her own work helped me to think more creatively, and this book is better for her insights. Sarah Easterby-Smith, too, read the entire manuscript and was, as ever, unreasonably enthusiastic about everything. I promise to reciprocate.

Christopher Hamlin graciously commented and allowed me to grill him on various subjects over food and e-mail. So too, Sally and Colin

Foxhall, Ian Henderson, Kate Smith, Neil Pemberton, and Mike Brown read other chapters, and I am very grateful for their suggestions. The ideas and enthusiasm of people working in convict and maritime studies have been a real inspiration; these include Hamish Maxwell-Stewart, Kirsty Reid, Ian Duffield, Tim Causer, and, in particular, Clare Anderson.

Parts of chapters 1, 3, 4 and 6 have benefited enormously from the remarks of anonymous reviewers for *Social History of Medicine, Journal of Imperial and Commonwealth Studies* and *Weather, Climate and Society*.

The History of Medicine Committee at the Wellcome Trust generously funded my three years' doctoral research, and the Menzies Centre for Australian Studies and Manchester University awarded me grants to undertake further research. I would therefore also like to thank Kirsten McKenzie, Alison Bashford, Robert Aldrich, Emma Christopher, Frances Clarke, and Samia Hossain for welcoming me to Sydney and making me think long and hard about historical perspectives from the other side of the world.

A huge number of participants at seminars and conferences at King's College London; Wellcome Unit for History of Medicine in Oxford; Sydney University; London School of Hygiene and Tropical Medicine; the Centre for the History of Medicine at Warwick; Mater Dei Institute, Dublin; Northumbria University; Department of History and Philosophy of Science in Cambridge; University College Dublin; Centre for the Social History of Health and Healthcare, Glasgow; and Institute of Naval Medicine, Gosport have given valuable feedback and asked thoughtful questions about my papers at various stages. Thank you.

It was a joy to spend time working at the Institute of Naval Medicine in Gosport, and I thank Jane Wickenden for her hospitality and generosity with the historical collections, and for her infectious enthusiasm for nineteenth-century naval surgeons. I would also like to acknowledge librarians and archivists at the Wellcome Library, British Library, The National Archives of Great Britain, the National Archives of Ireland, the Maritime Museums in Greenwich, Sydney and Liverpool, the National Libraries of Ireland and Australia, the Public Record Office of Northern Ireland, and the State Archives of New South Wales and Tasmania.

In 2010, Ludmilla Jordanova and Paul Readman in the History Department at King's College London backed me just when I really needed it. I thank them wholeheartedly for their welcome, and their patience, and also Keren Hammerschlag, Richard McKay, Rosie Wall, and the members of the reading group with whom it has been a pleasure to begin new projects.

Above all, I would like to thank Andy, who is a superstar. This book is dedicated to the memory of John and Christine Foxhall, and Dorothy Maureen Butler.

Abbreviations

ADM	Admiralty Records
ANMM	Australian National Maritime Museum (Sydney)
AONSW	State Archives of New South Wales (Sydney)
AOT	State Archives of Tasmania (Hobart)
CLEC	Colonial Land and Emigration Commission
CO	Colonial Office Records (when TNA)
CO	Convict Office Correspondence (when NAI)
CON	Convict Conduct Records
CSO OP	Chief Secretary's Office, Official Papers
DL	State Library of New South Wales, Dixson Library
FCO	Foreign and Commonwealth Office Collection
GPO	Government Prisons Office
HO	Home Office Records
HRA	*Historical Records of Australia*
KCL	King's College London, Special Collections
ML	State Library of New South Wales, Mitchell Library
MMM	Merseyside Maritime Museum
NAI	National Archives of Ireland (Dublin)
NLA	National Library of Australia (Canberra)
NMM	National Maritime Museum (London)
PCOM	Prison Commission Records
PRONI	Public Records Office of Northern Ireland (Belfast)
TNA	The National Archives (London, Great Britain)

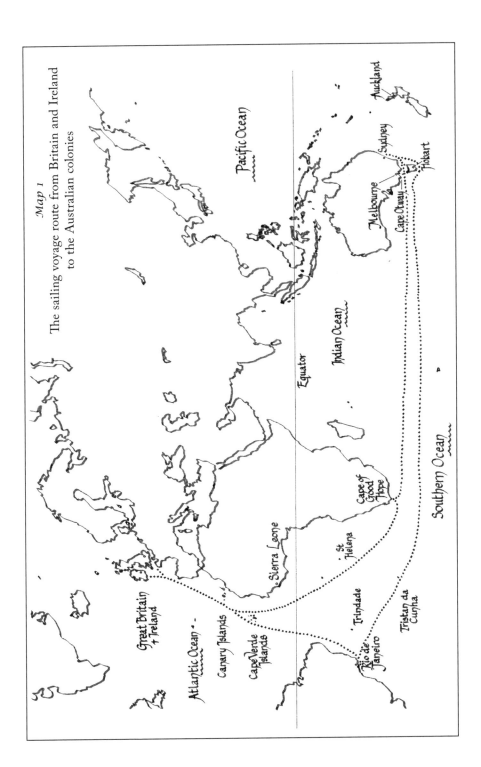

Map 1
The sailing voyage route from Britain and Ireland
to the Australian colonies

Introduction

In 1837, a twenty-nine-year-old woman named Mrs Bateup pleaded to be allowed onto the emigrant ship *Augusta Jessie* with her family. She had received government assistance to emigrate to New South Wales, but when the vessel's surgeon-superintendent, naval surgeon Thomas Galloway, later entered Mrs Bateup's case in his journal, he explained that she was a woman of a 'delicate constitution' who had suffered from influenza just before the voyage. She was 'evidently consumptive' on embarkation, but Galloway had relented and allowed her passage after hearing the woman's 'earnest entreaty to be permitted to proceed, in expectation that the voyage would give her a chance of recovery'.[1]

What did it mean for people like Mrs Bateup, and the surgeons who watched over them, to take a sailing voyage to Australia in the first half of the nineteenth century? Mrs Bateup's story begins to take us beyond a lingering assumption that poor emigrants and convicts who did not or could not write eyewitness accounts of their time at sea were simply 'cargo', their experiences unknowable, the ocean simply a space to cross, and the voyage a time to endure.[2] Mrs Bateup left no letters or diary but this fragment makes it clear that her travels were more than simply a means to an end. The Bateups were a large family of farm labourers from southern England who had sold all of their belongings in order to emigrate to Australia. If her family's initial decision to emigrate had been an economic one driven by the promise of government assistance and plentiful work in the colony of New South Wales, by the time they arrived at Portsmouth harbour, the prospect of going to sea itself held real meaning. It offered Mrs Bateup's only chance of recovering her health.

Voyages did not just deliver emigrants and convicts, they made them into colonists. This book shifts the focus of the history of maritime health in the belief that we can piece together a rich and analytically revealing account not just of what it was like for individuals to be at sea, but also that helps us to see how voyages to Australia partook of colonialism. Until now, we have often used evidence from the accounts left by literate emigrants and wealthy passengers to support the argument that voyagers largely came to share the surgeons' beliefs about the importance of governmental regulation and stringent maritime sanitary measures in the nineteenth century.[3] These hygienic endeavours led to the containment of disease and lowered rates of mortality at sea. The figure of the increasingly professional Victorian doctor, battling conditions and ignorance, is at the heart of historical accounts that explain declining maritime mortality.[4] These are important insights, but recent studies of land-based history have also made it clear that public health was never apolitical, or driven solely by a humanitarian desire to improve conditions.[5] Elsewhere, too, colonial historians have shown repeatedly that medicine was a colonial tool and a 'discourse of settlement', as much as it was about tackling illness.[6] When we shift the terms of analysis to what people did on and said about ships that sailed between Britain and its colonies, and how they understood their relationship with the ocean around them – rather than counting how many people lived or died – we begin to see how surgeons at sea, and the convicts and emigrants they supervised, became intimately involved in the meaning and in the processes that shaped colonialism.

It is precisely because voyages occur in the spaces between metropole and colony that they provide an invaluable opportunity to bring these two spaces together.[7] Doing so prompts us to ask some important but hitherto neglected questions. What did people believe about health at sea, and how did it change as they moved from here to there/there to here? What did medical authority mean for surgeons, and for those over whom they held that authority? What did voyages do for British colonialism, and what was medicine's value to those projects? How did voyages help migrants to place themselves as their worldview expanded, and how do they therefore help us to understand the British sense of its colonial self?

Sailing ships and the people who journeyed on them were the lifeblood not just of Australia, but of colonies in general. Ships were sources of labour, news, goods and food, ideas and government orders, but they also induced great anxiety. Most importantly, voyages were not separate from the social, political, cultural, and environmental contexts through which they began, passed, and ended. Through the experiences of people who travelled, I see voyages as assemblages: medical concerns, military priorities, social hierarchy, penal reform, mass migration, colonial politics, and geographical knowledge and environmental experience all jostled together.[8] As assemblages, voyages bound the British nation-state to its Australian colonies in more complex, important – and indeed, *interesting* – ways than we have hitherto realised.

People

There are good reasons for combining the histories of British and Irish convicts and emigrants. Overwhelmingly, they came from the same social background, the labouring poor.[9] In many ways, the experience of steerage emigrants who could not afford to pay for a passage more closely mirrored the experience of convicts than of cabin and second-class passengers. During the late 1830s, convicts and emigrants used the same ships (though on different voyages), with the same surgeons. Ships were a rich mix of people with different reasons for travel. Aside from the sailors, for example, colonial officials, missionaries, and paying passengers often sailed on convict ships, creating conflicting demands. One surgeon, facing a violent outbreak of scurvy among the convicts, complained bitterly about his captain, who shortened the ship's sails – thereby prolonging a convict voyage – because 'he had some timid lady passengers on board'.[10]

Around a thousand women – the wives of convicts – emigrated with their families to Australia on female convict vessels. Mary Owens was one of these women, and she 'laboured under great depression of mind from a strong presentiment that she will never reach [New South] Wales'. During the voyage Mary developed consumption. Believing that her suckling baby was the cause of the rapid development of her symptoms, the surgeon weaned the baby, to 'considerable benefit'. We can only speculate as to what Mary thought about the removal of her child, but we do see something of her feelings about the voyage. She remained in her berth and refused to take the air on deck until, a week after the surgeon's first entry, she died 'tranquil and rather comatose'.[11] Although her husband was at the other end of the voyage, Mary could not believe that the voyage had an end, and she refused to yield to Linton's insistence that the sea air would do her good. Where, also, might we place the women who experienced 'great depression of spirits' because they had been forced to emigrate although their 'views of future prosperity did not accord with those of their husbands'?[12] Surgeons sometimes heeded invalid convicts' requests to go to sea, but they also enforced the compulsory vaccinations to which emigrants had to submit if they were to be allowed to embark. Such examples remind us that the distinctions among freedom, coercion, and force, particularly with regard to colonialism and migration, can be unclear and contingent.[13]

Bringing convicts, government-assisted emigrants, sailors, soldiers, children, wealthy passengers, missionaries, and naval surgeons into a single analysis shows how and why being at sea meant different things to different people, and tells us something new and important about health, environment, and the experience of colonialism. Shared maritime experiences such as seasickness, curiosity about strange maritime creatures, and fear when a person fell overboard could bring people together. But the motivations for travel, comparative knowledge of health, perceptions of environment, and relationship with medical authority were shaped by differences in class, gender, life history, and social status. It is important to realise where experiences were shared, and where they diverged.

Because naval surgeons played such a key role in recording the voyages of poor people, their accounts – contained in the medical journals that they submitted to the colonial governor at the end of the voyage – necessarily shape the histories that we can write.[14] This book is, therefore, as much about the ideas, priorities, and the worldviews of the medical men who superintended these voyages as it is about the convicts and emigrants under their care. The British colonial government collated an extraordinary amount of material about convict and emigrant voyages to Australia in the first half of the nineteenth century, but until recently historians have left these medical journals largely unexamined.[15] Surgeons' accounts of convict and emigrant voyages certainly contain a wealth of evidence about mortality and sickness, not to mention a mass of often indecipherable medical shorthand, and they are important records of nineteenth-century power relationships. But if we look more closely we see that when surgeons engaged in practices of inspection, vaccination, post-mortem examination, and medical experimentation, it is hardly surprising that convicts, emigrants, and those who shared their spaces often responded not by accepting medical authority, but with resistance, concealment, and mistrust.

When brought into conversation with other sources, including letters, diaries, newspaper reports, government inquiries, maps, and contemporary literature, these journals become rich historical sources that give us a real sense of the sounds, smells, and sights of the sea, of what it was like as a place, what maritime isolation allowed surgeons to do, and the problems it caused. Even the relative formality of individual case notes reveals a rich seam of vernacular knowledge about health at sea: a glimpse of the hopes, fears, and regrets of convicts and government emigrants. Their words are mingled with, and often distorted by, the surgeon's words. Nevertheless, they are there, and they tell us something of how convicts and emigrants spoke of and about their bodies and related their illnesses to the world around them, the lives that they had left behind, their understanding of a strange present, and the future that they imagined before them. At the back of each journal, beyond the case notes and nosological tallies of disease, each surgeon had a relatively unconstrained epistolary space, the pages of 'General Remarks', where he wrote of the circumstances and events of the voyage, his frustrations and observations, his excuses for failure, and his recommendations for future success. The surgeons' journals reveal their own professional and personal priorities, their prejudices and obsessions, certainly, but they are also a window onto the sea and into the world of people who did not write, and from whom we have traditionally heard little. These people are important because they formed the majority of the colonists who sailed to Australia in the first half of the nineteenth century.

Oceans

Maritime history has enjoyed a surge in popularity: scholars consciously identify with Atlantic, Indian or Pacific ocean frameworks, at the same time as they acknowledge that such designations are inherently unstable and contested.[16] Ships are instruments in grand imperial schemes, or laboratories for sanitary practice, and oceans are highways or theatres.[17] Some scholars have written influential accounts of the social, racial, and political significance of seas and ports.[18] Others have written richly of the ocean's potency; Jonathan Lamb has explored the psychological and corporeal destabilisation of the British self in the South Pacific, and Clare Anderson emphasises the importance of the concept of crossing the 'kala pani', or 'black water', in Indian Ocean convict transportation histories.[19] Some of the richest maritime histories have been studies of individual voyages, particularly of those involved with the slave trade, while the concept of the 'middle passage' has proved a powerful way to explore the 'social and cultural transformations that resulted from the transport of people around the globe'.[20]

This book is shaped by my conviction that it matters that voyages occurred at sea. Such a comment may seem obvious, but paradoxically, much of the extant maritime literature pays little attention to the nature of the ocean. Water has become a social, cultural, or economic surface across which ships travelled. Oceans are theatres for, rather than actors in, history. In Philip Steinberg's words, the modern sea is 'an empty space to be crossed by atomistic ships'.[21] Oceans, with their winds and waves, storms, calms, and creatures have receded from view.[22] One explanation of this trend is as an understandable reaction to the romanticised idea of the sailor pitted against the elements. This is an image, Marcus Rediker argued in 1989, which 'has distorted the reality of life at sea by concentrating on the struggle of man and nature to the exclusion of other aspects of maritime life, notably the jarring confrontation of man against man'.[23]

Another explanation for the relative neglect of the sea as a material place is that scholars have become more interested in networks and nodes than in the influence of deep structures.[24] The historiographical focus on networks has afforded valuable insights into maritime colonialism, and the ways in which historians have pieced together colonial networks that linked Britain, Africa, South America, oceanic islands, and Australia have certainly had a formative influence on the chapters that follow.[25] But if we ignore the nature of the sea in such an important era of imperial expansion, we are missing something very important. People like Mrs Bateup were not unthinking pawns in a demographic, economic, or imperial game; so what did it mean to go to, and be at, sea? How did all the people who sailed to Australia make a place for themselves in this historical space?[26]

Historians, of course, have paid considerable attention to the close relationship between people, health, and environment, and there is a rich and growing body of work that embeds health and social struggles in diverse everyday environments.[27] That we have not yet used these insights to come to grips with the maritime world is perhaps more surprising, given Charles Rosenberg's oft-repeated assertion that, in the nineteenth century, 'the body was seen, metaphorically, as a system of dynamic interactions with its environment. Health or disease resulted from a cumulative interaction between constitutional endowment and environmental circumstance.' Thus, bodies were 'always in a state of becoming' and they were 'always in jeopardy'.[28] There are few historical situations where the environment was as physically and mentally challenging, for so many people, as the journey from Europe to Australia in the nineteenth century, and perhaps none that are so well preserved in archives. Illness could result from exposure to weather, mental anguish, fear, homesickness, nutritional deprivation, vapours, miasmas, poor ventilation, overcrowding, exposure to the moon, moral and economic poverty, heat, cold, or the transition between different climates. The importance of being *at* sea often derived from the different rhythms, frustrations, and accumulated problems associated with travelling south, of moving *through* storms and calms, of passing Sierra Leone and the Cape of Good Hope, of experiencing four seasons in as many months. Tropical climate made the insides of ships unbearable and forced surgeons to relax rigid rules about locking women below at night. Storms disrupted vaccinations and post-mortem examinations.

One of the questions I was asked as I worked on this project, a question that has stuck with me and shaped this book, is whether the history of ships is the same as the history of the sea.[29] The answer is no. Histories of people on ships are not the same as histories of people at sea, and we need to write both. Ships have certainly proved suggestive, but their histories can be constrained by the enclosure that governs physicality on board, and by the confinement conditioning the characteristics of individual ships as theatres, cultural microcosms, laboratories, and prisons. What happens when we (as ships do) let the sea leak in? The more I thought about the sea, the more I noticed it everywhere in contemporary accounts. In order to understand the obsessive concern with scraping, fumigating, and ventilating sailing vessels, we need to understand how contemporaries worried constantly that the ocean's airs and waters permeated every fibre of the ship's structure, with powerful consequences, both good and bad.

The ocean environment changed constantly during the course of a twelve-thousand-mile voyage; the transition from the tropics to the cold, wet weather of the southern oceans, for example, correlated too precisely with outbreaks of scurvy for it to be a mere backdrop. Again and again, the presence of the maritime environment shaped the experience of voyaging through the associations made with islands and coasts, in its heat, calms and storms, strange lights in the sky, and sharks that circled to forewarn of sickness and death. Surgeons struggled to reconcile the contrasting dangers associated with being inside and outside the ship, while sailors teased emigrants that strange things always happened 'in these parts'. Was exposure to the sun's rays, the night's dews, or a soaking downpour in the fresh air of the deck a greater evil than stifling confinement in the crowded, ill-ventilated spaces below? The sultry atmosphere off the African coast seemed to give one ship's sails a jaundiced appearance. In another voyage, the terror of a severe Southern Ocean storm seemed to precipitate the death of a frail woman. As they sailed the world's seas, ships gained their own reputations and life histories; they too became sickly or healthy in relation to their environment.

Chapters

While *Health, medicine, and the sea* is attentive to change over time, it is primarily maritime geography that propels the narrative. Each of the chapters contributes to tracing the journey, beginning in the ports of the British Isles and ending in Australia. The first chapter charts the changing political, social, and geographical character of Australian departures over the first half of the nineteenth century by examining the conflicts that emerged in the days around embarkation as medical men sought to assert their own understanding of what voyages should be, and who should travel. The business of departure was tense, chaotic messy, and confusing: no one simply left land behind when they stepped onto a ship.

On leaving the ports, estuaries, and harbours of Britain and Ireland, ships' captains negotiated the adverse winds of the English Channel and the Irish Sea before steering into the Atlantic and heading south-by-south west across the heavy swells of the Bay of Biscay. Chapter 2 introduces debates about the internal spaces of the ship. For surgeons and commentators, these were worryingly unreformed spaces permeated by moistures; sweat, breath, waves, and bilge water poisoned the atmosphere. The sight of islands such as Madeira, under clear skies and in fair breezes, reassured surgeons and travellers that they were sailing through a healthy climate, but as they reached the tropics, the maritime environment changed again. Chapter 3 dwells in the tropics, where the experience of calms reinforced and extended preconceptions about the coast of West Africa across the space of the sea. In this region the heat, unpredictable weather patterns, and sailors' equatorial traditions destabilised surgeons' authority and their attempts to maintain standards of propriety and discipline. Sailors turned maritime and medical authority upside down, dowsing passengers and mocking the surgeon's obsession with dryness in their rituals of 'crossing the line'.

The geographical organisation of the narrative invites us to appreciate the shared elements of voyaging, as well as the points where experience diverged, and to understand why these are significant in terms of larger themes in nineteenth-century social, colonial, and medical history. The three final chapters emphasise these convergences and divergences. Chapter 4 turns to convicts, to show how scurvy became resurgent as British prison committees steadily reduced prison dietary rations during the 1820s and 1830s. Going further still into the voyage, the Cape of Good Hope remained, as it had been in the eighteenth century, intimately linked to surgeons' expressions of regret and of relief about scurvy, but the disease itself seemed to have changed. From the archetypal maritime scourge, scurvy had become a penal disease. Despite their frustrations, the isolation of the ocean and the vulnerability of convicts' bodies offered surgeons an invaluable opportunity for medical experimentation during the 1840s.

Bringing convicts and emigrants back together, Chapter 5 explores how a series of questions about authority, class, gender, and social status mediated medical relationships as the pressures of the voyage accumulated. Themes of mistrust, cooperation, and coercion emerged in many different ways during the voyage, but together they are central to showing how surgeons' everyday relationships with convicts and emigrants fed into their attempts to carry out vaccinations and post-mortem examinations, and, in doing so, to gain the colonial status many of these medical men craved. In Chapter 6 we arrive in Australia, where, as emigrants became immigrants, the uncertainties of government responsibility combined with a poisonous political atmosphere to raise questions about eligibility and the conditions of admittance to their new colonial society. After 1828, the colonial authorities used the maritime quarantine line only against emigrants, and not convicts. Such a strategy, so clearly entangled in colonial conceptions about immigration, delineated why the experience of voyaging to Australia was not always a shared one.

Individual stories are at the centre of analysis throughout, but in addition to the main chapters, two short narratives stand alone to recount two individual voyages to Australia. The first, after Chapter 2, is about Eliza Baldwinson, a young female convict from London, transported in 1832, whose story we know from penal records. The second, after Chapter 5, uses Henry Wellings' steerage diary, and the map of the world that he sketched, to trace the voyage of a father from Salford who emigrated on the *David McIvor* in 1857. I hope that these narratives will tie together some of the themes that flow through these chapters and show the significance of being at sea for individual travellers. Understanding how people evaluated and re-evaluated their knowledge of health as they reacted to their ever-changing environment, and how medical authority played out in practice, gives us an important insight not just into the creation of medical knowledge across time and place, but into the British sense of its colonial 'self' in the nineteenth century. In many ways, not least environmental, voyages became tests of colonial fitness, and they helped to shape what British colonialism came to be in the nineteenth century.

Notes

1 TNA, ADM 101/76/4, Journal of surgeon Galloway on Emigrant Ship *Augusta Jessie* (1837). Case 16, Mrs Bateup, 12 July 1837. Mrs Bateup died at sea. A month into the voyage, whilst on deck, she began to spit blood. For five days, the surgeon wrote, she continued 'low, but cheerful', until a fit of coughing 'carried her off in a few minutes'.

2 Babette Smith, *Cargo of Women* (Kensington, NSW: New South Wales University Press, 1992); Sian Rees, *The Floating Brothel: the Extraordinary True Story of an Eighteenth-Century Ship and its Cargo of Female Convicts* (New York: Hyperion, 2002).

3 For a useful discussion of the biases in these written accounts see Andrew Hassam, *Sailing to Australia*: *Shipboard Diaries by Nineteenth-Century British Emigrants* (Manchester: Manchester University Press, 1994) p. 11.

4 Robin Haines, *Doctors at Sea: Emigrant Voyages to Colonial Australia* (Basingstoke: Palgrave Macmillan, 2005); Kim Humphery, 'A New Era of Existence: Convict transportation and the authority of the surgeon in colonial Australia', *Labour History* (Australia) 59 (1990), pp. 59–72; David Boyd Haycock and Sally Archer (eds) *Health and Medicine at Sea 1700–1900* (Woodbridge: Boydell Press, 2009); Alan Brooke and David Brandon, *Bound for Botany Bay: British Convict Voyages to Australia* (London: The National Archives, 2005).

5 Christopher Hamlin, *Public Health and Social Justice in the Age of Chadwick: Britain, 1800–1854* (Cambridge: Cambridge University Press, 1998), p. 21.

6 Warwick Anderson, *The Cultivation of Whiteness: Health and Racial Destiny in Australia* (New York: Basic Books, 2003), p. 4; David Arnold, *Colonizing the Body* (London, Berkeley and Los Angeles: California University Press, 1993).

7 Ann Laura Stoler and Frank Cooper, 'Between Metropole and Colony: Rethinking a research agenda', in *Tensions of Empire: Colonial Cultures in a Bourgeois World* (Berkeley and Los Angeles: University of California Press, 1997), pp. 1–56.

8 For a useful definition of assemblage see Stephen J. Collier and Aihwa Ong, *Global Assemblages: Technology, Politics and Ethics as Anthropological Problems* (Oxford: Blackwell, 2005), p. 12.

9 For convicts as labourers see Stephen Nicholas, *Convict Workers, Reinterpreting Australia's Past* (Cambridge: Cambridge University Press, 1988); Deborah Oxley, *Convict Maids: The Forced Migration of Women to Australia* (Cambridge: Cambridge University Press, 1996); Ian Duffield and James Bradley (eds), *Representing Convicts: New Perspectives on Convict Forced Labour Migration* (Leicester: Leicester University Press, 1997).

10 TNA, ADM 101/29/10, Journal of surgeon James Syme on convict ship *Gilmore* (1843), General Remarks.

11 TNA, ADM 101/79/5, Journal of surgeon Charles Linton on transport ship *Thames*, taking women and children from Cork to New South Wales (1826), Case of Mary Owens, 9 March 1826.

12 TNA, ADM 101/79/2, Journal of surgeon Harry Goldney on Freight Ship *Sir George Seymour* (1847). General Remarks.

13 Emma Christopher, Marcus Rediker and Cassandra Pybus (eds), *Many*

Middle Passages: Forced Migration and the Making of the Modern World (Los Angeles and London: University of California Press, 2007), p. 8.

14 Antoinette Burton, 'Archive Stories: Gender in the making of imperial and colonial histories', in Philippa Levine (ed.) *Gender and Empire* (Oxford: Oxford University Press, 2004), pp. 281–293.

15 The National Archives at Kew (TNA), ADM 101, contain over six hundred surgeons' journals, including some from government-assisted emigrant voyages. Oxley, *Convict Maids*, pp. 17–33, discusses most fully the sources available for researching convicts.

16 Jerry H. Bentley, 'Sea and Ocean Basins as Frameworks of Historical Analysis', *Geographical Review* 89:2 (1999), pp. 215–224; Marcus Vink, 'Indian Ocean Studies and the "New Thalassology"', *Journal of Global History* 2:1 (2007), pp. 41–62.

17 There have been a series of recent edited collections about the sea, including Jerry H. Bentley, Renate Bridenthal and Karen Wigen (eds), *Seascapes: Maritime Histories, Littoral Cultures and Transoceanic Exchanges* (Honolulu: University of Hawaii Press, 2007); David Cannadine (ed.), *Empire, the Sea and Global History: Britain's Maritime World, c. 1760–1840* (Basingstoke: Palgrave Macmillan, 2007).

18 Paul Gilroy, *The Black Atlantic* (Cambridge, MA: Harvard University Press, 1993); Marcus Rediker, *Between the Devil and the Deep Blue Sea: Merchant Seamen, Pirates and the Anglo-American Maritime World, 1700–1750* (Cambridge: Cambridge University Press, 1987); Marcus Rediker and Peter Linebaugh, *The Many-Headed Hydra: The Hidden History of the Revolutionary Atlantic* (Boston; Beacon Press, 2000); Greg Dening, *Mr Bligh's Bad Language: Passion, Power and Theatre on the Bounty* (Cambridge: Cambridge University Press, 1992).

19 Clare Anderson, *The Indian Uprising of 1857–8: Prisons, Prisoners and Rebellion* (London and New York: Anthem Press, 2007), esp. chapter 5; Jonathan Lamb, *Preserving the Self in the South Seas, 1680–1840* (Chicago: University of Chicago Press, 2001).

20 Robert W. Harms, *The Diligent: A Voyage through the Worlds of the Slave Trade* (New York: Basic Books, 2002); Emma Christopher, *Slave Ship Sailors and their Captive Cargoes* (Cambridge: Cambridge University Press, 2006); Christopher et al., *Many Middle Passages*, p. 2.

21 Philip E. Steinberg, *The Social Construction of the Ocean* (Cambridge: Cambridge University Press, 2001), p. 105.

22 For one historian who does emphasise materiality see Richard Drayton, 'Maritime Networks and the Making of Knowledge', in David Cannadine (ed.), *Empire, the Sea and Global History: Britain's Maritime World, c. 1763–c. 1840* (Basingstoke: Palgrave Macmillan, 2007), pp. 72–82.

23 Marcus Rediker, *Between the Devil and the Deep Blue Sea*, p. 5.

24 Fernand Braudel, *The Mediterranean and the Mediterranean World in the Age of Philip II*, 2 vols, trans. S. Reynolds (New York: Harper and Row, 1972).

25 Kerry Ward, *Networks of Empire: Forced Migration in the Dutch East India Company* (Cambridge and New York: Cambridge University Press, 2009).

26 Paul Carter, *The Road to Botany Bay* (London and Boston: Faber and Faber, 1987), p. 294.

27 James Boyce, *Van Diemen's Land* (Melbourne: Black Inc., 2008); Michelle Murphy, *Sick Building Syndrome and the Problem of Uncertainty* (Durham, NC: Duke University Press, 2006); Karl Jacoby, *Crimes against Nature: Squatters, Poachers, Thieves and the Hidden History of American Conservation* (Berkeley and Los Angeles: University of California Press, 2003); Conevery Bolton Valencius, *The Health of the Country: How American Settlers Understood Themselves and Their Land* (New York: Basic Books, 2002).

28 Charles Rosenberg, 'The Therapeutic Revolution: Medicine, meaning and social change in nineteenth-century America', in Morris Vogel and Charles Rosenberg (eds) *The Therapeutic Revolution: Essays in the Social History of American Medicine* (Philadelphia: University of Pennsylvania Press, 1979), pp. 3–25, p. 5.

29 I would like to acknowledge and thank David Arnold for posing this question.

1

Problems of departure

The British government first sent convicts to New South Wales in 1787, after the War of Independence had ended the possibility of banishing them to the American colonies.[1] From the first fleet until the system finally ended in 1868, 163,000 men and women colonised the Australian colonies as convicts. The majority came from the British mainland, around a quarter from Ireland. Much smaller groups also travelled from the Caribbean, South Africa and the Indian Ocean, reflecting Australia's role in a global imperial system of forced migration. The first convicts landed in New South Wales. From 1803 they were sent to Van Diemen's Land, and later still to Moreton Bay, Port Phillip, Norfolk Island and Western Australia. After 1815 the system expanded, and the greatest numbers of convicts sailed during the 1820s and 1830s; in this period around one-third of British assize or quarter sessions sentences resulted in an order that the felon be transported or that a death sentence be commuted to transportation. Of these, between two-thirds and three-quarters actually made the voyage to Australia. During the 1830s around 43,000 male and 7,750 female transportees made the voyage from Britain and Ireland to Australia, at the same time as Australia began to attract substantial numbers of free emigrants.[2]

In the first decades of convict transportation, ship owners were responsible for hiring surgeons, whose responsibilities in relation to the ship's master were ill-defined. Most of these surgeons took only one voyage, and for the vast majority we know little more than their name. Historians have yet to seriously re-assess William Redfern's contemporary estimation that these early surgeons were 'devoted to inebriety', but it is clear that many took colonial appointments. The surgeon of the *Coromandel* (1802), Charles Throsby, was one of the first permanent settlers in New South Wales. In the colony, he gained several medical appointments, was appointed a magistrate, and became a prominent landowner and explorer.[3] Jacob Mountgarrett, the surgeon of the *Glatton* in 1803, became colonial surgeon at Risdon Cove in Van

Diemen's Land, and witnessed what would become known notoriously as the Risdon massacre.[4] On some ships there appears to have been no medical supervision at all. Although, after the disastrous experiences of the Second Fleet (1789–90), the government appointed naval agents to oversee the convicts' embarkation, the experiment was abandoned by the beginning of the nineteenth century.

The early colonial governors of New South Wales had often despaired of the state in which convicts arrived. In 1802, for example, Governor King complained that the convicts from the *Royal Admiral* were 'in a state of great debility', and unlikely to 'ever recover the strength of men', while the whole of the convicts of the *Hercules* and *Atlas* were either 'dead or in a dying state'.[5] In 1814, when the *Three Bees*, *General Hewitt* and *Surrey* all disembarked convicts in a terrible condition, colonial frustrations reached a head. Determined to 'avert the recurrence of such Calamities' for the future, Governor Lachlan Macquarie asked his colonial surgeon, William Redfern, to investigate the state of the three recently arrived convict ships. As he sent Redfern's report back to Britain, Macquarie angrily complained that 'the principal part' of the crew and convicts of the *Surrey* had been 'in a wretched and deplorable state of disease'.[6]

William Redfern had been a naval surgeon, but he started his colonial career in 1801 as a convict, after he was transported for his role in the 1797 naval mutiny at the Nore. By 1802, Redfern had gained a post as assistant surgeon on Norfolk Island, and Governor King issued him with a free pardon a year later. Having returned to Sydney in 1808, Redfern attracted the powerful patronage of Lachlan Macquarie. Redfern's inquiry into the three disastrous voyages makes no suggestion that there had been a surgeon on board the *Three Bees*. Four days after leaving Ireland on 27 October 1813, it anchored in Falmouth, a port on the south-western tip of the English mainland, where bad weather forced the convicts to remain below decks for a further five weeks, until 7 December. Here, it was 'exceedingly Cold and the Prisoners Suffered Severely'.[7] Finally, the *Three Bees* sailed into the Atlantic winter. During wet and cold weather fires were used to warm and dry the ship's prison, but while the ship was anchored in Rio de Janeiro in February, a case of 'Common Ship fever' appeared. Later in the voyage scurvy, which had 'long been lurking' among the prisoners, broke out. By the time the *Three Bees* arrived in Sydney, nine men had died, and fifty-five of the convicts were sent to the colonial hospital. Seven more men died in the colony.[8]

With such apparently straightforward evidence of medical neglect, Redfern recommended that convicts must be adequately clothed and that transports should not depart in winter. Attention must be paid to hygiene, to ensuring the proper allocation of rations, and to ventilation, fumigation, and fresh air. Redfern 'respectfully' suggested that the British government select naval surgeons – 'men of abilities, who have been accustomed to sea practice' – who, as officers, would have full power 'to exercise their judgment', without being subordinate to the ship's master.[9]

Historians have seen Redfern's report of 1814 as a foundational moment in the history of Australian and maritime public health; Redfern's name has entered the fabric of Australian culture and a suburb of modern Sydney takes the surgeon's name. From 1815, the Admiralty assigned a qualified naval surgeon to every convict ship departing from Britain and Ireland. The surgeon would not interfere with the sailing of the ship and, in turn, the captain and crew would not interfere with the management and discipline of convicts. The surgeon-superintendent's authority now encompassed all aspects of moral discipline and medical care, and during the 1830s the model was also extended to Australia-bound emigrant vessels.[10] Mortality declined rapidly under the naval surgeons' superintendence. Crude death rates for convicts at sea fell from an average of 11.3 per thousand people per month in the years before 1814, to 2.4 per thousand per month between 1814 and 1868.[11] Put more simply, this means that while ten or more convicts might die during an average voyage before naval surgeons routinely superintended voyages, after 1814 deaths fell to a usual rate of one, two, or three. Many surgeons made it clear that they expected to lose none.

This largely apolitical narrative of sanitary and disciplinary progress is appealing, but mortality figures tell only a fraction of the medical history of the Australian voyage. With many of its surgeons in need of work now that the Napoleonic Wars had ended, the British government could afford to accede to Redfern's requests, but the emergence of medical authority at sea is a much more complex history. Apart from being an important and fascinating history in its own right, it also has profound implications for our understanding of the role of medicine in Australian colonisation. It is a story of conflicting penal, medical, professional, and colonial priorities encompassing different government departments in a changing geographical space. As this chapter will begin to demonstrate, surgeons struggled with convicts, emigrants, British and Irish prison officials, colonial agents, and new diseases, not to mention their own medical peers and bruised egos. Moreover, the convicts and emigrants over whom surgeons held authority never just left their life histories behind them. They too brought their own hopes, fears, priorities, and knowledge to the voyage. The days of departure were messy, frustrating, and fraught with sometimes irreconcilable tensions. What was the purpose of the voyage? What was at stake in the act of leaving? Who should be allowed, or made, to undertake the voyage to Australia? These questions were and are important, and they are not questions to which sanitation alone could provide answers.

The surgeon who oversaw the beginning of the *Three Bees*' voyage in Ireland saw the problem of diseased or elderly convicts distinctly differently to William Redfern, who witnessed its end in Sydney. In September 1813, Dr Harding, the Medical Officer for Cork, visited a convict in the city gaol who had been sentenced to transportation to New South Wales. The man, named only as 'Haly', was 'very bad spitting blood'. 'I think he will fall into a consumption,' Harding predicted in his journal. Although Haly was 'still bad' two days later, Dr Harding was sure that the man's health would improve during the several months' voyage to Australia. 'I am convinced it is the very best remedy,' he concluded.[12] On 16 September, the doctor sent Haly to the *Three Bees*, a sailing vessel hired by the British government, which now lay anchored in the Cove of Cork (modern-day Cobh), a huge natural harbour on the Irish south coast a few miles away from the gaol. Finally, on 27 October 1813, the *Three Bees* weighed anchor and sailed south into the Celtic Sea with 219 convicts, bound for New South Wales.[13]

Dr Harding had been sure that Haly would 'mend', and that going to sea was the 'very best remedy'. When, over a year later, the Inspector General of Prisons in Ireland received Macquarie's report about the state of the convicts, he vigorously defended Dr Harding: 'There is Employed an Eminent Physician of great experience at Cork, who during the embarkation examines them, sees them cloathed, cleansed, and selected that none unfit by age or infirmity should proceed on the voyage,' Foster Archer wrote. Archer pointed out that Ireland did not have any hulks for the confinement of invalids, 'nor a general Depot at Cork Harbour where the sick or convalescent might with safety be committed'. Persons afflicted with fever or dysentery 'are taken up to the City Gaol of Cork which has neither Court Yard or airing Ground attached, here they remain till death or recovery ensue'. Archer asked whether the old and sick should remain in Irish prisons 'in iniquity' to corrupt other thoughtless and 'inexperienced' young convicts.[14] Archer's angry defence of Harding reveals acute tensions between British and Irish administrators about the practical administration of the convict system, but it also illustrates that the medical debate that surrounded Redfern's report was as much about *who* should go to sea in the first place as it was about what should happen to them during the voyage, or after they arrived.

Haly's voyage for health

As Dr Harding sent Haly to the *Three Bees* in Cork in the autumn of 1813, the invalid prisoner became more than a convict sentenced to transportation beyond the seas: somewhat incongruously to our modern eyes, Haly also became a traveller for health. Dr Harding's confidence that Haly's voyage might improve his health seems at best naïve, at worst wantonly ignorant of the practical realities of early nineteenth-century voyaging, but the recommendation that invalids should travel in an attempt to cure chronic diseases such as consumption and asthma was becoming an increasingly popular practice.

Physicians had recommended a 'change of air' as medical treatment for centuries. Once Britain was no longer at war with France and Spain, European resorts such as Vichy, Pau, and Nice became an appealing prospect and physicians eagerly promoted Mediterranean, mountain, and spring-water resorts to take advantage of a growing stream of wealthy tourists and invalids.[15] Colonists also flocked to colonial spas, hill stations, and healthy islands. It is not unreasonable to identify, as Eric Jennings has done, a 'cult of temperateness' among enervated colonial officials who sought climatic and hydrotherapeutic relief in the tropics.[16]

Within this general enthusiasm for medical travel, the idea of the medicinal sea voyage held a particularly powerful romantic appeal. Ebenezer Gilchrist's *The Use of Sea Voyages in Medicine* (1756) affirmed that a 'vivifying principle' contained in air 'abounds most at sea'. Sea air is 'so much purer, milder and more highly cherishing', Gilchrist enthused.[17] *The Use of Sea Voyages* had been reprinted in several editions throughout the middle of the eighteenth century, and nineteenth-century writers repeatedly quoted Gilchrist as they insisted that invalids must go further than the fashionable beaches, piers, or baths of coastal resorts. The sick needed to go to sea.

In 1832, in one of the first systematic studies of English industrial and trade-related diseases, Charles Turner Thackrah classed sailors among workers who 'approach nearest to the perfection of the physical state ... healthy and robust, hardy and enterprising, living well, and enjoying good air and exercises, their diseases are few'.[18] A few years later, James Clark – who would later become physician to Queen Victoria – emphasised that the voyage remedy 'must be pursued for a long period'.[19] Another writer explained that because sea voyaging engendered 'an almost constant muscular exertion ... of so gentle a character' it invigorated the body without exhausting 'the living energies'.[20] The idea of the voyage for health began to appear in popular maritime literature. First published in 1840, Richard Henry Dana's *Two Years before the Mast* explained that the author had taken a voyage in the hope that 'plenty of hard work, plain food and open air' would cure a weakness of his eyes, 'which no medical aid seemed likely to remedy'.[21] Observations about the vigorous health and strength of sailors provided further evidence to support the medical promotion of sea voyaging.

The enthusiasm for the sea voyage was not universal, and even some writers who believed in the prophylactic potential of the sea warned that consumptives in the latter stages of disease should not be sent to sea in the vain hope of a miraculous cure.[22] As early as 1804 Thomas Trotter, an influential naval surgeon and writer, condemned physicians who ordered a change of air for their patients simply 'to relieve the ennui of medical admonition in a tedious illness'.[23]

Nevertheless, the promise of a cure for a chronic illness is a powerful thing. Australia was certainly at the end of a very long voyage. Moreover, contemporary medical opinion also held that Australia's soil and climate might offer immunity to diseases such as consumption. The naval surgeon Peter Cunningham was one of the earliest writers to promote Australian emigration by proclaiming the 'extraordinary healthfulness' of the New South Wales climate and promising cure, or at least relief, from 'European' phthisis.[24] From a 'distasteful penal colony with a bizarre, evil or humorous environment', J.M. Powell has argued, the 'cult of the ocean voyage' contributed to the new idea that Australia might prove to be 'an inviting place for white settlement'.[25] By the 1860s, Samuel Dougan Bird would argue that the effect for invalids of the Australian voyage 'is sometimes marvellous ... carried along without effort, he is exposed to the complete and continuous alterative of constantly breathing the pure, stimulant, ozoniferous, and yet soothing air of mid-ocean'.[26] As British doctors migrated to Victoria, the trend for invalid voyaging accelerated into the final decades of the nineteenth century.[27]

Voyaging convict and emigrant invalids

Evidently, then, we need to take the fashion for medicinal voyaging seriously as part of the nineteenth-century medical history of Australian migration, but it is also clear that therapeutic sea voyages were not designed for convicts like Haly, and it is difficult to see how we might reconcile 'voyages for health' with the history of a physically and mentally demanding process of colonisation that necessitated healthy, productive minds and bodies. In 1803, for example, the

Calcutta founded the colony of Van Diemen's Land. In studying this foundational moment, historians have observed that almost all of the convicts were skilled in trades suitable to starting a colony: shoemakers, sawyers, carpenters and fishermen, as well as soldiers, wives, and children. They had been hand-picked, and the ship also carried the hunting dogs that were crucial for survival in a wild new environment.[28] Yet James Hingston Tuckey, a naval officer who wrote an account of the *Calcutta*'s journey, also described how 'between England and Teneriffe, we lost four convicts by death'. Two of these convicts 'had been embarked in the last stages of consumption, vainly hoping that a warmer climate might restore their healths'.[29] With evidence of such apparent care in the selection of these convicts, the presence of consumptives on such an important voyage seems entirely contradictory to the received narrative of the *Calcutta*'s purpose. Did early nineteenth-century doctors really believe that sending sick convicts to sea would improve their health enough to make them useful colonists? Or do these decisions in fact lead us into a much larger debate about what exactly Australian voyages were for, and who had the authority to decide?

When we look, we find that surgeons did often sent invalid convicts to sea *for*, rather than *despite*, their health. Perhaps more surprisingly, the convicts themselves often played a part in the decision. Ann Thomas, suffering from 'pectoral affection', was taken forward to board the convict ship *Mellish* in 1830 'at her own earnest solicitude, and with a hope that her complaint would be benefited by removal from the confinement of a prison'. Ann's case notes reveal that she had spent three months in the Westminster Hospital in London for pneumonia. She had been discharged a few days before her arrest, and 'was more or less affected [by disease] during the whole of her confinement in Newgate'. Ann attributed the attack on the *Mellish* that brought her to the ship's surgeon to 'her catching cold on coming on board'.[30] In 1849, James Deegan also was taken onto the *Hyderabad* 'at his own request'. The surgeon had reported him as unfit to go on the voyage but Deegan 'entreated me to take him'.[31]

Some men and women found that they were able to use the promise of improved health at sea as a way to exert some level of agency over the terms under which their sentence of transportation occurred and what it meant to their sense of self. Recognising this agency makes us think more carefully about how some individuals might have come to terms not just with sickness, but also with the punishment of transportation, but it is also clear that convicts did not, and could not, make decisions about their health independently of the penal imperatives that governed this episode in their lives. Often, a desire to go to sea says as much about the experience of imprisonment in places like Newgate gaol in London as it does about the curative potential of the maritime environment itself.

The existence of debates about the idea of the 'voyage for health' also begins to explain why departure was so often a defining moment for naval surgeons as they began to make claims to authority in the first half of the nineteenth century. In 1843 surgeon Thomas Dunn of the *Waverley* recorded that Michael Duffy '*stated* to me … that he had been suffering from distressing pain of the lumbar and right ingroinal regions for several weeks in gaol, but that he was advised to conceal his complaint from me as the only chance he had of recovering his health, depended on going to sea'.[32] At first glance, this seems a straight-forward record of a conversation, but the surgeon's words contain a distinct level of ambiguity about who believed what. Did Duffy believe his health would recover? Did the surgeon of the gaol really 'advise' in the sense of a recommendation that Duffy conceal his illness, or was it more like a threat? Earlier in the journal, Dunn's case notes record that the voyage to New South Wales 'had been represented to him to be the only certain means of restoring his health'.[33] For the gaol surgeon, the medically fashionable promise of the cure was a way to justify his decision to send away a sick prisoner, and a carrot with which to persuade Duffy to play his own part in the deception: when asked by the naval surgeon, Duffy 'denied the existence of any complaints'. Duffy may well have come to believe the gaol surgeon's promises, and to hold out some hope for the voyage, but experience soon confirmed otherwise. For his part, Dunn, the *Waverley*'s surgeon, absolved himself of blame for Duffy's death by repeating his account of the other men's collusion in a prominent position in his journal. 'I need scarcely remark', Dunn continued, that 'the motion of the ship only tended to hasten the final event.'[34] By no means all surgeons believed that a voyage could cure, yet Michael Duffy and invalids like him alert us to a key theme that runs through *Health, medicine, and the sea*: political expediency and motives of defensive self-interest always shaped how surgeons accounted for their medical decisions. Naval surgeons only received their pay after they had safely landed an acceptable number of convicts in good health in the colonies. They were always mindful of the need to ensure the blame for sickness always lay elsewhere.

Inspections: concealment and conflict

From 1815, when a naval surgeon received a letter of appointment to a convict ship he proceeded to Deptford, where, on the bank of the River Thames, a few miles to the east of London, a huge dockyard flanked by storehouses contained rum, ropes, cables, bedding, and clothing for the Royal Navy. Here, the private vessels which had been hired by the government for the Australian voyage were fully fitted out by the contractor.[35] The Medical Storekeeper at the Royal Victualling Yard provided the surgeon with his surgical instruments, his cases of medical supplies, and a certificate which he must deliver to the colonial Governor in Australia in order that he should receive his pay and a return passage. As the sailors prepared convict vessels for departure, they breeched the guns, stowed the casks of rations (after their quality had been checked by the surgeon), and pumped water into the forehold.[36] A military guard of around fifty men embarked from the barracks of Deptford or Chatham, often bringing their families with them, and attracting curious crowds as they marched through the streets.[37] Then the crew weighed anchor and headed east along the tidal reaches of the Thames.

A few miles downstream, the ships usually received their first convicts at Woolwich or Chatham from the prison hulks that lined the banks of the Thames estuary (Map 2). Converted from captured vessels and old Navy warships, these hulks included *Discovery*, *Ganymede*, *Justitia*, *Fortitude*, *Warrior* and *Retribution*. Boys came from *Euryalus*. Convicts from Millbank penitentiary in London, other prisons around the country, and, by the 1840s, Pentonville also embarked at Woolwich. Other empty transports continued to the open sea, round the Kent peninsula, and into the English Channel before receiving convicts from the *York* and *Leviathan* hulks at Gosport and Portsmouth, another important naval port. From the 1840s, transports also called at Cowes, on the Isle of Wight, and at Plymouth to receive prisoners from the new prisons at Parkhurst, Portland, and Dartmoor.

Around a quarter of convict transports left the British mainland without convicts and sailed to Cork in Ireland, where convicts came initially from the city gaol and later from a depot (1817) and hulk (1822) in Cork Harbour. Cork had become an important port in the early modern period, trading butter, beef, and sailcloth to the Royal Navy and to Britain and its colonies.[38] During the Napoleonic Wars, the British fortified the harbour and used it as a strategic point from which to cover the western entrance of the English Channel. Transportation from Ireland to Australia began four years later than from Britain, in

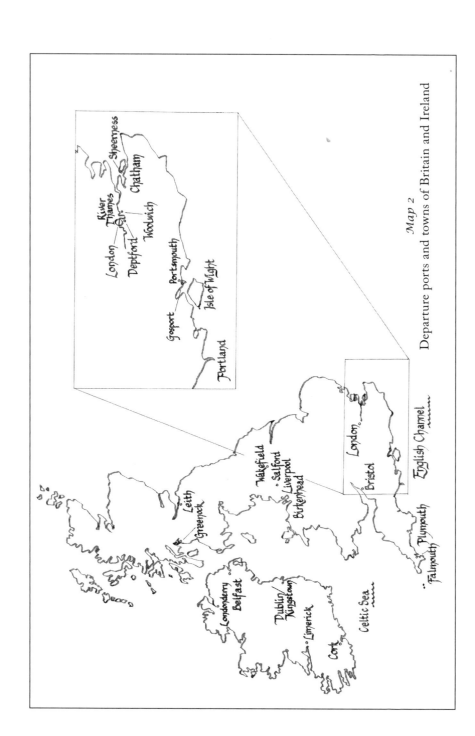

Map 2
Departure ports and towns of Britain and Ireland

1791. In these early decades, convicts from county prisons in the north and east of Ireland travelled first from Dublin to Cork by sea, an often rough and miserable passage in small boats. By 1825, convict transports anchored near Dublin to take convicts directly from the *Essex* hulk in Kingstown harbour, Newgate, Kilmainham, and, from 1836, the Grangegorman female depot.

In all of these ports, in Britain and Ireland, surgeons inspected the men or women who had been chosen for the voyage. The muster of convicts from the hulks and prisons was a crucial, tense moment in which members of the medical profession faced off across courtyards and decks, and the presence of unwell, frail, or elderly convicts posed a particular source of friction. In 1830, George Fairfowl complained that it was impossible to pick out every case of sickness as convicts lined up before their embarkation:

> The examination of the convicts … is very unsatisfactory, for the men being anxious to get away, and the surgeon equally anxious to get rid of bad or troublesome cases, both the parties from whom the naval surgeon expects to receive information are interested to conceal any symptom of disease. Many therefore were approved who ought never to have been brought forward for examination, and even some of those I had rejected were embarked – a piece of ingenuity not found out until too late to be remedied.[39]

As we have already seen, when Foster Archer received surgeon Redfern's report in 1815 he complained bitterly that Ireland's gaols would become schools of corruption. The question of whether some convicts were too old or sick to travel remained particularly acute in Ireland. In 1833, the Inspector General of Irish Prisons, Dr Edward Trevor, over-ruled the naval surgeon Andrew Henderson, who objected to the state of prisoners from the *Essex* hulk in Kingstown Harbour, just outside Dublin. 'I never in the course of my experience have seen so many miserable looking human beings together at any one time,' Henderson wrote. When Henderson voiced his concerns aloud, and warned that he expected to lose at least fifteen of the convicts during the voyage, the Irish Agent for Transports, who was also present at the muster on the *Essex*, had acknowledged that he too 'had never seen prisoners at any former muster look so bad'.[40] Although apparently most heated in Ireland, similar arguments occurred in all the places where surgeons received convicts. Only a few weeks after Andrew Henderson's argument with Dr Trevor in Dublin, another naval surgeon complained that the surgeon of the hospital hulk at Chatham in the Thames had instructed a convict to 'conceal his illness under threat of severe punishment', when it came to the inspection.[41]

Far from being an emerging profession united in a quest to improve their position and status, medical men who spent their time at sea had very different priorities than their colleagues in either Britain or the colonies. These simmering tensions about the embarkation of invalids boiled over when the *Lord Lyndoch* arrived in Van Diemen's Land in August 1836. Although the passage of four months was relatively quick, there had been five deaths and 138 cases of illness out of 330 prisoners. When George Arthur, Lieutenant Governor of Van Diemen's Land (1824–36), read the surgeon's journal from the *Lord Lyndoch*, his attention focused on two convicts who had been allowed to embark with consumption. The governor concluded that the fates of James Smith and George Manders had been 'inevitable under any circumstances'. Arthur was a rigorous defender and promoter of the transportation system, and an ardent supporter of the system of assigning convicts to colonists as labour. It angered him that chronically sick prisoners 'should be embarked and placed in a situation only likely to add to and aggravate their suffering and misery'.[42] Although his account is wrapped in the language of compassion, it is clear that invalids could have no place in Arthur's vision of a productive society based on colonial labour. The surgeon's journal from the voyage revealed that James Smith had complained of 'frequent purging attended with griping pains' within days of embarking. Smith told the surgeon that he had been 'in delicate health' for two years and 'in the hospital all the time he was in Chatham'.[43] Manders too had complained of symptoms of phthisis shortly after embarking. The surgeon called on the convicts' words to support his version of the events.

Colin Arrott Browning (who was rapidly making a name for himself as one of the naval surgeons most dedicated to making a medical career in convict transportation) inquired into the case of the *Lord Lyndoch* for the Admiralty. He repeated his colleagues' earlier complaints that 'there is, on the part of the officers of the Hulks, whose business it is to bring forward the Prisoner for inspection with a view to embarkation, *a disposition to impose upon the Surgeon of the Transport*, men in a state of health, which renders them quite unfit for the voyage'. In addition to the two cases of consumption, Browning pointed out that 'two of Mr Lawrence's worst cases of scurvy had for their subjects, toothless worn out old men'. Other convicts, too, 'appeared to be of a delicate habit of body'.[44]

Andrew Robertson, the surgeon of the *Fortitude* hulk at Chatham, who had sent the convicts to the *Lord Lyndoch*, took the accusations personally, and denied 'most emphatically' and with 'just indignation' that he had embarked any prisoner direct from his hospital to the waiting vessel. However, Robertson also argued as a matter of principle that Governor Arthur's proposal not to allow any prisoners who had previously suffered disease to be exposed to the hardship of the Australian voyage would 'in a short period render the hulks at home floating hospitals'. There were 'numerous' chronic diseases 'which affect the constitution but which will not prevent the prisoner from being landed safe at any of the Colonies'. Robertson reminded the Admiralty that its own instructions stated that the criterion for selecting convicts was only whether the voyage was likely to 'destroy' their life.[45]

John Ward's account of the pre-embarkation examination from the perspective of a convict describes a hulk surgeon's repeated attempts to get rid of a sick man. In September 1839, while Ward was on the convict hulk *York* in Portsmouth harbour, 'a ship came to take 240 men'. Although nine Australian transports had come and gone since Ward arrived on the *York*, this was the first time he had been mustered for inspection. During the inspection the 'ship's Doctor' pulled Ward by the elbow and said: 'I cannot take a man like this.' At the time, Ward had been suffering from a severe cough. Having been refused for the voyage, Ward was ordered 'to change clothes with another man who was glad enough to go in my stead'. Ward recognised that he suffered from consumption, but two months later the hulk officials mustered him again. This time, the naval surgeon passed him as fit and Ward embarked onto the *Mangles*, bound direct for Norfolk Island.[46]

Throughout the period, suspect invalids like Ward were a constant battleground for naval surgeons who sought to assert their own ideas about which convicts should or should not travel. These arguments became particularly urgent as wider political questions about Australia's future reached a climax. Naval surgeons' continual complaints about the levels of deception and ingenuity demonstrated during embarkation inspections, and the apparent complicity of convicts who hid their illnesses, reinforced a recurring theme in criticisms of the transportation system. As John Ward's description of the man who had been 'glad enough to go' suggests, it had become clear to contemporaries that some convicts wanted to be transported to Australia.

In the late 1830s colonies were emerging from penal settlements. Sydney, in particular, was firmly integrated into global maritime networks by the 1820s. Convict transportation had reached its peak, and the continuing visibility of the unfree labour supply jarred with the need to fashion an image of respectable development, and colonial pretensions to self-government. During the 1830s, growing opposition to both transportation and slavery, Kirsten McKenzie has written, 'spoke to an increasing acceptance of the philosophy of the economic and social virtue of free labour'.[47] In 1837 the British government convened a Parliamentary Committee to inquire into the efficacy of transportation as a punishment and its effect on colonial society in New South Wales. The Committee was led by Sir William Molesworth and packed with supporters of free emigration, and its results were a foregone conclusion. The report condemned New South Wales society, McKenzie continues, as 'a veritable inferno of gender inversion, corrupted childhood, venereal disease and what were referred to as unnatural crimes between men'.[48]

The contradictions inherent in creating a free society from a penal settlement designed to instil terror were clear in May 1837, when Molesworth's committee called the naval surgeon Thomas Galloway to give evidence on the state of convict transportation to Australia. In answer to a question about whether convicts generally looked upon convict transportation as a severe punishment, Galloway answered that he believed that convicts 'think it is desirable to be sent out, and I believe many of them got themselves into scrapes for the purpose of being transported … from hearing of the fine country they were to go to'.[49] Nevertheless, Galloway's evidence also attested to the naval surgeons' ongoing struggles with health at sea. Galloway admitted, from the experience of five previous voyages to Australia, that convicts generally arrived at the end of the voyage in worse health than they had been at the beginning.

For naval surgeons, convict transportation had become one of their main sources of full, paid employment after the end of the Napoleonic Wars. As the following chapters make clear, these voyages also provided important opportunities for medical and scientific experimentation. But, as the system came under sustained attack during the 1830s, naval surgeons were still far from confident about their position. The ongoing conflicts about invalids with their medical peers in Britain and with the colonial authorities were symptomatic of broader struggles over professional status, pay, and their unfavourable position relative to army surgeons at this period.[50] For historians looking back to the 1830s, it has seemed apparent that the surgeons' increasing medical authority over convicts led to a decline in shipboard mortality, and that it was only natural that the British government should take these lessons and apply them to emigrants. Yet Galloway's evidence hints that naval surgeons working in 1837 were by no means confident either in their medical authority or in their power to improve overall health at sea, not least because they were witnessing a deeply disturbing re-emergence of scurvy among convicts during this decade. For surgeons, it was not obvious that this was a good moment for them to take responsibility for an entirely new group of migrants bound for Australia.

Schemes for emigration

In 1831 the British government introduced the first formal schemes of government emigration to Australia, using funds from colonial land sales to finance all or part of a steerage passage.[51] From 1834, the amended Poor Law allowed parishes to raise money from landowners and rate-payers, in order to assist the emigration of their parishioners, and the Colonial Office stationed half-pay naval officers in a number of ports to oversee emigration.[52] Initial numbers of emigrants were very small. After the government established a new Land and Emigration Committee, with T.F. Elliott as its Agent General, emigration expanded rapidly. Between 1836 and 1840, 28,985 immigrants arrived in New South Wales from Britain, of which 22,642 (85 per cent) were assisted by these government and bounty schemes. Within three years the numbers of immigrants were three times those of arriving convict transportees, and by 1840, as the British government suspended convict transportation to New South Wales in the wake of Molesworth's reports, new emigrant arrivals outnumbered their convict compatriots by four to one.[53]

When surgeon Thomas Galloway was summoned to give evidence to the Parliamentary Select Committee in the spring of 1837, he had just been appointed as one of the first naval surgeons to take responsibility for the superintendence of an emigrant voyage to Australia. Before departure, his duties included selecting suitable candidates for government assistance. Once Galloway had filled his quota, he would then accompany the emigrants to New South Wales. When he was called to give evidence in London, it interrupted his tour of southern English counties to recruit married couples under the age of 30, skilled in agriculture and 'mechanical' trades such as carpentry and blacksmithing. As both selector and surgeon, Galloway was responsible for the emigrants' character as well as their physical health.[54]

In May 1837 Galloway met the emigrants at Portsmouth, where the *Augusta Jessie* awaited its new passengers. The British government had simply adapted the vessel to accommodate a new class of people. Between 1837 and 1840, hired ships such as the *Augusta Jessie* were fitted out for emigrants at Deptford almost exactly the same as they were when used as convict ships. At the end of the voyage the surgeons returned the same journals to Sir William Burnett, the Director

General of the Admiralty Medical Department. Indeed, many of the
emigrant journals from these years still had the instructions for convict
ships pasted inside. The *Augusta Jessie* had a busy Australian career, and
on its return to England in 1838 would refit immediately for two more
voyages with convicts.

Just as the convict transports did, the ships hired for the conveyance
of emigrants sailed from Deptford. To a casual observer standing on
the banks of the Thames, only the presence of a military guard made
it obvious whether a ship was destined to carry emigrants or convicts.
From Deptford, the ships sailed to a series of ports around England,
Ireland, and Scotland where the previously selected emigrants awaited
notice that their vessel was ready to depart. It was at this point that
one of the first major differences between emigration and convict
transportation emerged. When we compare the geography of the ports
used for convict departures (Cork, Dublin, London, Portsmouth) with
those used by emigrants, we see that from the beginning government
emigration was far less reliant on the coastal military infrastructure
of the British Isles than was the system of penal transportation.
Around a third of these emigrant vessels embarked their emigrants
from Gravesend, well beyond the prison hulks in the Thames estuary.
Other vessels sailed from Bristol; from Limerick, Dublin, Cork and
Londonderry (now Derry) in Ireland; and from Greenock, Leith, Loch
Foyle and the Isle of Skye in Scotland.

Furthermore, because emigrants made their own way to the ships,
unrestrained by the institutional mechanisms that delivered convicts,
they brought a new character to the problems of departure in the
late 1830s. Without the presence of a mediating figure bound to take
responsibility for any emigrants the naval surgeon might deem unfit to
travel, it was much more difficult for surgeons to reject emigrants who
had committed everything they had financially, and also emotionally
and physically, to their Australian voyage. For many emigrants, as for
the consumptive Mrs Bateup whom we met in the Introduction as she
pleaded with surgeon Galloway to be allowed to embark the *Augusta
Jessie*, there simply was often nowhere, and nothing, to which they
could return.

Subsequent to their selection for the voyage several weeks earlier,
many emigrants travelled over long distances to reach their port. They
were liable for their own costs, and often with little money for food or
accommodation. The effects of events that might appear to be minor
mishaps in the days, weeks or months before a voyage lingered, and
re-emerged as causes of illness in their conversations with surgeons. In
1839 Mrs Baker got wet as she travelled from Hastings to Gravesend,

and had slept in her wet clothes. She suffered from diarrhoea with fever for three days before presenting herself to the surgeon.[55] Another woman, Mrs Burr, explained to the surgeon that she too had been 'much exposed to inclement weather', in this case during her previous work in the fields as a hop gatherer. Mrs Burr admitted that she had concealed her complaint at embarkation in order that she would not be refused passage.[56] A young boy came to the *Augusta Jessie* from 'the marshy flat in the neighbourhood of Rye' (a village on the English south coast), where he and his father had both been subject to intermittent fevers. These complaints returned in the cold, damp, maritime atmosphere, while other children brought scarlatina, measles, and eye disorders to the early days at sea.[57]

One emigrant stated that the evening before his embarkation on the *Lady Nugent*, he had been exposed to heavy rain as he travelled from Rolvendon, a small village in Kent. He had been 'obliged to remain in a cart during the night in his wet clothes', and in the morning 'he was subject to cold shivering with entire loss of appetite'.[58] We know a great deal about the imperial careers of travelling Victorians, but the common threads that weave through these accounts give us a glimpse of how experiences related to health shaped the meaning and experience of travel for people who were totally unaccustomed to, and largely unprepared for, a migrant life. Even the shortest of everyday journeys – let alone a voyage to Australia – carried significance. Emigrants brought the everyday pathologies of nineteenth-century labouring life, and their understanding of this world, to the first few days at sea. Although this was often a profoundly topographical and environmental knowledge based on their former lives in fields and villages, and the roads and weathers that they had encountered on their journey to the ship, it was also a knowledge that surgeons understood, and to a large extent shared. When Thomas Galloway reflected on the start of the *Prince Regent*'s voyage in 1839 – his second with emigrants – he wrote that the people had been 'in general healthy' when they arrived at their port of departure. However, 'the lateness of the season, together with the stormy weather to which they were exposed in travelling to Gravesend laid the foundations of diseases which soon showed themselves'.[59]

Irish departures

Wherever surgeons received convicts in Britain and Ireland, they continually requested that emigrant and convict vessels should not be allowed to depart in the autumn and winter. For both convicts and emigrants, the isolated rural terrain and unpredictable weather of Ireland posed particular problems before even getting to sea. In 1839, one emigrant surgeon recorded that two young children had died of diarrhoea after getting cold on the journey to the ship as they travelled for nearly eighty miles in 'a common cart in very cold weather ... [F]rom the general excitement consequent on getting on board, and subsequently sea-sickness and want of proper care, the disease got too far advanced to be checked.' Perhaps sensing that he might have implicated himself in this explanation, he reiterated that 'everything I could do for them was done'.[60]

The effects of exposure to weather were also a central theme in correspondence about convict ships from Ireland. When the *Augusta Jessie* left Kingstown harbour in October 1839, the weather had been typical of the maritime autumn; winds from the south and north-west brought rain for a week after the convicts boarded the transport. One of the convicts, Patrick Wilson, believed that the pain in his back and limbs, as well as his troublesome cough, was the result of his 'recent exposure to raw boisterous weather'. The surgeon noted that the convict had already been transported once before, which accounted 'for Patrick's extraordinary degree of anxiety and mental depression' as the *Augusta Jessie* lost sight of the Irish shore. Such effects were only temporary, and within ten days the surgeon reported that all of the convicts had recovered from the effects of 'sea sickness and expatriation'.[61]

In 1844 the owner of a steamship offered to transfer prisoners from the depots in Dublin to the waiting ships in Kingstown harbour, but would only allow the convicts to travel on the open deck. The Convict Office rejected the proposition because the distance was 'so far that the convicts would be exposed to wet' and there was 'no possibility of being able to supply them with dry clothes upon them reaching the ship'. Within two months, however, the Convict Office had changed its mind. It now reported that the use of a steam tug 'obviated all the disagreeable consequences' that had attended sending convicts by road, and saved the troops 'a long hurried march from the depot'. By 1845, the Convict Office's focus had shifted from the meteorological problems of the harbour to those of the convicts' overland journey: 'The removal of convicts from distant parts of the Kingdom in open jaunting carts coming out of warm prisons in bad weather without any covering save what they wear in their cells, leaves them liable to cold and other diseases.' Moreover, 'sailing from Ireland in a tempestuous season produces an early seasickness most detrimental, whereas if ships sailed from Ireland in moderate weather the convict would become inured to the sea by degrees & better fitted for the long voyage'.[62]

Far from being banal, these observations about the Irish weather make an important geographical point about the experience of Australian voyages. Like many of their contemporaries, surgeons often commented on cultural and national differences between English, Scottish, and Irish people, as well as between those from cities and rural areas. For example, Andrew Henderson described the Irish character as 'a complete tissue of inconsistencies ... and constantly brooding over their misfortunes', but did believe that 'the Irish were in general better scholars than the English'.[63] In 1844 John Munn explained that 'on proceeding to sea most of the prisoners were very severely affected with sea sickness ... some of the old men in particular from the interior of Ireland, never having even seen the sea or a ship before suffered extremely, and were in such a state of despondency that I was afraid they would sink altogether'. These men 'required much nursing and encouragement to enable them to bear up against their position', and to the loss of their tobacco.[64] A few years later, Charles Smith observed that the Irish women suffered 'from grief and depression of spirits at leaving their friends and native country, the more delicate were sea-sick and unable to use the common rations and it became necessary to support them with medical comforts and wine'.[65] Surgeons' statements clearly reflected prevalent contemporary cultural assumptions about 'Irishness', as they did paternalistic ideas about women and children.[66] Nevertheless, it is also important to recognise that many of these reflections contained more subtle observations about the terrain of nineteenth-century Ireland and about the maritime reality of sailing from Cork or Dublin.

The vessels that left southern English ports had more options for anchoring in a chain of natural harbours and sheltered ports stretching several hundred miles from Kent in the east to Falmouth at the far western tip of the British mainland. Convicts and emigrants who left Ireland's south coast, on the other hand, immediately faced the unpredictable gales of the Celtic Sea and the huge swells that rolled across the vast, open expanse of the North Atlantic Ocean, with only Falmouth as a realistic option for shelter.

The intimacies of past lives

From a sharp downpour in an open cart to the most protracted of chronic illnesses, everyone brought something of their old life with them when they embarked on a voyage to Australia. If the character of the sea profoundly affected the experience of voyaging from the very start, the more intimate details from a person's past life also helped to explain their mental and physical constitution, and their prospects for health at sea. This was as true of sailors and soldiers as it was of emigrants and convicts. In 1838 Jonathan Boorman, an emigrant, embarked on the *Lady Nugent* in 'a debilitated habit of body'. As a butcher, he had led 'a very irregular life and was for many years a habitual drunkard'.[67] A young woman on the emigrant ship *Mandarin* 'had been for a long time previous in the most abject poverty and when she came on board she found a facility of getting good food which nothing could induce her to abstain from'.[68] Eleanor Stephenson, although 'of naturally good constitution', had been 'much reduced by close attendance (often 16 hours a day) in a cloth manufactury, where she first had an epileptic fit, about three months back'.[69] When the *Blenheim* left Kingstown harbour in September 1848, four of the military guard were suffering from syphilis, but the surgeon found in general that the soldiers' health was worse than that of the convicts. Several of the military men suffered from bronchitis and consumption, and most of them 'were young recruits, raised in Ireland and probably most of them suffered from the late disastrous famine and fever'.[70]

The naval surgeon's instructions made it clear that he was to give the crew and military guard the benefit of his medical assistance when needed, though he was not allowed to interfere in any way with the navigation of the ship. In turn, the ship's officers and crew no longer had any authority over the management of emigrants or convicts. In these first few days on the empty ship, before emigrants or convicts embarked, the sailors, privates, and officers of the military guard often took it upon themselves to seek treatment for venereal diseases. While until the late eighteenth century the Admiralty had enforced a fine of twelve shillings upon sailors who needed treatment for the pox, the frequency with which sailors and soldiers appeared on sick lists within a few days of embarkation suggests that they now saw an Australian voyage as an opportunity to receive a free and uninterrupted course of medical treatment.[71]

In 1840 one surgeon stated simply that 'on our passage across the Bay of Biscay, and towards Madeira, the cases put on the sick list were chiefly syphilitic amongst the guard and catarrhal amongst the prisoners'.[72] So too, when their cases involved women, surgeons often recorded numerous cases of venereal disease in their sick-list entries and summary tables, but made no further comment on them in individual case notes. Some surgeons removed sailors, soldiers, and convicts with venereal diseases back to shore, but the vast majority were confident (even if such confidence was misplaced) that a regime of mercurial treatment could successfully treat both primary and secondary symptoms of syphilis in a month or two.[73] On the other hand, it is also true that many women were not able, or perhaps did not try, to hide that they had undergone previous courses of mercurial treatment in prison. During the first three weeks of the voyage of the female convict ship *Australasia* in 1849, for example, the surgeon entered eight cases of syphilis on the sick list but reserved his detailed case notes for cases of fever, dysentery, and bronchitis.

In the ports and military garrisons of the British Empire, 'prostitution, crime and mobility formed a heady trio of prejudices', Philippa Levine has written. Joy Damousi, too, has argued that venereal diseases invited comments about the circumstances of the life that a person left behind, particularly for women.[74] It is important to note, therefore, that in the first half of the nineteenth century, before the Contagious Diseases Acts, the majority of surgeons did not routinely fill their journals with 'outbursts of hatred, disgust and loathing' that would characterise debates later in the century.[75] For most naval surgeons, the environmental – rather than the moral – causes and implications of disease occupied the vast majority of their journal space. In the first half of the nineteenth century, before the fears aroused by debates about the Contagious Diseases Acts, naval surgeons appear relatively disinterested in venereal diseases. They did not seem to see them as a real opportunity for medical enquiry (as, for example, disinfection, scurvy, and cholera were) or as a potential source of professional conflict that would threaten their reputation at the end of a voyage (as invalidity, consumption, and fevers were). So long as surgeons' medicine chests were well stocked with mercury, they seem to have treated venereal diseases as another legacy of the lives that people brought with them to the start of a voyage. On emigrant voyages, the issue was almost entirely absent. This is not to say that these naval surgeons did not encounter emigrants with venereal diseases, nor that they did not share contemporary assumptions about morality and respectability, but it reminds us again that surgeons' medical journals served a particular purpose. Journals are not simply transparent windows onto voyages. Perhaps they are better likened to salt-and-limpet-encrusted port-holes.

The 1840s: change and divergence

In 1840 the newly created Colonial Land and Emigration Commission (CLEC) took over governmental supervision of emigration as New South Wales began making rapid progress in the transition from a penal colony to a free society. With a shrinking pool of surgeons, and increasing commitments in West Africa, the Navy was as reluctant to commit its surgeons for the purposes of emigration as the CLEC was to pay the costs of employing them when private surgeons would do the job more cheaply.[76] For their part, surgeons seem to have found the care of so many nursing mothers and children that emigrant voyages involved to be quite tedious. One complained that 'the duty of Surgeon-Superintendent of an Emigrant ship is arduous and harassing, particularly at the commencement of the voyage when he has to bring into order and regularity a mass of people totally unaccustomed to such habits and unable to appreciate the importance of cleanliness'. Another wrote that the government's preference for selecting married couples with children was 'an error', because the children 'have not strength enough' to bear the change of climate and diet.[77]

In 1839, after the Molesworth Committee's conclusions condemned New South Wales society, the nature of convict voyaging was also changing. The British government suspended convict transportation to the colony and instead focused its penal attention on Van Diemen's Land, which now received an 'avalanche' of convicts. In just four years, from 1840 to 1844, the island's convict population increased by 40 per cent as over sixteen thousand convicts arrived.[78]

Even as they withdrew from direct involvement with emigration, naval surgeons increasingly invested in a vision of the convict voyage as a space of educational and moral reform, and an opportunity to undertake their own medical and disciplinary experimentations. By the 1840s, surgeons routinely set up schools on convict ships to teach convicts, particularly the youngest, to read and write. On the *Mountstuart Elphinstone* George Moxey employed twenty-nine tailors to sew trousers from 'grey frieze and buck'.[79] By the 1840s, religious instructors accompanied many convict voyages. One of the most striking pastimes was the creation of ships' newspapers. On the *Pestonjee Bomanjee*, for example, the surgeon described the convicts' weekly journal as a vehicle for preparing them for their 'advent in that beautiful country where, it is hoped, you will retrieve the errors of your past life'. Handwritten, and distributed week by week, the newspaper would '[indicate] the advance you make in correct reasoning and feeling'.[80]

If surgeons were increasingly confident about their practices at sea, penal reforms back in Britain were creating new medical problems that manifested from the very beginning of the voyages. Faced with the ongoing problem of what to do with its convicts, in 1842 the British government opened Pentonville prison, proclaimed as the model of the 'separate' system of solitary confinement and the 'portal to the colonies'. Over the previous decade, reformers had introduced designs for confinement in separate cells. In Pentonville, convicts would undergo a regime of imprisonment designed to instil religion and moral reform through exacting calculations of punishment, reflection, and labour, spending the vast majority of the day in their own cell. After this probationary period they would sail to Australia, where, with tickets of leave that allowed them to work, they would provide colonial labour. Observers soon began to notice the mental and physical effects that such extreme confinement had on prisoners. When Pentonville first opened, the surgeon of the *Wye* hospital ship at Chatham warned publicly that early experiments with solitary confinement had rendered many convicts 'more fit for an hospital than for dockyard labour'.[81] Later, Thomas Archer's *The Pauper, the Thief and the Convict* (1865) described 'something peculiarly blank and hopeless about the smooth and bare surface of the cell-walls, something terribly unsympathetic in the rigid monotony of unbroken order which is stamped upon each small detail of the prison furniture'.[82]

As Frank Dikotter has argued, penal realities often 'had little to do with ambitious plans on paper'.[83] The naval surgeons who received prisoners destined for Australia were among the first of Pentonville's critics. In November 1844 the *Sir George Seymour* transported the first group of Pentonville convicts to Port Phillip and Van Diemen's Land.[84] John Hampton, the surgeon, had previously superintended two other convict voyages. On the *Sir George Seymour*'s arrival in Australia, Hampton remarked on the 'superior quality' of its convicts. Here was a group of 'useful and efficient workmen' who were 'well worthy of the establishment from which they were received and deserving the attention of all who are interested in the success of reformatory penal discipline'.[85]

Hampton had received 345 men from Pentonville, all of whom had undergone separate confinement for periods varying from fifteen to twenty-two months. Hampton's endorsement of the convicts' 'superior quality' says more about his belief in the success of his voyage regime and his own investment in a career in the convict system (a year later, Hampton became comptroller of convicts in Van Diemen's Land) than it does about the good effects of Pentonville, because his account of the *Sir George Seymour*'s departure paints a very different picture. 'The sudden change from extreme seclusion to the noise and bustle of a crowded ship', he wrote, 'produced a great number of cases of convulsions, attended in some instances with nausea and vomiting in others simulating hysteria, and in all being of a most anomalous character.' Hampton laid the convicts down on the deck in the fresh air and gave them mild stimulants, but so many 'novel and alarming cases caused doubts as to the prudence of sailing, not only until the convulsions ceased, but until it was seen whether the men were otherwise in a fit state to commence a long voyage'.[86]

Other naval surgeons soon corroborated Hampton's reports of convulsing convicts. Ten months later, on the *Stratheden*, nineteen men suffered from convulsions immediately after their embarkation. All had spent between eighteen and twenty months in solitary confinement in Pentonville.[87] When the Medical Officer for Pentonville visited the convict ship *Eden* in September 1848, he too admitted that 'of the 193 Prisoners from Pentonville on board, there had been nineteen cases of convulsive fits, and less violent symptoms in great number'.[88] As convicts left the tightly regulated solitary spaces of the new prison cells, their bodies betrayed the complex physical and mental effects of penal reform.

As we have seen, naval surgeons often complained about the hidden diseases of convicts, but here in the 1840s was an entirely new problem. This was not an unfitness caused by exposure to bad weather, consumption, or invalidity, but an institutionalised unfitness, inherent in the very fabric of prisons such as Pentonville. This was an unfitness revealed suddenly and violently as convicts collapsed on the crowded decks of ships after leaving their cells. Nevertheless, it appears that surgeons' complaints went largely unremarked as penal transportation as a whole became mired in scandal and its termination became inevitable. Amid the hysteria surrounding allegations of homosexuality, male transportation to Van Diemen's Land was suspended in 1846, although women, particularly from Ireland, continued to arrive. In Port Phillip too, colonists increasingly opposed the arrival of Pentonville's 'exiles'.[89]

Cholera

Men who left solitary confinement in the 1840s displayed some remarkable and disturbing symptoms of the effects of their imprisonment, but they were not the only convicts to collapse in the days following departure from Britain. Surgeons of convict ships had first encountered epidemic cholera in 1831. The diagnosis 'cholera', or 'cholera morbus', had long been a catch-all term for a variety of seasonal acute bowel disorders and diarrhoeas, but 'malignant' or 'Asiatic' cholera had travelled through Persia, Russia, and the Baltic coast.[90] Many contemporaries identified Sunderland as its British point of entry, but some naval surgeons believed that the disease with which they were dealing had entered Britain by the infected ships that arrived at the Medway quarantine station in the Thames in the summer of 1831. This was, of course, the same estuary in which thousands of convicts were housed in hulks.[91] In 1831, surgeon John Stephenson had his first experience with the new disease on the convict ship *Katherine Stewart Forbes*. He had described the cholera cases as 'perfectly appalling'. Out of twenty-one cases, thirteen had appeared 'desperate'. Stephenson countered the violence of the disease with bold therapeutics. For one patient he used hot baths and vigorous rubbing: 'strong friction usually abated the pain' and was 'constantly kept up'. Stephenson administered opium, mustard rubs, blisters, bleeding, calomel, spirits of ammonia and aether. He applied 'nearly boiling' water to another patient's feet in an attempt to draw the poison out.[92]

The following year, this time on the convict ship *Waterloo*, Stephenson again encountered cholera, and he remarked that its character was the same as he had witnessed on the *Katherine Stewart Forbes*. Like many other surgeons and physicians around the country, Stephenson pondered the nature of this new disease and saw an opportunity to contribute his opinion to the politically charged arguments about whether or not cholera was contagious. Initially, he had 'tended to favour the doctrine of contagion', but he had changed his mind after observing that many men had remained healthy even when they had worn the clothes of and slept under the blankets of dead patients (in defiance of his order that they be destroyed), which satisfied him that cholera was not contagious.[93]

In his *Waterloo* journal Stephenson described how he allowed the mother and wife of one of the convicts – a man named Robert Coney – on to the transport to say goodbye to him as the sailors prepared to weigh anchor. 'Whilst talking with them on deck', Stephenson explained, Coney had been 'suddenly seized with vertigo, universal tremor, nausea and vomiting, and such a state of weakness that he was unable to support himself'. Coney was taken below and in less than an hour 'had every symptom of malignant cholera'. During the night, he died.[94] Stephenson was clearly interested in cholera as one of the most pressing political and medical debates of the day, but his intimate account of Robert Coney's collapse on the deck of the *Waterloo* as he bade farewell to his wife is also revealing of cholera's significance. Coney's inability to support himself indicated the emotional rupture he experienced as he was removed from loved ones, and signalled the onset of cholera. For contemporary commentators, collapses like these helped to explain how cholera so often attacked those people who were seasick, weak, drunk, or melancholy. After the second 1848–49 epidemic, the General Board of Health's *Report on the Epidemic Cholera* explained that a person's 'weakened vital stamina' suddenly gave way to cholera when 'specific acts of intemperance in food or drink, over-fatigue, or perhaps sudden alarm, have destroyed the resisting power'.[95] The violence of cholera seemed to reveal the underlying mental and physical state of the person.

Coney's collapse also makes us rethink our historians' emphasis on epidemic cholera using the metaphors of mass migration, military invasion, social crisis, colonial disorder, Malthusian purging and industrial modernity that fill the pages of cholera's literature.[96] Perhaps most persistently, however, cholera's commentators have described a 'migrant' disease on the move, an invading disease of immigrants' arrival. Alan Kraut writes of a disease that 'sailed' into New York and other American ports. Charles Rosenberg suggested that it 'swept like revolution', a pestilence that 'often flared up among immigrant barge and steamboat passengers, debilitated by long sea voyages, hungry, dirty, and huddled together on decks so crowded that even the sick could not lie down'.[97] John Snow described cholera as a disease that 'travels along the great tracks of human intercourse, never going faster than people travel, and generally much more slowly'. Here was a disease of sea ports and of 'intercourse with the shore'.[98] Nevertheless, when Horatio Gates Jameson wrote that cholera liked to ramble in 'mud and mire, and crowded houses, and low places', he hinted at a much less rampant history, one often lost amid cholera's close association with 'otherness'.[99] In emphasising cholera's association with arrival on a huge scale, we have perhaps missed the extent to which contemporaries knew that cholera was also a disease that revealed very intimate things about estuaries and ports of departure.[100] By 1848, cholera also confirmed that there was something profoundly troubling about the effects of solitary confinement on the health of convicts.

Despite the problems in Van Diemen's Land, the British government was still determined to find somewhere that would accept its convicts. In 1848, Lord Grey attempted to re-introduce transportation to New South Wales. The *Hashemy* would be the first convict ship to sail to New South Wales in a decade. The angry crowds that greeted its arrival in Sydney are well known, but the *Hashemy*'s departure, which coincided with the return of epidemic cholera in the autumn of 1848, was equally traumatic.[101] The *Hashemy*'s surgeon, Colin Arrott Browning, received 237 convicts from four different English prisons who had crossed the estuary in small boats. Most of the men came from Wakefield and Pentonville, both prisons that used separate cells. One man came from London's Millbank penitentiary, and twenty-five juveniles from Parkhurst, the boys' prison on the Isle of Wight. Many had spent time in two or three prisons. As Browning questioned them about the circumstances of their removal from their individual cells, the Pentonville prisoners reported that in preparation for the voyage they had undergone 'association' over a period of twenty-three days for two hours each day before they embarked the transport. Association was supposed to allow convicts to readjust to social contact, but as the men from Pentonville reached the *Hashemy*, Browning described how their 'power of thinking, their common sense, and in a peculiar degree their *memory*, appeared to have been left behind them buried in their cell'.[102] The men demonstrated an 'absolute incapacity to render themselves useful to the community either at home or in the colonies'.[103] In the two months that the *Hashemy* remained anchored off the English south coast Browning dealt with 193 cases of cholera, of which fourteen men died.[104]

On 13 December Browning wrote to the Director General of the Medical Department of the Navy describing the scenes on the *Hashemy*'s deck:

> Prisoners, when embarked from the cells in which they have long been solitarily confined are liable for several days after their embarkation to be affected with *syncope* and *convulsions*, sometimes *hysterical*, sometimes *epileptic*, or resembling those of epilepsy … One, two three, & even sometimes *four* at one time were carried out of the prison, and laid on the deck under the influence of the affections just specified.... The *cause*, it appears to me, is to be found in the *suddenness* and *extent* involved in the change of the embarkation of the prisoners from their solitary cells, unseasoned, unprepared by social intercourse for the period of a required number of weeks, previous to them being sent on board the transport.[105]

Browning found it 'difficult to imagine a body of 239 men and boys placed in circumstances *more favourable to the appearance of cholera* amongst them and more unfavourable to its arrest and removal'. Restating a common naval surgeons' plea that prisoners should embark from a healthy locality during a season likely to ensure favourable weather, Browning otherwise paid little attention to epidemic cholera. Primarily, Browning saw cholera as collapse at the end of a chain of illness that resulted from the anguish, dislocation, and protracted mental and physical deprivation caused by prolonged or solitary imprisonment. The extreme regime of separate confinement had left the men 'ill-prepared' to 'endure [cholera's] violence' or 'to recover from its effects on the entire frame'.[106]

When the first of the *Hashemy*'s convicts showed the symptoms of cholera, Browning requested the assistance of two doctors from the shore whom he assembled in his cabin 'in order that we might act consistently and not *injure* our patients by counteracting each others practice, to *agree* on a mode of treatment to which we should adhere'.[107] The Admiralty had established huge hospitals on the English south coast at Gosport and Plymouth during its expansion in the middle of the eighteenth century.[108] Browning knew that he could utilise all of the facilities of the Navy's Royal Haslar hospital, the hospital hulk *Unite*, and the quarantine ship *Menelaus*. Accordingly, he instructed the ship's master to steer for the naval base of Gosport. When cholera broke out on the female convict ship *Cadet* in 1848, the surgeon similarly ordered that the ship put in to Plymouth, where the Navy provided an assistant surgeon to help.[109]

Convicts who sailed away from Britain may have experienced a personal rupture, even collapse, but politically they remained within a coherent governmental system. Even when ships were racked with cholera, penal and military infrastructures overlapped. From land to sea, and back to land, the British government remained responsible and liable for the health of convicts until the end of their sentences. This observation is important because, as we will see, the reality for emigrants became very different.

Liverpool

As naval surgeons grappled with the problems of new penal systems and cholera in the late 1840s, New South Wales and Van Diemen's Land had both entered a severe economic depression. With little demand for labour, free migration to Australia had virtually ceased after the first peaks of the late 1830s. In 1846 and 1847, gross numbers of free immigrants to New South Wales were below a thousand.[110] Britons still migrated in great numbers during this lull, but overwhelmingly they went to North America.[111] For this reason, while cholera became a huge problem in cities like New Orleans and New York, it had little effect on discussions about Australian migration until the 1850s.[112] Indeed, in January 1849 the *Maitland Mercury* summarily dismissed rumours that a recent immigrant had brought cholera to New South Wales as a false alarm 'only raised by the wonder hunters for want of something else to talk of'.[113] As far as Australian colonists were concerned, cholera, like the Irish famine, had been 'lost in transit'.[114]

While convict transportation relied on the naval infrastructure of the British and Irish southern ports, the focus of emigration very soon shifted to other ports in the West and North, including Bristol, Southampton, Belfast, and, most importantly, Liverpool. The city's merchants had initially grown rich by trading slaves and cotton. In the first half of the nineteenth century the estuary of the river Mersey, flanked by Liverpool on the north bank and Birkenhead to the south, had become the hub of a massive, chaotic, and ill-regulated commercial North American emigrant trade. During the late 1840s – the years of the Irish famine – the Mersey's authorities struggled to balance the rapidly increasing importance of the estuary's international connections with their fears about the influx of migrants, typhus fever, and cholera.[115] Between 1849 and 1853, 1,241,000 people arrived in the Mersey from Ireland, of whom nearly half were paupers. To cope, Liverpool's authorities, and the ship-owners who profited, had developed slick systems for processing and sending migrants onwards.[116]

In 1851, when Edward Hargraves proclaimed that he had discovered gold in New South Wales, the Mersey became the new main port of departure for Australian migrant voyaging. The Gold Rush ended any possibility of resuming convict transportation to Van Diemen's Land and Port Phillip (from 1853, only Western Australia would continue to accept convicts until the system ended for good in 1868), and it attracted a flood of free migrants from the British Isles, Europe, America, and China.[117] The effect on Liverpool was huge and immediate. In 1852, the CLEC constructed a depot in Birkenhead capable of holding four thousand emigrants at a time. In 1854 alone, 127 ships took 41,000 emigrants to Australia from the Mersey.[118] Shipping companies vied with each other for business by promising ever-faster voyages, on ever-larger ships. On some days, an inspector could receive sixteen notices in one morning to clear ships for departure.[119] Although many emigrants still received government assistance to pay for their passage, for the first time a majority of labouring people paid their own fares to Australia, even as those fares more than doubled, from £10 in 1851, to £23 in 1853.[120] The trade no longer bore much relation to the government schemes of the late 1830s, but grew instead from a booming commercial enterprise with only a veneer of government regulation once ships had left the sight of land.

On 18 February 1854, William Dooly wrote from Liverpool to 'Betty' in Ireland to say that the family had received a draft for twenty pounds, and a certificate to guarantee their passage to Australia.[121] For several years, William had planned his emigration, along with a woman called Ann Jane – probably William's sister – and with the assistance of a sister who already lived in Adelaide.[122] On 17 June, William wrote again to Betty to confirm that he and Ann Jane would 'sail from a place called Birkinhead [*sic*] on the other side of the river from Liverpool. I am not sure yet how soon the ship will sail after that but we shall have to live in the depot untill she is ready for sea.' William sent enough money to pay for Ann Jane's passage from Belfast across the Irish Sea on the Wednesday night ferry. 'I will meet her at the boat next morning,' he wrote.[123] On 26 June, William and Ann Jane crossed the Mersey to the Birkenhead emigrant depot to await the *Dirigo*.

After lying in the estuary off Birkenhead for nine days, the *Dirigo* finally set sail on 6 July 1854 with over five hundred passengers, including William and Ann Jane Dooly, bound for Port Adelaide.[124] Shortly afterwards, several of the passengers came down with a fever, from which two infants, a young boy, a 13-year-old girl and a man died. By the second evening of the voyage, the health of the passengers had deteriorated. It was clear that fever had become cholera. The next morning, as the ship arrived in Cork, Ann Jane Dooly died. In a letter to the family in Ireland, William explained that he had attended upon Ann Jane 'with several young women all the day and night but we could not save her'.[125] Captain de Courcy, the government emigration officer for Cork, hired the 'only available hulk' in order to separate the twelve sick passengers from those who remained healthy, but with such limited facilities, de Courcy explained, that he had 'no means of accommodating healthy passengers here'. After a hurried exchange of telegraphs, de Courcy ordered the *Dirigo*, and all the emigrants who appeared healthy, back to Liverpool under the tow of a steamboat, the *Minerva*.[126] Just four days after it first departed, the *Dirigo* returned to the Mersey. As the ship reached the dock gates at Birkenhead the Customs authorities ordered the Captain to anchor in the middle of the estuary, and placed the vessel in quarantine.[127]

From London, the Secretary to the Colonial Land and Emigration Commissioners directed that the healthy emigrants could return to the emigration depot, but provision for the sick 'must be made outside the depot'.[128] Lieutenant Prior, the Government Emigration Officer for Liverpool, reported that the local Birkenhead Improvement Commissioners had 'refused to allow the *Dirigo* to be brought into dock'. Prior forced the Birkenhead Commissioners to accept the emigrants by threatening to land the people if the parish did not provide accommodation for them.[129] On 13 July, the Birkenhead Commissioners 'at last determined to erect an iron house on a piece of ground outside the [emigrant] depot' for the reception of the sick, but a 'rabble' of Birkenhead residents then threatened to pull the structure down.[130] The *Liverpool Mail* of 15 July reported that 'an unfounded rumour prevailed' on Wednesday evening, that 'a number of the residents of the north of Birkenhead were determined by force to oppose the landing of the sick emigrants in the township'. To prevent violence, the *Mail* continued, 'the boatmen belonging to Woodside ferry were armed with bludgeons and other weapons, but fortunately they were not called upon to use them'.[131] Finally, the Birkenhead Commissioners agreed to admit twenty-two patients from the *Dirigo* into the parish fever hospital. However, they 'respectfully' suggested that

> when disease breaks out in an emigrant ship after she has commenced her voyage she ought not to be allowed to return to the port from which she sailed when that would cause considerable and unnecessary delay in procuring assistance and relief to the passengers ... There can be no doubt that if the necessary relief had been afforded at Cork the disease would have been much less virulent, and that many lives would have been saved.[132]

Beneath the language of relief and welfare, the question of who should be responsible for the *Dirigo*'s emigrants was at the heart of these discussions.

On a local level, the arguments about the *Dirigo* stemmed directly from ongoing battles in Liverpool and Birkenhead about migration and disease that had drained local resources for nearly a decade. The *Liverpool Standard*, for example, identified an English family from Southampton as the bearers of disease. The *Dirigo* outbreak had 'been clearly traced to sufferers who, having forsaken another emigration port and come to Liverpool, have unconsciously brought with them the seeds of disease and death, and disseminated these amongst their hapless fellow-travellers'.[133] However, the *Dirigo* also helps us to understand the changing nature of Australian voyaging and, importantly, the divergent histories of departure. In the act of departing, the *Dirigo*'s emigrants became outsiders who were now somewhere else's problem. When they left land, emigrants could no longer rely on the governmental structures and systems – represented most clearly by the emigrant depot – that were designed to ensure their welfare. Their political and social status, and their right to belong anywhere, became very uncertain. These issues would re-emerge on the emigrants' arrival in Australia.

Conclusion

We have already come a long way from Dr Harding's decision in 1813 to send the Irish convict Haly on the *Three Bees*, in the hope that the voyage might improve his health. When the British government first made naval surgeons responsible for all aspects of the health and discipline of convicts at sea in 1815, these medical men stepped into a rapidly expanding and evolving process of global migration. As surgeons sought to define the parameters of their authority and the purpose of the convict voyage, the character of the Australian colonies, and the streams of people who went there, also changed. In the 1830s, the first substantial waves of government-assisted emigrants coexisted with the peak of transportation, and there was little to differentiate between the two schemes. By the 1850s these had become, in the political and geographical sense, very different. As the focus of convict transportation shifted to Van Diemen's Land in 1840, and the initial wave of free emigrants declined, naval surgeons withdrew from emigration. Instead, they saw their interests served best by aligning themselves with convict transportation. This investment offered opportunities for medical and disciplinary experimentation, even as surgeons openly criticised penal reforms on land, a theme to which we will return in subsequent chapters.

By the 1850s, the commercial port of Liverpool dominated the massive Australian emigrant trade, and convict transportation was in terminal decline, but even then the question of what the Australian voyage was for remained at the fore of medical decisions about who should travel.

In May 1851, the Chair of the Select Committee on the Passengers' Act asked John James Lancaster, MD, Medical Officer for Liverpool, about his policies for rejecting sick emigrants. Lancaster had confirmed that either he or one of his colleagues inspected every ship leaving Liverpool. He rejected emigrants for typhus, ophthalmia, or the 'ordinary eruptive diseases of childhood'. When asked 'Do you reject [passengers] for consumption?' Lancaster replied categorically: 'No; it is not an infectious disease.'[134] Lancaster admitted, however, that an inspector did often reject a person who looked 'delicate' or bore the external signs of 'pauperism'.

In December 1852 one emigrant observed the ritual of the emigrants' medical examination in Liverpool. The Emigration Commissioner refused to allow a second woman to embark because she was 'in a sickly state of health'. She, and her husband, 'were obliged to take their luggage and return' to the shore. And yet, the Commissioner allowed a cabin passenger, so ill 'in consumption' that he had to be carried on board, to remain because he was travelling to Australia 'to recover his health'.[135]

In December 1851, the naval surgeon R. Whitmore Clarke listed forty-one female convicts from Grangegorman government female prison whom he had refused to accept on to the *John William Dare*. Clarke explained his strict rationale: it was in 'the interest of the colony' to select only 'the young and healthy'.[136] He rejected two of the women for debility, two others for their age, and four for both 'age and debility'. In total, Clarke rejected seventeen out of the forty women for being weak, debilitated, wasted, consumptive, too old, or simply 'totally unfit'.

Tracing the politics and problems of disease at sea from the moment of departure begins to make it clear that health at sea was never just about inspecting for infectious diseases, or about the surgeon's authority to enforce standards of hygiene and cleanliness. For many reasons, departure was often a messy, protracted affair, but it is precisely this messiness that illuminates the medical, political, colonial, and professional tensions that shaped maritime health and medicine. If, as one historian has written, the concept of cholera 'could be shaped and reshaped to serve the needs of whoever sought to depict it', the same was no less true of a problem like invalidity, a constant reminder that the purpose of Australian voyaging was never entirely clearly defined.[137] Even after the chaos and bustle of the fitting out and the embarkation inspections had subsided, arguments, delays, returns to port, exchanges of rations, and the return of people who were 'unfit' blurred the distinction between the politics and problems of land and sea. These were not simply mundane or messy inconveniences that distracted surgeons from getting on with their role of maintaining health at sea; on the contrary, they defined and shaped it. Whether about cholera, syphilis, invalidity, or convulsions, the life histories that people brought to sea, the decisions surgeons made at departure, and the language they used to justify them, bore fruit during the long weeks at sea.

Notes

1 From 1615, the English government sent convicts overseas as a commutation of capital punishment. In 1718 the Transportation Act made a sentence of transportation a secondary punishment in its own right, along with hard labour and incarceration in a house of correction. For the early history of transportation to America see Abbot Emerson Smith, *Colonists in Bondage: White Servitude and Convict Labour in America, 1607–1776* (Gloucester, MA: Peter Smith, 1965).

2 A.G.L. Shaw, *Convicts and the Colonies* (London: Faber and Faber, 1966), p. 148.

3 Charles Bateson, *The Convict Ships 1787–1868* (Glasgow: Brown, Son & Ferguson, 1985), p. 179.

4 James Boyce, *Van Diemen's Land* (Melbourne: Black Inc., 2010), pp. 38–39.

5 Governor King to Lord Hobart, 30 October 1802, *Historical Records of*

Australia (Sydney: Library Committee of the Commonwealth Parliament, 1916) Series 1: Volume 3, p. 583 (hereafter *HRA*).

6 Governor Macquarie to the Commissioners of the Transport Board, 24 March 1814, *HRA* 1:9, p. 244, and 1 October 1814, *HRA* 1:9, p. 275.

7 Surgeon Redfern to Governor Macquarie, 30 September 1814, *HRA* 1:9, pp. 274–293 (hereafter Redfern's Report), p. 278.

8 Redfern's Report, *HRA* 1:9, p. 279.

9 Redfern's Report, *HRA* 1:9, p. 291.

10 Kim Humphery, 'A New Era of Existence: Convict transportation and the authority of the surgeon in colonial Australia', *Labour History* (Australia) 59 (1990), pp. 59–72, pp. 63–64.

11 For quantitative calculations for convict voyages see John McDonald and Ralph Shlomowitz, 'Mortality on Convict Voyages to Australia, 1788–1868', *Social Science History* 13:3 (1989), pp. 285–313; for comparative figures and discussion see Hamish Maxwell-Stewart and Ralph Shlomowitz, 'Mortality and Migration: A survey', in David Boyd Haycock and Sally Archer (eds), *Health and Medicine at Sea, 1700–1900* (Woodbridge: Boydell Press, 2009), pp. 128–142. For emigration see Robin Haines, 'Medical Superintendence and Child Health on Government-assisted Voyages to South Australia in the Nineteenth-Century', *Health and History* 3:2 (2001), pp. 1–29.

12 National Archives of Ireland (NAI), Chief Secretary's Office OP 399/11, Doctor Harding, Journal for Attendance on Convicts, 1812–1813, 14–16 September 1813.

13 Bateson, *The Convict Ships, 1787–1868*, pp. 48–49, 382–383; Redfern's Report, p. 279.

14 NAI, OP 1815/439/5, Foster Archer, 'Observations on Governor Macquarie's Dispatch to Earl Bathurst and also on the remarks made thereon by the Right Hon'ble Lord Sidmouth' (n.d. 1815).

15 On travelling for health, see Clark Lawlor and Akihito Suzuki, 'The Disease of the Self: Representing consumption, 1700–1830', *Bulletin of the History of Medicine* 74 (2000), pp. 459–494, p. 471; Vladimir Jankovic, 'The Last Resort: A British perspective on the medical south', *Journal of Intercultural Studies* 27:3 (2006), pp. 271–298. On the seaside see Alain Corbin, *The Lure of the Sea: The Discovery of the Seaside in the Western World, 1750–1840* (Cambridge: Polity Press, 1994); John K. Walton, *The English Seaside Resort: A Social History, 1750–1914* (Leicester: Leicester University Press, 1983).

16 Eric T. Jennings, *Curing the Colonizers: Hydrotherapy, Climatology and French Colonial Spas* (Durham and London: Duke University Press, 2006), p. 37–8; Harriet Deacon, 'The Politics of Medical Topography: Seeking healthiness at the Cape during the nineteenth century', in Richard

Wrigley and George Revill (eds), *Pathologies of Travel* (Atlanta: Rodopi, 2000), pp. 279–297; Dane Kennedy, *The Magic Mountains: Hill Stations and the British Raj* (Berkeley, Los Angeles and London: University of California, 1996), pp. 19–38.

17 Ebenezer Gilchrist, M.D., *The Use of Sea Voyages in Medicine, and particularly in a Consumption: with Observations on that Disease*, new edition (London: T. Cadell, 1771), pp. 63–64.

18 Charles Turner Thackrah, *The Effects of Arts, Trades and Professions ... On Health and Longevity: With Suggestions for the removal of many of the Agents which produce disease and shorten the duration of life ... Second Edition, Greatly Enlarged* (London: Longman, Rees, Orme, Brown, Green, & Longman, 1832), pp. 7, 22.

19 James Clark, *A Treatise on Pulmonary Consumption Comprehending an Enquiry into the Causes Nature Prevention and Treatment of Tuberculous and Scrofulous Diseases in General* (London: Sherwood, Gilbert and Piper, 1835), p. 332.

20 William Sweetser, *A Treatise on Consumption; Embracing an Inquiry into the Influence Exerted upon it by Journeys, Voyages and Changes of Climate* (Boston: T.H. Carter, 1836), p. 173.

21 Richard Henry Dana, *Two Years before the Mast: A Personal Narrative of Life at Sea* (New York: Harper and Brothers, 1842), p. 6.

22 James H. Pickford, M.D., *Hygiene, or, Health as Depending upon the Conditions of the Atmosphere, Foods and Drinks, Motion and Rest, Sleep and Wakefulness, Secretions, Excretions and Retentions, Mental Emotions, Clothing, Bathing, &c.* (London: Churchill, 1858), p. 260.

23 Thomas Trotter, *Medicina Nautica*, 3 vols, vol. 3 (London: Longman, Hurst, Rees, and Orme, 1804), pp. 334–335.

24 Peter Cunningham, *Two Years in New South Wales* (Sydney: Angus and Robertson, 1966), p. 94, cited in Warwick Anderson, *The Cultivation of Whiteness: Science, Health and Racial Destiny in Australia* (New York: Basic Books, 2003), p. 16.

25 J.M. Powell, 'Medical Promotion and the Consumptive Immigrant to Australia', *Geographical Review* 63:4 (1973), pp. 449–476, pp. 451–453.

26 Samuel Dougan Bird, *On Australasian Climates and their Influence in the Prevention and Arrest of Pulmonary Consumption* (London: Longman, 1863), pp. 25, 31.

27 Powell, 'Medical Promotion', pp. 455–462; Linda Bryder, '"A Health Resort for Consumptives": Tuberculosis and immigration to New Zealand, 1880–1914', *Medical History* 40 (1996), pp. 453–471.

28 Marjorie Tipping, *Convicts Unbound: The Story of the Calcutta Convicts and their Settlement in Australia* (Melbourne: Viking O'Neill, 1988), discussed in Boyce, *Van Diemen's Land*, pp. 25–27.

29 James Hingston Tuckey, *An Account of a Voyage to Establish a Colony at Port Philip in Bass Strait* (London: Longman, Hurst, Rees, and Orme, 1805), p. 33.

30 TNA, ADM 101/53/2, Journal of surgeon John Love on female convict ship *Mellish* (1830), General Remarks and Case 1: Ann Thomas.

31 TNA, ADM 101/35/6, Journal of surgeon L.T. Cunningham on male convict ship *Hyderabad* (1849), Case 13: James Deegan.

32 TNA, ADM 101 73/7, Journal of surgeon Thomas R. Dunn on convict ship *Waverley* (1843), General Remarks (emphasis added).

33 TNA, ADM 101 73/7, Dunn, Journal on *Waverley*, Case 3: Michael Duffy.

34 TNA, ADM 101 73/7, Dunn, Journal on *Waverley*, General Remarks.

35 Bateson, *The Convict Ships*, pp. 13–22.

36 For an account of departure see 'Charles Picknell's Journal' in Anon, *The Kains: Female Convict Vessel* (Adelaide: Sullivan's Cove, 1989), pp. 11–12.

37 State Library of New South Wales, Mitchell Library, Mss 1524, Reminiscences of James Cripps (1848–59), Chapter 1st: Departure from Chatham.

38 R.F. Foster, *Modern Ireland, 1600–1972* (London: Penguin, 1989), p. 201.

39 TNA, ADM 101/2/6, Journal of surgeon George Fairfowl on convict ship *Andromeda* (1830), General Remarks.

40 TNA, ADM 101/65/2, Journal of surgeon Andrew Henderson on convict ship *Royal Admiral* (1833), Report on Scurvy: Causes.

41 TNA, ADM 101/73/3, Journal of surgeon John Stephenson on convict ship *Waterloo* (1833), Case of Thomas Emerson, June 1833.

42 TNA, ADM 105/36, Report of Lieutenant George Arthur re health of convicts upon the *Lord Lyndoch* (1837).

43 TNA, ADM 101/44/3, Journal of surgeon James Lawrence on convict ship *Lord Lyndoch* (1836), Case 3, James Smith; Case 13, George Manders; General Remarks.

44 TNA, ADM 105/36, Colin Arrott Browning to John Montague regarding the report into the sickness on board *Lord Lyndoch*, 21 September 1836 (emphasis in original).

45 TNA, ADM 105/36, Andrew Robertson, Letter regarding sickness on the *Lord Lyndoch*, 27 April 1837.

46 National Library of Australia, Canberra (NLA), MS3275, Diary of John Ward including voyage to Sydney on convict ship *Mangles* (1841–1842), entry dated September 1839, pp. 106–107, 113.

47 Kirsten McKenzie, *Scandal in the Colonies* (Melbourne: Melbourne University Press, 2005), p. 122.

48 McKenzie, *Scandal in the Colonies*, p. 124–125; John Ritchie, 'Towards Ending an Unclean Thing: the Molesworth Committee and the abolition of transportation to New South Wales, 1837–1840', *Historical Studies (Melbourne)* 17:3 (1976), pp. 144–164.

49 United Kingdom, House of Commons, Evidence of Thomas Galloway, *Report from the Select Committee on Transportation* 1837 [518], p. 183.

50 Mark Harrison, "'An Important and Truly National Subject'": The West Africa Service and the Health of the Royal Navy in the Mid Nineteenth Century', in David Boyd Haycock and Sally Archer (eds) *Health and Medicine at Sea, 1700–1900* (Woodbridge: Boydell Press, 2009), pp. 108–127, p. 110.

51 These had been preceded by experiments with Irish emigration to Upper Canada in 1823 and 1825 when 2,000 Irish labourers became known as 'Peter Robinson's settlers'. For government experiments with schemes of government emigration from Scotland and Ireland to Canada in the 1820s see Marjory Harper and Stephen Constantine, *Migration and Empire* (Oxford: Oxford University Press, 2010), pp. 16–21.

52 Fred H. Hitchins, *The Colonial Land and Emigration Commission* (Philadelphia: University of Philadelphia Press, 1931), pp. 17–23.

53 Robin Haines, *Emigration and the Labouring Poor* (Basingstoke: Palgrave, 1997), p. 261. For an overview of the mechanisms of assisted migration see Eric Richards, 'How did Poor People Emigrate from the British Isles to Australia in the Nineteenth Century?', *Journal of British Studies* 32:3 (1993), pp. 250–279, pp. 250–256. The vast majority of these Australian migrants travelled in steerage, a voyage which cost around £30 in 1828, £18 in 1836, and fell to £10 in 1851.

54 Evidence of Thomas Galloway, *Report from the Select Committee on Transportation*, pp. 178–179.

55 TNA, ADM 101/78/9, Journal of surgeon Thomas Galloway on emigrant ship *Prince Regent* (1838–9), Case 1: Mrs W. Baker.

56 TNA, ADM 101/78/9, Galloway, journal on *Prince Regent*, Case 2: Mrs E. Burr.

57 TNA, ADM 101/76/4, Journal of surgeon Thomas Galloway on emigrant ship *Augusta Jessie* (1837), Case 3: James Roots; TNA, ADM 101/78/9: Galloway, journal on *Prince Regent*, General Remarks.

58 TNA, ADM 101/77/10, Journal of surgeon G. Roberts on emigrant ship *Lady Nugent* (1838), Case 1: G. Pile.

59 TNA, ADM 101/78/9: Galloway, journal on *Prince Regent*, General Remarks.

60 TNA, ADM 101/76/7, Journal of surgeon John Patchell on emigrant ship *Crescent* (1839–1840), General Remarks.

61 TNA, ADM 101/6/6, Journal of surgeon Thomas Dunn on the convict ship *Augusta Jessie* (1839–1840), Abstract of the daily journal; Case 5: Patrick Wilson.

62 NAI, CON LB 22, Convict Office, Outgoing Letters, 20 July and 25 September 1844, 28 January 1845.

63 TNA, ADM 101/65/2, Journal of surgeon Andrew Henderson on convict ship *Royal Admiral* (1833), Report on Scurvy: Causes.

64 TNA, ADM 101/25/3, Journal of surgeon John Munn on convict ship *Emily* (1844), General Remarks.

65 TNA, ADM 101/20/3, Journal of Charles Smith on convict ship *Duke of Cornwall* (1850), General Remarks.

66 David Fitzpatrick, '"A Peculiar Tramping People": the Irish in Britain, 1801–1870', in W.E. Vaughan (ed.), *A New History of Ireland*, Vol. 5: *Ireland under the Union, 1801–1870* (Oxford: Oxford University Press, 1989), pp. 623–657.

67 TNA, ADM 101/77/10, Journal of surgeon G. Roberts on emigrant ship *Lady Nugent* (1838), Case 4: Jno Boorman.

68 TNA, ADM 101/78/2, Journal of surgeon Edward Leah on emigrant ship *Mandarin* (1838), Case 9: Elizabeth Arthurs, and General Remarks.

69 TNA, ADM 101/76/5, Journal of surgeon James Scott, M.D. on emigrant ship *Bussorah Merchant* (1839), Case 5: Eleanor Stephenson.

70 TNA, ADM 101/12/5, Journal of surgeon T.R.H. Thomson on convict ship *Blenheim* (1848–9), Case 2: Owen McCabe.

71 Guenter Risse, 'Britannia Rules the Seas: The health of seamen, Edinburgh, 1791–1800', *Journal of the History of Medicine and Allied Sciences* 43 (1988), pp. 426–446, p. 430.

72 TNA, ADM 101/46/7, Journal of surgeon Alex McKechnie on convict ship *Mandarin* (1840), General Remarks.

73 Syphilis and gonorrhoea were not clinically distinguished until 1879, and there was little clinical agreement about the nature of the disease, or its stages. Philippa Levine, *Prostitution, Race and Politics: Policing Venereal Disease in the British Empire* (New York and London: Routledge, 2003), p. 66.

74 Levine, *Prostitution, Race and Politics*, p. 187; Joy Damousi, *Depraved and Disorderly: Female Convicts, Sexuality and Gender in Colonial Australia* (Cambridge: Cambridge University Press, 1997), p. 30.

75 Levine, *Prostitution, Race and Politics*, p. 46.

76 Robin Haines, *Doctors at Sea: Emigrant Voyages to Colonial Australia* (Basingstoke: Palgrave Macmillan, 2005), pp. 77, 89–90.

77 TNA, ADM 101/76/6, Journal of surgeon James Smith on emigrant ship *Charles Kerr* (1838–9), General Remarks; TNA, ADM 101/78/2, Journal of surgeon Edward Leah on emigrant ship *Mandarin* (1838), General Remarks.

78 Shaw, *Convicts and the Colonies*, p. 300.

79 Public Record Office of Northern Ireland (PRONI), 560/2, John Martin, Journal of voyage from Ireland on the convict ship *Mountstuart Elphinstone* to Australia, 1849–1850, entry for 10 July 1849.

80 'Introduction', *The Pestonjee Bomanjee Journal* no 1 (28 April 1852), ML, A1831/CY1267.

81 United Kingdom, House of Commons, Medical Report of the Fortitude Convict Hulk, *Convicts, Two Reports of John Henry Capper* 1843 [113] xlii, 8.

82 Thomas Archer, *The Pauper, the Thief and the Convict* (London: Groombridge and Sons, 1865), p. 211.

83 Frank Dikotter and Ian Brown (eds), *Cultures of Confinement: A History of the Prison in Africa, Asia and Latin America* (C. Hurst & Co: London, 2007), p. 9.

84 Bateson, *The Convict Ships*, p. 395.

85 TNA, ADM 101/67/10, Journal of surgeon John S. Hampton on convict ship *Sir George Seymour* (1844–1845), General Remarks.

86 TNA, ADM 101/67/10, Hampton, journal on *Sir George Seymour*, General Remarks.

87 TNA, ADM 101/69/6, Journal of surgeon Henry Baker on convict ship *Stratheden* (1845–6), General Remarks.

88 TNA, PCOM 2/88, 'Minutes of a Convened Meeting of the Commissioners for the Government of Pentonville Prison', 30 September 1848, Pentonville Prison Minute Book (1848).

89 Boyce, *Van Diemen's Land*, p. 236–243; Reid, *Gender, Crime and Empire*, pp. 204–246.

90 For discussion of the different choleras see George S. Rousseau and David Boyd Haycock, 'Coleridge's Choleras: Cholera morbus, Asiatic cholera and dysentery in early nineteenth-century England', *Bulletin of the History of Medicine* 77:2 (2003), pp. 298–331, p. 300.

91 TNA, ADM 101/29/6, Journal of surgeon James Hall on convict ship *Georgiana* (1832–3), General Remarks.

92 TNA, ADM 101/40/3, Journal of surgeon John Stephenson on convict ship *Katherine Stewart Forbes* (1832), Case 1: Joseph Massam; Case 2: Henry France.

93 TNA, ADM 101/73/3, Journal of surgeon J. Stephenson on convict ship *Waterloo* (1833), General Remarks.

94 TNA, ADM 101/73/3, Stephenson, Journal on *Waterloo*, Case 2: Robert Coney.

95 United Kingdom. *Report of the General Board of Health on the Epidemic Cholera of 1848 & 1849* 1850 [1273–5] xxi, Appendix A, p. 4.

96 Erin O'Connor, *Raw Material* (Durham and London: Duke University Press, 2003); David Arnold, *Colonising the Body* (London, Berkeley and Los Angeles: University of California Press, 1993), pp. 159–199.

97 Alan M. Kraut, *Silent Travelers: Germs, Genes and the Immigrant Menace* (Baltimore and London: Johns Hopkins University Press, 1994), p. 31;

Charles E. Rosenberg, *The Cholera Years: The United States in 1832, 1849 and 1866* (Chicago: University of Chicago Press, 1962), pp. 101–103.

98 John Snow, *On the Mode of Communication of Cholera*, 2nd edn (London: John Churchill, 1854), p. 2.

99 Horatio Gates Jameson, *Treatise on Epidemic Cholera* (Philadelphia: Lindsay and Blakiston, 1855), p. 277.

100 See for example A.C. MacLaren, 'On the Origin and Spread of Cholera in the 8th District of Plympton St. Mary, Devonshire', *Journal of the Statistical Society of London* 13:2 (1850), pp. 103–134.

101 McKenzie, *Scandal in the Colonies*, pp. 174–179; Shaw, *Convicts and the Colonies*, pp. 324–326.

102 TNA, ADM 105/36, *Hashemy* correspondence, Report of Colin Arrott Browning on cholera on board the *Hashemy*, December 1848, p. 4.

103 TNA, ADM 101/32/5 Journal of surgeon Colin Arrott Browning on convict ship *Hashemy* (1848–9), General Remarks.

104 DL, MS Q19/ CY 2824, Log of Captain Ross on *Hashemy* (1848–1849); TNA, ADM 101/32/5 Browning, Journal on *Hashemy*, General Remarks.

105 TNA, ADM 105/36, *Hashemy* Correspondence, Letter from Colin Arrott Browning to William Burnett, 13 December 1848 (emphasis in original).

106 TNA, ADM 105/36, Browning, Report on Cholera, pp. 16, 27–29.

107 TNA, ADM 101/32/5, Browning, Journal on *Hashemy*, General Remarks and Nosological Table.

108 Mark Harrison, *Medicine in an Age of Commerce and Empire* (Oxford: Oxford University Press, 2010), p. 19; David McLean, *Surgeons of the Fleet: The Royal Navy and its Medics from Trafalgar to Jutland* (London and New York: I.B. Tauris, 2010), p. 9.

109 TNA, ADM 101 15/3, Journal of surgeon Bowman on convict ship *Cadet* (1848–1849), General Remarks.

110 Noel George Butlin, *Forming a Colonial Economy: Australia 1810–1850* (Cambridge: Cambridge University Press, 1994), p. 22.

111 For emigration to America see Elizabeth Jane Errington, *Emigrant Worlds and Transatlantic Communities: Migration to Upper Canada in the First Half of the Nineteenth Century* (Montreal and Kingston: McGill-Queen's University Press, 2007); Charlotte Erickson, *Leaving England: Essays on British Emigration in the Nineteenth Century* (Ithaca, NY: Cornell University Press, 1994); William E. van Vugt, *Britain to America: Mid-Nineteenth-Century Immigration to the United States* (Urbana: University of Illinois Press, 1999); for a forceful critique of the treatment of Irish emigrants by 'the banditti of the Victorian business world' see Robert Scally, 'Liverpool Ships and Irish Emigrants in the Age of Sail', *Journal of Social History* 17:1 (1983), pp. 5–30.

112 Rosenberg, *The Cholera Years*, pp. 101–105.

113 'Colonial News. Port Phillip', *The Maitland Mercury and Hunter River General Advertiser* (20 January 1849), p. 4

114 Patrick O'Farrell, 'Lost in Transit: Australian reaction to the Irish and Scots famines, 1845–50', in Patrick O'Sullivan (ed.) *The Meaning of the Famine: The Irish World Wide*, Vol. 6 (Leicester, 1997), pp. 126–139.

115 Gerry Kearns, 'Town Hall and Whitehall: Sanitary Intelligence in Liverpool, 1840–1863', in Sally Sheard and Helen Power (eds) *Body and City: Histories of Urban Public Health* (Aldershot: Ashgate, 2000), pp. 89–108, p. 98.

116 J. Matthew Gallman, *Receiving Erin's Children* (Chapel Hill and London: University of North Carolina Press, 2000), p. 28. Cormac Ó Gráda calculates that between the mid-1840s and 1850s over a million people permanently migrated from Ireland as a result of the famine. Cormac Ó Gráda, *Black '47 and Beyond: The Great Irish Famine in History, Economy and Memory* (Princeton: Princeton University Press, 2000), p. 106; Frank Neal, 'Liverpool, the Irish Steam Ship Companies and the Famine Irish', *Immigrants and Minorities* (1986), pp. 28–61, pp. 34–35.

117 Haines, *Emigration and the Labouring Poor*, p. 261; Paul A. Pickering, 'The Finger of God: Gold's impact on New South Wales', in Iain McCalman, Alexander Cook and Andrew Reeves (eds) *Gold: Forgotten Histories and Lost Objects of Australia* (Cambridge: Cambridge University Press, 2001), pp. 37–51, p. 38.

118 Graeme J. Milne, *Trade and Traders in Mid-Victorian Liverpool* (Liverpool: Liverpool University Press, 2000), p. 191.

119 United Kingdom, House of Commons, *Report from the Select Committee on the Passengers' Act; with the Proceedings of the Committee, Minutes of Evidence, Appendix and Index* 1851 [632] xix, pp. xiv–xvi.

120 Andrew Hassam, *Sailing to Australia: Shipboard Diaries by Nineteenth Century British Emigrants* (Manchester and New York: Manchester University Press, 1994), p. 9.

121 PRONI, D1384/12, Letters of the Dooly family regarding their emigration to Australia, 'William Dooly to Betty', 18 February 1854.

122 The ship's register names Ann Jane as a 31-year-old single woman, and William as a single man. State Library of South Australia, Passenger Lists 1847–1886 GRG 35/48a http://www.theshipslist.com/ships/australia/dirigo1854.htm (accessed 22 June 2011)

123 PRONI, D1384/15, Letters of the Dooly family regarding their emigration to Australia, 'William Dooly to Betty', 17 June 1854

124 See Haines, *Doctors at Sea* for an account of the *Dirigo*'s voyage, pp. 110–113.

125 PRONI, D1384/17, Letters of the Dooly family regarding their emigration to Australia, 'William Dooly to Betty', 19 July 1854.

126 United Kingdom House of Commons, Letter from Capt de Courcy, R.N. to S. Walcott, *Emigrant Ship 'Dirigo'* 492 [1854] xlvi, p. 4.

127 Lt Prior to S. Walcott, Esq. 10 July 1854, *Emigrant Ship 'Dirigo'*, p. 4

128 S. Walcott to Lieutenant Prior, 10 July 1854, *Emigrant Ship 'Dirigo'*, p. 7.

129 Lt Prior to S. Walcott Esq., 11 July 1854, *Emigrant Ship 'Dirigo'*, p. 8.

130 Lieut. Prior to S. Walcott, Esq, 13 July 1854, *Emigrant Ship 'Dirigo'*, p. 12.

131 *Liverpool Mail*, 15 July 1854, p. 5.

132 Ambrose Wahn to Secretary to the Colonial Land and Emigration Commissioners, 21 July 1854, *Emigrant Ship 'Dirigo'*, p. 22.

133 *Liverpool Standard and Commercial Advertiser*, 18 July 1854, p. 5.

134 United Kingdom, House of Commons, *Report from the Select Committee on the Passengers' Act*, xix, p. 142.

135 The 1849 Passenger Act exempted cabin passengers from medical inspection. ANMM, MS KAT, Diary of Richard Hall on the ship *Kate*, Liverpool to Melbourne, Dec 1852–April 1853, Tuesday 6th December.

136 NAI, GPO Letter Book 2/1215, R. Whitmore Clarke to the Admiralty re refusal to accept 40 female convicts intended for embarkation, 24 December 1851.

137 Catherine J. Kudlick, *Cholera in Post-Revolutionary Paris: A Cultural History* (Berkeley: University of California Press, 1996), p. 11–12.

2

Steaming ships

Three days after the cholera-stricken *Dirigo* returned to the Mersey estuary in July 1854, 116 of the passengers signed a memorial, which they presented to the Colonial Land and Emigration Commissioners. The statement objected that the *Dirigo*'s surgeon had allowed diseased passengers to embark, and described how initial cases of fever seemed to modify, worsen, and develop into cholera within the confines of the ship. The *Dirigo* was, the memorial explained,

> quite unfit for us passengers to proceed in, as she is at all times damp, and very much given to leakage. We have the opinion of many of the sailors as to the above-mentioned fact, together with our own experience … We were on board for fourteen days, and during that length of time she was constantly wet; and we consider that the damp state of the ship tended greatly to the progress of the disease we had amongst the passengers.[1]

Beyond the depots and lodgings of the frenetic Mersey estuary, the medical inspections, and the politics of departure, the statement asserted that the *Dirigo* had played its own part in the unfolding cholera drama. As land receded, the micro-world of the ship took centre stage with surprising speed. Within the material structure of the damp and leaking vessel, disease appeared to change form. The passengers' memorial turned the hierarchy of official knowledge on its head. It was not the medical authority of the ship's surgeon, or of the emigration Commissioners, that proved 'the above-mentioned fact' of the *Dirigo*'s unsuitability, but the opinion of the sailors.

Historians of maritime mortality have argued that we should understand nineteenth-century ships as 'working laboratories' for the implementation of sanitary regimes. Captain Cook's ship, Alain Corbin has suggested, was the first 'hygienic city in miniature'.[2] Other historians have described emigrant and convict voyages as 'laboratories for investigating the effectiveness of public health initiatives' and for

implementing measures to reduce mortality.[3] Using the language of
laboratories and hygiene has allowed historians to fit nineteenth-
century voyaging into the history of the emergence of modern public
health in Britain and Australia, and into discussions about declining
mortality in the nineteenth century. These arguments are predicated on
the metaphor of ships as self-contained objects within which surgeons
could develop general rules for disciplining people. Yet, in equating
maritime managerial techniques to contemporary developments in
factories, prisons, and schools, these discussions overlook two important
points: first, ships had by and large been bypassed by these kinds of
spatial reform. Second, unlike institutions on land, health at sea was
always about the overwhelming presence of water.

In the nineteenth century, we might certainly argue that sailing ships
were analogous to prisons, but they were analogous to *old* prisons. Ships
were persistent reminders of the confined spaces of an earlier era: slave
ships, crowded prisons, 'Black Assizes' and the 'Black Hole of Calcutta'.
Surgeons, writers, and inventors continually insisted on the importance
of ventilation to remedy these evils because the pathological internal
spaces of ships actively contributed to the production and development
of disease at sea.[4] As they feared the unreformed cellars, slums, and
tenements of contemporary Britain and Ireland, the medical profession
also drew on long-standing ideas about the pathological potential of
confined space so as to warn that the overcrowding of migrants and
convicts in the steerage decks of sailing ships could produce disease.

Ships were not just ill ventilated; they also drew in, held, and exuded
moisture in myriad forms. Sailing ships were made of porous materials
such as wood and canvas. Casks of food and water leaked and rotted.
Livestock – sheep, pigs, chickens – added to the polluted atmosphere.
Salt water, and the effluvia of breathing, excreting bodies, impregnated
the timbers that formed the keel, decks, partitions, and cabins. Ships
carried ballast and bilge water from which noxious odours emanated
with little chance of escape. A sailing voyage was a constant battle
against wetness and stagnation; the surgeon's battle was with the
obstinately permeable ship that sailed *through* the sea, as much as it was
with emigrants who travelled *over* it.

In a period when ideas about health and disease were profoundly
environmental, people who travelled on ships understood that they
entered into a heightened organic relationship with their environment.
Changing sanitary and medical knowledge certainly played an
important part in this understanding – in the shift from sulphurous
fumigation to the sprinkling of Burnett's zinc fluid, for example – but
they could not eradicate the fundamental problems of ships that moved

through unpredictable maritime localities. This chapter argues that a cumulative ecological interaction defined by a spectrum of moisture extending from human breath to the rolling waves formed the primary basis on which surgeons, commentators, and travellers understood their prospects for health in ships.

Analogies of unreformed ship space

In the middle of the eighteenth century, Sir John Pringle explained that the pathological potential of the internal spaces of the sailing ship was exactly analogous to the prisons of land. Pringle explained that 'fever is proper to every place that is the receptacle of crowded men, ill aired or kept dirty, or what is the same, wherever there is a collection of putrid animal steams, from dead or even diseased bodies'.[5] Pringle elaborated further on the specific dangers of ships: 'besides the number of men, and confined air, as an additional ferment, the corruption of the bildge [*sic*] water, is not only a main cause of the sea scurvy, but often concurs in crowded ships, to raise a fever of the hospital or jayl kind'.[6] Dirt, sweat, and the pungent odours of exhalations impregnated the air, walls, and floors of spaces occupied by too many bodies. Fevers preyed on people who were already weakened by overwork, anguish, previous illness, malnutrition, or other constitutional debility.

Pringle's ideas about diseases in crowded spaces played an important role in the emergence of a new way of understanding disease – particularly fevers – in terms of population.[7] These changing ideas about fevers, confinement, and disease would become integral to new ideas about institutional design and spatial organisation.[8] The eighteenth-century English prison reformer, John Howard, based his condemnations of English prisoners on observations that more prisoners and debtors died of 'gaol-distemper' than were executed.[9] The 1774 'Act for preserving the Health of prisoners in gaol and preventing the gaol distemper' emphasised the need to provide washing facilities and proper ventilation and cleaning in order to prevent disease.[10] Prisons, hospitals, and asylums were spatially reconfigured and rebuilt in the eighteenth and nineteenth centuries. New nineteenth-century hospitals, for example, were built in airy places, and had large floor-to-ceiling windows that allowed light and through-draughts.[11]

For obvious reasons, sailing ships could not be reconfigured and redesigned, and therefore could not benefit from the medical advantages of these kinds of total spatial reform. Take, for example, Alfred Russel Wallace's 1898 description of sailing ship design. Wallace agreed that there had been a 'gradual improvement' during the nineteenth century, which had culminated in 'our magnificent frigates for war purposes and the clipper ships in the China and Australia trade'. Yet, there had been no change in the fundamental principles of sailing ship design; 'the grandest three-decker or full-rigged clipper ship was but a direct growth, by means of an infinity of small modifications and improvements, from the rudest sailing boat of the primeval savage'.[12] As they got bigger and confined ever-greater numbers of people on multiple decks, ship spaces became in some ways more, not less problematic.

In his report into the causes of disease on convict ships (1814), William Redfern extolled the virtues and necessity of '*air*, the great Pabulum of Life, without which existence can scarcely be maintained for a minute'.[13] In the *Surrey*, in which an 'infectious fever' had killed fifty persons including the captain and his first and second mate, the poison generated by the close confinement of the convicts in their ocean prison had 'diffused its malignant influence through every part of the ship and spared none who came within the sphere of its action'. In future, Redfern argued, every effort should be directed towards preventing the generation of this 'subtle, malignant and indescribable poison … it is to be regretted that those ships, which are the subject of this investigation have most miserably failed'.[14] As he endeavoured to explain the generation of this 'most subtle poison', and looked backwards into Britain's penal and imperial history, Redfern found that the Black Hole of Calcutta of 1756 and the Old Bailey Assizes of 1750 provided meaningful comparisons to the inside of convict ships.

During the siege of Fort William in Calcutta in 1756, in a room traditionally used by the East India Company as a prison, Indian soldiers had imprisoned a group of Europeans. John Holwell, who claimed to have been a prisoner in the Black Hole, described 'one hundred and forty six wretches, exhausted by continual fatigue and action … crammed together in a cube of about eighteen feet, in a close sultry night, in Bengal'.[15] 123 people allegedly died from suffocation in that night. The veracity of Holwell's and other accounts has long been questioned, and in the eighteenth century the event seems to have aroused little sustained interest. By the middle of the nineteenth century, however, Victorian literature reflected a growing obsession with the idea of the Black Hole. What Linda Colley has described as a 'partly bogus piece of imperial history' became the 'great crime' that shamed British colonial power in India.[16] However, in the decades before it gained such popular cultural and political resonance as a Victorian imperialist myth, the idea of the Black Hole had already become a salient trope in medical discussions, appearing in public health treatises and common parlance to describe air corrupted by the exhalations of human bodies and putrefying vegetable or animal matter.[17] In the 1820s, Thomas Southwood Smith and Charles McLean both used the Black Hole of Calcutta to support their scathing critiques of quarantine.[18] The overseers of the Cork workhouse named the solitary confinement room the 'Black Hole', and in 1837 a Sydney newspaper described the cells of Campbelltown gaol as equalled only 'in the comforts enjoyed by its inmates, by the Black Hole of Calcutta'.[19] In Liverpool, in 1843, Henry Duncan described Irish cellars housing up to thirty lodgers as presenting 'a picture, in miniature, of the Black Hole of Calcutta'.[20] Redfern's use of the term in 1815 suggests that the Black Hole already provided an unambiguous analogy to describe the generation of disease.

Lest his readers remain unconvinced, Redfern also compared the convict ships to the infamous Old Bailey Assizes in 1750. This was one of a series of 'Black Assizes' in London, so called for a fatal infection that spread from the prisoners to the members of the court and the wider public. Sixty people died of a fever that allegedly swept through the open door of the prison and into the court-room during a trial.[21] Alain Corbin has suggested that the differences between 'that terrible jail fever, produced in stenches', and 'pure and simple suffocation' were ill defined.[22] I would argue that the analogies were no less useful for blurring such boundaries. The imagery of Black Holes, Assizes, and gaol fevers mingled mythology, medical theory, imperial history, and class fear. Ideas about confined spaces were about crowded bodies, but they were also always about unreformed spaces. Similar analogies appear in the official contemporary discussions of ship interiors throughout the period. In 1849, the Board of Health's *Report on Quarantine* described ships as moveable cellars. It equated sailing vessels with 'the dirtiest courts on shore', that would be 'condemned as unfit for habitation' under the government's Public Health Act, passed only a year earlier.[23]

If we jump to the British summer of 1852, the tenacity of these analogies becomes clear. As news of the Australian gold fields travelled the world, the CLEC chartered eight American-built double-decked sailing ships. Five of these ships sailed to the colony of Victoria. Another two ships sailed to South Australia, and the *Beejapore* sailed to Sydney. Each left the Mersey with more than 750 passengers, mainly government-assisted emigrants. Although such massive ships had successfully taken emigrants across the Atlantic with less loss of life than smaller ships, this proved not to be the case on the Australian route.[24]

The *Ticonderoga* arrived outside Port Phillip harbour on 1 November 1852. This had been a remarkably fast passage of sixty-four days. During the voyage, out of 811 passengers, there had been 102 deaths, and a further sixty-eight of the *Ticonderoga* emigrants died in the quarantine station at Nepean Head, Port Phillip.[25] Victoria's Lieutenant-Governor La Trobe visited the double-decked emigrant ship *Ticonderoga* at the Nepean Head quarantine station on 18 December 1852. He accused the British government of a policy of 'manifest expedience' in using such large ships to convey 'large bodies of emigrants'. He continued: 'I scarcely think that any further such examples as that afforded by the *Ticonderoga* would be necessary to demonstrate the mistake that has been made.' La Trobe believed that 'no ordinary exertion and abilities could suffice to introduce at once system and order and overcome that repugnance to cleanliness and fresh air which distinguishes certain classes of the labouring population of Europe'.[26] The ship had become 'little more than a floating pest-house', La Trobe concluded.

An anonymous correspondent of Melbourne's *Argus* further reminds us that the terms of these debates about ships owed a great deal more to eighteenth-century qualitative narratives of illness than to new quantitative methods. The 'Observer' explained that he had been on business in the area:

> being a sea-faring man and curious to know the state of the vessel which had been the scene of such unparalleled disease I went on board, and very soon ceased to be surprised at anything which had taken place on board this ill-fated vessel. The miserable squalid appearance of the passengers at once attracted my attention, and on looking down the hatchway, the smell and appearance of the between decks was so disgusting, that though accustomed to see and be on board of slave vessels, I instinctively shrank from it.[27]

The 'Observer's' disgust at the situation below the hatchways recalled Olaudah Equiano's description of the inner decks of the slave ship as 'so crowded that each had scarcely room to turn himself, [which] almost suffocated us. This produced copious perspirations, so that the air soon became unfit for respiration, from a variety of loathsome smells, and brought on a sickness among the slaves of which many died.'[28]

In Britain, when news of the disastrous voyages arrived in Britain early in 1853, a *Times* editorial took up the case of the double-decked ships. Blaming the outbreak of disease on the close packing of emigrants, the writer requested that 'we should like to see the line between the accommodation afforded to an emigrant on his voyage to a British colony, and that accorded to a negro by a Spanish pirate on his way to Cuba a little more sharply defined'.[29] Perhaps the *Ticonderoga* reminded colonists a little too sharply of the intense debates of the 1830s and 1840s that had compared convict transportation to slavery. The *Argus*' 'Observer' asked why such a ship had been 'allowed to come and vomit her diseased and dying freight in the midst of an over-crowded city?'[30] Even as ships doubled in their capacity, analogies to slave ships, Assizes, and Black Holes retained meaning as the messy practicalities of global voyaging revealed the reductive inadequacies of spatial calculations.

Three of these voyages from 1852, during which over 250 more emigrants had died, primarily of typhus and scarlatina, provoked letters to *The Times* in London and to Australian newspapers, and became the subject of an official inquiry. In the Select Committee's Report, the CLEC Officers in Liverpool explained that they had calculated the cubic space per passenger in relation to the height between decks and the ship's tonnage in order to decide the numbers of emigrants they could embark. The Commissioners firmly believed that 'passengers shipped with a careful regard to the means of ventilation, and having at least the superficial space, and on average, more by one-fourth than the cubical space required by the law, would receive no injury to their health'.[31]

Numerical representations, statistics, charts, tables, and laws created new forms of abstract knowledge about urban and institutional population densities; one historian has argued that the first half of the nineteenth century witnessed 'a new organisation of space and of bodies in space'.[32] From early on, these calculations translated naturally into shipping. In 1788, the Dolben Act had limited the number of slaves per ton, and a further Act of 1799 prescribed a minimum of eight square feet per slave.[33] From 1803, the Passenger Acts defined the number of passengers ships could carry, using similar criteria.[34] However, calculating the numbers of passengers that individual ships could hold proved contentious. Referring to the *Marco Polo*'s charter party (the contract of hire made between the CLEC and the ship's owner), the Immigration Board calculated that the CLEC had embarked 749½ statute adults; this was 48½ statute adults (children counted for half) more than the charter party had specified. The representatives of the CLEC replied that the figure of 701 in the charter party figure was equal to 5 per cent fewer adults than that ship could carry under the provisions of the Passenger Act. The CLEC argued that the legal complement allowed was in fact 738½ statute adults. It had then gained a further extra eleven spaces by reducing the 'excessive' crew of seventy to fifty-nine. Suffice it to say, the Emigration Commissioners were confident that all of the ships which arrived in Melbourne in 1852 had met government requirements for the volume of cubic space allocated to each emigrant.[35] In a letter to *The Times*, Robert Rankin, the Chairman of the Shipowners' Association of Liverpool, also angrily refuted suggestions that a 'system of packing' had been used in embarking the emigrants on such ships.[36]

The Commissioners firmly believed that the migrants had not been overcrowded and that therefore the causes of disease during the voyages must lie elsewhere. The Commissioners noted that many of the emigrants had suffered a 'whole night's drenching rain' on the steamer from Glasgow to Liverpool before embarking on the *Wanata*. They also suggested that the 'badness' of the drinking water during the voyage constituted a 'serious evil'. A very large proportion of this water had been 'quite unfit for use, being full of a slimy gelatinous substance, resembling frogspawn'. This, too, should share the blame for disease. Shifting the focus of blame to the surgeon, and to the emigrants, the Commissioners said that although they had strictly prohibited the 'unhealthy' practice of washing (rather than dry scraping) the decks of the ships, this appeared to have continued during the voyages.[37] The Commissioners also pointed to the poor health of the emigrants on the *Wanata*, and argued that Irish and Highland labourers were 'of a class' more susceptible to disease than the passengers in private ships. Being 'far less cleanly, healthy and well-fed' than the average English emigrants, they were 'far more liable to contract and propagate disease'. In the case of the *Bourneuf*, the Commissioners suggested that 'the extent of the mortality is in part ascribed to the insurmountable objection of the Irish and Scotch parents to the medical treatment of their children'. Much of the evidence and testimony collated in the Parliamentary Reports also focused on the ill-effects of allowing greater numbers of children on to the ships. In February 1853, the Emigration Commissioners undertook to employ no more double-decked ships and to return to earlier, more stringent rules about children.[38]

As the Commissioners for Emigration cast around for causes of disease they seized on common assumptions about the moral and social failings of the emigrants, but it was in the problems of water that they found their most consistent excuses. Drenching rain, slimy drinking water, and the constant dampness of washed decks introduced wetness in different forms. The impossibility of controlling water – as much as people – was a key factor that consistently thwarted attempts to regulate health on a carefully quantified basis.

Reputations

When the emigrant ship *Garrow* arrived in Sydney on 2 March 1839, Sir George Gipps explained to Lord Glenelg, the Colonial Secretary, that measles and whooping cough had appeared soon after the vessel left Ireland. Typhus fever had then appeared during the latter part of the voyage. Five deaths occurred on board and, when the vessel reached Sydney, seventeen cases of typhus fever remained, five of which the surgeon believed to be dangerously serious cases.[39] As we will see in Chapter Six, diagnosing typhus contained political as well as medical significance. The Sydney immigration agent declared that the *Garrow*'s immigrants were sick. The ship too was 'unhealthy', although in its dimensions it appeared to be a 'roomy and tolerably ventilated vessel'. The surgeon described a dangerous 'species of miasma' resulting from leaks in the *Garrow*'s hold. The leakage had compounded the problems of the green (i.e. damp and unseasoned) timber used to build the ship only a year earlier. The bowels of the ship had become 'very foetid'.[40] The *Garrow* had been packed with salt between the timbers, a traditional method of preserving wood. However, the practice drew in moisture and seemed to create the unhealthiest type of atmosphere. The Immigration Agent explained that because the ship was only a year old, the new wood used in its construction had 'greatly assisted in producing a dampness which was always present in opposition to every effort to avoid its evil effects'.[41]

Sixteen years later another 'salted' vessel, the emigrant ship *Constitution*, arrived in Sydney, again with many cases of fevers and also smallpox. The Agent for Immigration, noting that the Sydney Medical Board had previously objected to the use of salted vessels for emigrants, explained that 'whenever disease of a malignant character breaks out on board a vessel which has undergone the process of salting it invariably assumes a typhoid character'. Such malignant diseases were not only more obstinate and difficult to treat, but made all other passengers considerably more susceptible to infection 'by the infusion of poisonous gases they are compelled to breathe'.[42]

On arrival, colonial officials judged emigrants by the physical state of their vessel. In doing so, they often used the same language of worth and eligibility to describe ships as they did to assess the suitability of the people within them. The *North Britain*, for example, was 'not by any means an eligible' ship, and the *Heber* was 'discreditable'.[43] The arrival of 'healthy' ships also directly informed judgements about immigrants' potential contribution to colonial society. The *James Pattison* arrived from England 'in a particularly healthy state, and brought a very fine class of immigrants who were rapidly engaged'.[44] When the *Florist* arrived in Sydney in October 1839, the Agent for Immigration noted that she too was 'in the most extraordinary state of cleanliness and health'.[45] The surgeon, J.F. Hampton, repeatedly emphasised the 'really excellent health' of the emigrants in his journal, and reported that several of the members of the Emigration Board had 'stated that they had never before seen either an Emigrant or Convict ship in such order'. By 'quiet and patient perseverance', Hampton explained that he had 'succeeded in a short time in exciting a spirit of rivalry amongst the Emigrants about cleaning which lately rendered it difficult to make them stop cleaning … before twelve o'clock'.[46]

If officials could read the worthiness of people (and, as Hampton clearly believed, the quality of the surgeon) in the fabric of ships, then the worthiness of a ship was in turn reflected in the health of the people within her. Moreover, through successive journeys, vessels accumulated their own medical life-history, which depended in large part on the people and cargoes that had sailed in them. For example, as cholera spread through the *Hashemy* in the winter of 1848–49, the surgeon, Colin Arrott Browning, asked the ship's master, John Ross, to recall the recent journeys that the ship had made. Might there have been earlier cases of sickness in the ship that could explain such a sudden and disastrous outbreak of disease in the winter of 1848–49? Ross recounted that the present owners had purchased the *Hashemy* in November 1845. In 1846 the ship had sailed with a 'general cargo' for Madras and Calcutta. From Madras, the ship took three thousand bags of rice and 282 coolies across the Atlantic to Demarara, a voyage which had been, Ross emphasised, 'the only instance of a ship carrying Coolies from the East to the West Indies without a death during the voyage'.

Ross continued his account. In March 1847, the *Hashemy* arrived in London with a cargo of sugar and rum. After a period of 'necessary repairs', it then sailed to Port Phillip in Australia with 'general merchandise' and thirty-five passengers. Again, Ross emphasised that all had been well during the voyage. From there, the *Hashemy* sailed for China, Hong Kong, Singapore, and Madras in November 1847, finally embarking '7 officers, 2 ladies and 247 men and women' of Her Majesty's Fourth Own Regiment, before finally returning to London. Although the voyage was tedious, after five months the passengers were landed 'in much better health than when they embarked'.[47]

Richard Gamble, an Assistant Surgeon in the Army, had been the surgeon of the *Hashemy* during this five months' passage. He too was called on to testify regarding its condition and, like Ross, emphasised the ship's health:

During the whole period I had not even one solitary case of illness from any disease with the exception of some six or seven men who contracted disease in India and some from ordinary colds among infants. The crew were also free from any complaint. I also believe that never was a more healthy voyage performed by so many men after completing their Indian service.[48]

The *Hashemy* had sailed all around the world in the preceding few years, but had remained resolutely healthy throughout; there was nothing in the vessel's past to indicate why cholera broke out with such virulence in 1848, a fact that further confirmed Browning's certainty that the causes lay in the mental effects of Pentonville's cells.

The *Sir George Seymour* had a very different record. In 1844, the Admiralty hired the vessel as a convict ship to carry the first of the Pentonville exiles to Australia. After a bad start, when the convicts convulsed as they left their prison cells, the health of the ship's company had been very good during the voyage.[49] Unfortunately, the *Sir George Seymour* had then carried a cargo of oil, and had begun to leak. When, in 1847, it was hired to carry military pensioners and their families to New Zealand, the surgeon described the vessel as a 'freight ship', implying his belief that the vessel was ill-suited for the conveyance of passengers. Every morning the crew pumped for twenty minutes to expel 'a considerable quantity of water not varying with the state of the weather, extremely fetid, with an oily surface'. The surgeon also overheard that the ballast had been 'in a dirty state when taken on board'.[50] The *Sir George Seymour's* previous cargo lingered on, a poisonous residue with serious implications for the health of those groups of people who followed.

The body of the ship

The idea that ships were living beings was an old one. 'Were an animal to be formed the size of a large ship', Stephen Hales had mused in 1741, 'we are well assured by what we see in other Animals, that there would be ample provision made to furnish that Animal with a constant Supply of fresh Air, by means of large Lungs, which are formed to inspire and breathe out Air.' Hales had invented a ventilator, enabling ships to breathe. Powered by several men, the bellows system could expel up to 3,600 tons in an hour and provided the 'wholesome breath of life in exchange for the noxious air of confined places'. Hales explained that every twelve hours, 'nineteen Ounces and a half of Matter' perspired from a man in England. When multiplied by the number of people crowded into a ship, such large quantities of vapour, combined with the incessant stench of the bilge water and the 'hot stagnant, putrid unwholesome air in the Hold' of the ship, made it imperative to constantly renew this polluted air. The perspiration of people was one danger, but Hales explained that his ventilators would be of particular use in new ships 'on account of the greater Quantity of sappy Wreak which arises from new timber'.[51] A second inventor, Samuel Sutton, devised a fire and pipe system which burned the bad air inside the ship while sucking in fresh air from outside with a 'certain and uninterrupted effect'.[52] Neither invention was entirely successful; the Admiralty reported that Sutton's pipes were dangerous, while Hales' ventilator was bulky and demanded manual labour.[53]

In an intellectual environment stimulated by continuing discoveries about the constituents and vital qualities of air, there was no shortage of literature on the subject of good and bad airs.[54] The confinement of bodies loaded the air with the presence of animal or vegetable miasmas, and infectious matter could remain in beds, blankets, and any other articles that been in contact with the patient's body. At the same time, respiration vitiated or depleted air of its life-giving ingredients.[55] Vitiation was a normal result of breathing, but if the air was not replenished it became unusable. The vitiation of air was analogous to too many people trying to share food that provided only enough sustenance for one.[56] G.O. Paul explained that 'ten persons may suffer by confinement in a room, in which one might remain in health'. Henry MacCormac, Consulting Physician to Belfast General Hospital, explained the problem succinctly: 'We act upon the atmosphere, and the atmosphere acts, in turn, upon us … If we poison the atmosphere with the products of respiration and otherwise, the atmosphere so empoisoned, will poison us in turn.'[57]

In 1757, James Lind had explained that ships absorbed bad airs into their timbers. Lind suggested that 'a vapour constantly exhaling from the wood may be felt, and is often seen by candlelight in a well illuminated ship. It appears sometimes like a thin mist, and other times like a luminous stream.'[58] Although mechanical explanations of disease went out of fashion by the late eighteenth century as interest in the chemical properties of air grew, the sense that ships respired (if they did not actually breathe), and ideas about putridity, continued to hold great practical explanatory power. William Turnbull's influential handbook, *The Naval Surgeon* (1806), reiterated the dangers of wetness from ill-seasoned wood in new ships, and described the steams, moistures, and emanations of ships and the people in them. Water in the hold or sandy or earthy ballast soaked up the dampness that over time would seep back out.[59] In 1804, Thomas Trotter had attempted to prevent the 'quackery' that he considered rife amongst ships' captains in their lax attitudes towards cleaning their vessels. Trotter explained that 'the foul air which lodges in ships decks, where people live and sleep, is chiefly that portion of common air which is the *residuum* of respiration; we say chiefly because we shall afterwards find, that it is liable to be mixed with another kind, that sometimes rises from the hold or well'.[60] Adding fresh water in a misguided attempt at cleanliness only increased the dangers. Robert Finlayson's address to the captains of the Royal Navy (1825) described a similar 'morbid chain of humidity' that arose from the practice of washing the lower decks of ships, particularly in the tropics; the washing water, now saturated with vegetable and animal matter, ran into the lower department of a ship, where, below decks, the putrefying matter became the 'great common cause' of fevers.[61] William McDowell, the surgeon of the *Blenheim*, believed that the cases of dysentery were a result of the bad water, which had become 'glairy and thick emitting a most offensive putrid effluvia almost intolerable'.[62] Nearly a century after Hales' and Sutton's attempts at modernising ventilation, the same windsails, scuttles, ports, and hatchways still provided the main means of ventilating sailing ships. In calm or stormy weather – just when ventilation and dryness were most crucial – such simple openings and mechanical devices were of little worth.

As surgeons rubbed, bled, and purged human bodies, so they continued to scrub, pump, and ventilate the bodies of the ships to fight the constant ingress of water in myriad forms. F.F. Sankey's *Familiar Instructions in Medicine and Surgery* was particularly concerned with health at sea, and instructed its readers that 'all moisture or dampness should be dried up … Dry scraping and rubbing is therefore far preferable to any other mode of cleaning a deck in damp weather.'[63] During Australian voyages, surgeons ordered sailors to remove the hatches from the lower decks and insisted that convicts and emigrants air their bedding as well as their lungs above deck, while swinging stoves were hung below decks to fumigate, purify, and dry every nook of the dark hold. Emigrants and convicts did not sit idly by while the business of cleaning the ship went on. Of all the material paraphernalia of the maritime voyage, the holy-stone defines most clearly the physical relationship between people and their ships. Made from a block of sandstone, the holy-stone took its name from the practice of cleaning a ship on a Sunday, and because the person had to kneel to use it. On the *Asia*, 'the deck was never wetted but scraped and dry holystoned daily'.[64] When illness, particularly fevers, broke out on ship, these practices became more urgent, and repeated more often. It was vital to keep the ship as dry and the air as sweet as possible between decks; convicts and emigrants scraped, scrubbed, and rubbed their berths and decks. Some used hot sand to dry the planks in hot weather. Surgeons insisted that no clothes must be allowed below decks in a wet or dirty state, and appointed constables from among the emigrants to ensure 'regularity and cleanly habits'.[65] One surgeon enlisted the constable to search for the emigrants' clothes that he felt sure they had hidden below. When the surgeon discovered the garments, the emigrants complained that they that been scared of losing them overboard. Surgeon Campbell explained that 'it is of the utmost importance to the health of the people to keep everything dry below not even allowing the wet towels to be lying under their tables'. He added that 'such people as emigrants are so ignorant of those things the surgeon should personally inspect every nook and corner and make the people keep everything dry at all times'.[66]

When faced with the inadequacies of maritime ventilation, surgeons were forced to choose between exposing people to the bad weather or immersion in the impure air below. In 1835, even in the coldest of the southern latitudes, James McTernan ensured that all the convicts washed themselves every day and that the ship was carefully ventilated. McTernan's 'certain belief' in the salutary effects of his system overruled his 'feelings of compassion for their shivering limbs' as the convicts lined up on the deck in the cold weather. By insisting that the ship's hospital be constantly ventilated, McTernan believed he had ensured that there had been 'neither furious nor continued illness' during the voyage.[67] James Lawrence disagreed: his journal explained that making people go on deck in cold, stormy weather was 'injudicious'. Nevertheless, he acknowledged that his solution to the problem contained its own dangers. When people 'remain below in a close atmosphere ... unless the greatest attention is paid to dryness, cleanliness and ventilation, an animal miasm is generated which produces fever [amongst] those whose moral vital powers are depressed, or weak from the voyage, or from any other cause'.[68]

Exasperated by his attempts to ventilate the emigrant ship *Westminster*, Lawrence suggested that 'perhaps Dr Arnott's thermometer stoves would answer better, because they consume a small quantity of fuel and produce little smoke'.[69] Nowadays, Neil Arnott is best known as a friend of Edwin Chadwick, who, along with J.P. Kay and Thomas Southwood Smith, inquired into the causes of fever in London's East End in 1838. Their reports would become the medical foundation for Chadwick's famous *Report on the Sanitary Condition of the Labouring Population*

(1842).[70] Arnott was also a self-styled authority on ventilation, as much a man of business as of medicine.[71] In 1838 he had published *On Warming and Ventilating*, in which he provided detailed instructions and pictures for the construction of a stove to remove, through mechanical means, the 'deadly, though invisible poison' that built up in confined and crowded places. As he marketed his stoves Arnott drew, predictably, on the resonant scene of death in the Black Hole of Calcutta; these events, he explained, were 'the consequence of the confinement without ventilation, carried not very much farther than has been witnessed for a short time in some voluntary English crowds'. Warming and ventilation, Arnott assured his readers, could prevent and cure fevers and other diseases, the likes of which one could encounter in even the most apparently innocuous everyday spaces.[72]

As he warned about the dangers of poor ventilation, Arnott made his point by carefully mixing analogy and metaphor with detailed calculations. If a person made fifteen inspirations in a minute, he or she would vitiate three hundred cubic inches, or nearly one sixth of a cubic foot of atmospheric air. As this unusable air escaped, it mixed 'with several times as much'. Thus, each minute's breathing would render unfit for respiration 'at least two cubic feet under common circumstances'.[73] Arnott had originally designed two canvas funnels, one to admit fresh air, the other to remove bad air, during a brief stint as a surgeon on the East India Company ship *Surat Castle* between 1807 and 1811.[74] Although he left the sea for more lucrative private medical practice in London, Arnott continued to personally court naval surgeons in promoting his methods of ventilation. As Arnott walked the streets of London in 1838, looking with Kay and Smith for unsanitary fever haunts, his own ventilation crusade found an enthusiastic audience among surgeons at sea who battled with ineffective canvas funnels and the smoke from swinging stoves as they attempted to purify the air between decks.

By the 1840s, Arnott's pumps began to appear on naval warships, including the double-decked *HMS Anson*. In 1843, the government used the *Anson* as a convict ship. Its huge size enabled it to carry 506 male convicts, nearly double the usual number for one vessel.[75] The surgeon described how, during the voyage, 'the means of ventilation, were the air movers or pumps constructed according to the plan given to me by Dr Neil Arnott of London'. The pumps 'were kept in full and uninterrupted operation day and night; they could be plied in every variety of weather ... A single pump, worked by a boy for two hours without causing fatigue, exceeded in power the other forms of ventilating.'[76]

Disinfecting odours

Ventilation removed and replaced vitiated air but it did little to remove
the moistures that were at the heart of the problem with ships, particularly those foetid fluids in the water closets and bilges. Between 1827
and 1829, the Admiralty carried out a number of experiments using
chloride of lime. Supported by the testimony of naval surgeons, Fred
Fincham promised that his chloride of lime and soda would achieve the
same purifying results as vinegar, for one tenth of the cost.[77] Surgeons
reported that they had carried out experiments with 'Mr Fincham's
chloride' in East India Company ships, in Chatham, Deptford, and
Sheerness dockyards, in the naval hospitals at Plymouth, Haslar, and
Woolwich, and also tested bilge water and experimented with varying
quantities of the chloride on convict ships. One West Indiaman
commander wrote directly to Fincham, gladly reporting that chloride
of lime had a 'sensible effect on the effluvia arising from ... the bilge
water' and (more remarkably) 'rendered sweet and eatable fresh meat in
an advanced state of decomposition'.[78]

In the decades after the end of the Napoleonic Wars a newly
confident naval culture of scientific and medical experimentation
was emerging. In 1827 the Navy established a library and museum at
Haslar, and employed a full-time lecturer. The Admiralty librarian was
instructed to 'embrace all opportunities of pointing out the effects of
climate and of habit, and to explain the influence they produce both on
the minds and bodies of seamen'.[79] Between 1827 and 1830, attendance
registers reveal that naval surgeons attended weekly lectures on a whole
range of topics at the naval hospital in Haslar. Many of the surgeons
who regularly attended, including Andrew Millar, Edward Leah,
Alexander Bryson, and Frederick Le Grand, would be surgeons of
convict ships at some point in their career.[80]

The Navy had a long tradition of undertaking medical, surgical,
and victualling trials and of examining the effects of environment and
deprivation on the minds and bodies of its men. A newly invigorated
post-Napoleonic climate of intellectual exchange coincided with the
peak years of government involvement in Australian voyaging and
supported surgeons' enthusiasm for experimenting with various medical
and scientific practices, including vaccination, scurvy therapeutics,
and anatomical dissection.[81] Naval surgeons may have aspired to
gentility, but they were doing something fundamentally different
to the 'gentlemanly' scientists of grand, eighteenth-century imperial
exploration. Their experiments reflect a practical approach to the
requirements of a large-scale Navy that needed to function on a global

scale. In this context, convict and emigrant ships were useful, precisely because they carried so many people, superfluous to the business of military or navigation requirements, over such long distances.[82]

Convict-ship surgeons reported enthusiastically about chloride of lime's power to get to the very core of the problem of the ship. On the *Sovereign*, George Fairfowl ensured that the water closets were washed out three times a day, and each time sprinkled with the chloride of lime. 'The instantaneous action of this fluid upon ammonia and fetid animal effluvia renders it a very valuable article to the surgeon,' he reported.[83] Using the chloride of lime on alternate days enabled Obadiah Pineo to walk the length of the *Lord Lyndoch*, even in the middle of the night, when the ship was least well ventilated, 'without experiencing the slightest foul smell, not even from the water closets'.[84]

Chloride of lime could be poured into the deepest recesses to disinfect the most noxious liquids. Used as a whitewash, it brightened and sweetened the atmosphere. As if to illustrate the close parallels between the bodies of ships and of people (as well as the limitations of the maritime medical cabinet), some convict-ship surgeons also began to experiment with using the chloride as a medicinal treatment. Campbell France used a drachm of chloride of lime in a pint of water as an external application for ulcers. Henry Kelsall gave a similar treatment to more than twenty cases of ringworm.[85] A century after Hales had described the ship in animal terms, the bodies of ships and people were still, it seems, not so dissimilar.

With openings for pump wells, chain lockers, hatches, and port-holes, not to mention the inundations that accompanied rough weather, even sailing ships with the most water-tight of hulls and the most rigorous regimes of cleaning and purifying were constantly leaky. A continuous exchange of vapours and moistures took place between the inside and outside of ships. Surgeons appointed convicts and emigrants to monitor and empty water closets, and Obadiah Pineo posted a guard outside the water closet at all times. Concerns about the flows of water into and through the material structure of the ship intensified with the sure common knowledge that crowded bodies in confined spaces produced disease, as the miasmas that emanated from human bodies further loaded the air with impurities. One emigrant in 1852 feared that 'the heat and damp aided by perspiration from 250 persons ... produces a state of atmosphere which must be eminently productive of disease'.[86] The 'steams' breathed by the sick, the sweat of too many people, the effluvia of night buckets and the vapours from the ship's bilges all endangered health.

Reporting on the deaths of two women from the *Cadet* in 1848,

Captain Superintendent Nicholas of the naval hospital at Plymouth, suggested that the 'unfortunate' women had 'slept close to the vapours of the water closets'. He had seen this before; the cases resembled the first cases of cholera on board the *Justitia* hulk at Woolwich, where the disease appeared first in those who 'are stated to have slept close over the discharge of a highly offensive smelling drain'.[87] After Sarah Prosser's death, the dangers that had come at first from the vapours of the closet now emanated directly from the corpse. Susan Owens, another of the women on the *Cadet*, suffered from purging and vomiting. She had been nursing 'a weakly fretful child', but the hospital's surgeon also identified that her exposure to 'the foul examations and emanations from Sarah Prosser deceased' had made her sick. Prosser's body had physical and psychological consequences. Its presence 'seems to have exerted a very depressing influence on the convicts generally and yesterday evening an unusual number came to the sick bay complaining chiefly of derangement of the stomach and bowels', Henry Richardson reported.[88] Prosser's body had also exerted its influence over the surgeons. In his report the following day Richardson apologised to the Director General of the Admiralty's Medical Department that 'the depression that I myself experienced at the failure of all our means in the case of Prosser may have given a higher colouring to yesterday's report than the real circumstances of the case would fully warrant'.[89]

Under the powerful patronage of William Burnett, from 1848 naval surgeons began to replace chloride of lime with another new disinfectant, which also helped to prevent wood from rotting: 'Burnett's fluid'. This neatly packaged and branded substance was noticeably more modern than chloride of lime. In order to gain the naval surgeons' approval as chloride of lime had done, zinc chloride had to remove odours. After all, as Edwin Chadwick had famously said in 1840: 'all smell is, if it be intense, immediate acute disease; and eventually we may say that by depressing the system and rendering it susceptible to the action of other causes, *all* smell is disease'.[90] On the *St Vincent* in 1850, the surgeon declared that 'I cannot speak too favourably of the solution of Chloride of Zinc. I had daily opportunities of testing its effects as a Deodorizing agent.' With only two water closets for over two hundred women and their children, 'the odour emanating from them at times was extremely offensive ... so much so that the Prisoners occupying the Berths on each side of the ladder leading to the water closets were constantly affected with headaches'. The surgeon removed the offensive odour by pouring the solution of the chloride of zinc down the closets. When 'the effluvium' arising from so many women and children in warm weather became disagreeable it was again 'soon dispersed by sprinkling the dilute solution of Chloride of Zinc' around the decks.[91]

For surgeons, the effluvia of the water closets remained the litmus test. Nevertheless, Burnett was, of course, their Director-General, and surgeons must have felt little choice but to report in a gushingly positive way. Nevertheless, the substance's ability to remove odour was such a convincing indication of its efficacy that it also seems to have helped persuade convicts and emigrants to cooperate in surgeons' sanitary regimes. The surgeon of the *Blackfriar* sprinkled the zinc solution twice a day around the prison and water closets. 'So sensible were the prisoners of its utility in removing the disagreeable odours that after a short time they were regular in their attendance and as anxious to get the sprinkling stuff as I was to supply it.'[92]

Seminaries of infection

As urban reformers redesigned towns and cities along sanitary lines, and moved dangerous spaces such as hospitals and graveyards beyond the spaces of urban habitation, ships remained stubborn throwbacks to an earlier era. Surrounded by the ship, and beyond that the sea, the maritime hospital epitomised everything that was dangerous about bad airs. Like water closets, ships' hospitals demanded vigilance. This was not primarily a place of cure, but a space of containment, and its placement within the ship mattered. In his famous *Essay* of 1762, James Lind had condemned the common practice of allocating the fore-deck of the gun bay or the ship's hold to the sick. 'The most damp and unwholesome Part of a Ship' had too often proved to be 'a Seminary of Infection to her whole Company', he warned.[93] The term sick bay is, in fact, much more apt than hospital to denote the purpose of the space reserved for contagious illness at sea. The convict-ship surgeons' instructions of 1812 explained clearly the accepted function of the ship's hospital:

> As few complaints as possible, besides those that are infectious are to be conveyed to the hospital, which is chiefly intended for those labouring under fevers and fluxes, or such complaints as render confinement to bed necessary … When men with infectious complaints enter the hospital, you will take care to have their clothes stripped off, their hair cut off, and to cause them to be washed, if possible, in a bathing tub.[94]

When judge and royal commissioner John Bigge inquired into the effectiveness of convict transportation in 1822, he paid close attention to the circumstances of the voyage from Britain, and in particular to the placement of the hospital on convict ships. Bigge believed that the part of the ship currently devoted to the hospital should be used instead for punishment:

> [The bow] would indisputably form the best situation for a separate place of confinement for offenders, as all the inconveniences arising from bad or suspended ventilation, increased motion, leakage and opening of the sides of the vessel in bad weather, are necessarily felt there, in a greater degree than in the other parts of the ship.

Precisely these factors, Bigge observed, rendered the bow 'unfit for a hospital'.[95]

As the plan of the *Atlas* (Figure 1) shows, the sick berths at the bow of ships received the full vibrating, soaking force of the waves through the woodwork of the ship's hull. The ventilation scuttles could be opened in only the calmest seas if the sick were not to be inundated with salt water. Far forward of the nearest deck hatch, the bow benefited little from any breezes, and the most persistent air movements that did eventually waft into the hospital had already absorbed the effluvia from the bunks full of convict bodies. Bigge believed that the hospital had been placed in the bow in an attempt to protect the rest of the ship's company from its bad airs. 'It is asserted', Bigge continued (though by whom, he did not say), that 'the introduction of the hospital into the after parts of the ship, whereby it would be placed next to the crew and the guard, might augment the dangers of infection to them'.

Because convicts' lives were 'the least valuable' at sea, such reasoning went, it was of little consequence that convicts incurred 'the greatest risk' to their health by having the hospital in the bow. Yet Bigge believed that such a strategy was misguided. Confining the hospital to the dampest, least-ventilated part of the ship increased danger; it made the cure of infectious diseases more difficult, and thereby exposed a greater number of persons to their influence over the course of a voyage. Bigge believed that the present arrangement had developed without the consultation of any medical men. Confidently, he invited anyone with medical authority to sanction the present position of the hospital in the bow and counter his argument. Until then, Bigge would continue to believe that 'the object of security from any sudden violence of the convicts, has been preferred to that of security from the contagion of disease' in governing the placement of the hospital on ships bound for Australia.[96]

It is not clear whether Bigge's report was the catalyst for change, but by the middle of the 1830s, just at the time when emigrant vessels began

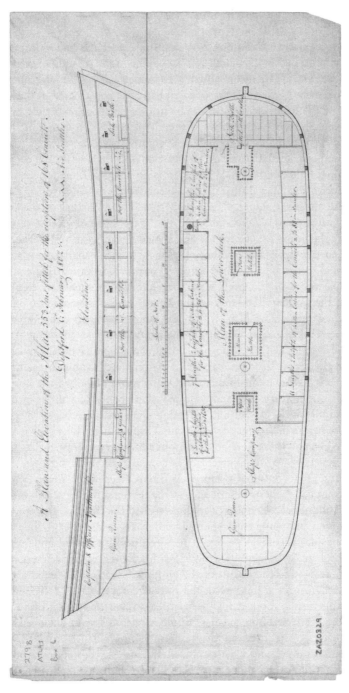

Figure 1 'A Plan and Elevation of the *Atlas*' (1802).

to sail regularly to New South Wales, ships' hospitals had indeed been moved. In 1834, on his fourth convict voyage to the Australian colonies, surgeon David Thomson noted a favourable change in the internal arrangement of the ship: the hospital had been constructed in the after part of the lower deck, which was 'in every respect preferable to the Bows of the ship where it was formerly placed'.[97] On emigrant ships, the placement of sick berths was a slightly more complicated matter than on convict ships. Vessels that carried only male or female convicts required only one hospital. Emigrant ships required one for men and another for women. In his diary, a second-class passenger drew a plan of the emigrant ship *Lord Auckland* which showed that of the three hatchways on the *Lord Auckland*, two were situated almost directly above the hospitals: one for the single men towards the bow of the ship and, further back, another above the single women's apartment with the hospital to the side. A third hatchway ventilated the married couples' compartment in the middle of the ship, which separated the men from the women. The bows in the *Lord Auckland* now accommodated the crew and young men, whilst the cabin passengers and the young women took the drier sections of the ship's stern.[98]

Nevertheless, if ships' hospitals occupied a more favourable position from the 1830s, their heat and foul air remained common themes in surgeons' explanations of disease. One surgeon described the hospital in his ship as 'very dark and confined, there being no scuttles or ports for admitting light and air, excepting the small one … only twelve inches square in the stern [of each deck], which might let a little impure air to escape'. These port-holes 'seldom admitted any fresh air, as there was generally a strong current of hot impure air from the lower deck rushing aft to find exit wherever it could'.[99] On the *William Nicol* in 1837, surgeon Roberts described how the febrile suffering of the women and children accelerated as the ship reached the tropics. 'The crowded condition, the number of young children and the uncleanly habits of the people in general produced between decks a loaded and impure atmosphere, with mephitic effluvia, which proved highly deleterious in every respect to the health of the children.' Sickness assumed a daily cycle: 'During the time when the passengers were upon deck, and all possible means adopted for free ventilation and circulation of air, the children confined from sickness would appear to revive,' but as evening approached, the between decks became unavoidably crowded, and the air became 'loaded with effluvia'. Because the hospital was on the same deck, it came 'under the full influence of all the impurities'. Each morning, Roberts wrote, the sick were 'quite exhausted, and for want of change of situation, no amendment could possibly take place'.[100]

Thus, the everyday business of health and sickness – of catarrhs and diarrhoeas, scurvy and consumption, and even of childbirth – did not routinely go on in the isolation of the ship's hospital but in the cabins, bunks, steerage quarters, prisons, and decks of ships. Every morning, surgeons made their way through the different compartments, where the sick or their messmates could request medical attention. In addition, everyday routines of washing, cleaning, and eating, of opening and closing hatches, of moving up and down from the cool air of the open decks to the heat of the decks below also provided subtle opportunities for the surgeon to make medical observations. In these crowded spaces, illness was part of the collective experience and quotidian events of voyaging.

For example, in 1837 the boatswain of the convict ship *Prince George*, a man named George Wells, came to the surgeon's attention when he explained that he had a 'bit of a headache'.[101] When the boatswain failed to report for duty the next morning, the surgeon initiated a search of the ship. A crewmate found Wells 'lying in his bed, under the forecastle'. As we have just seen, this 'small, ill-ventilated and crowded place', had been in previous decades the site of a ship's hospital, but now the sailors hung their hammocks here. Diagnosing typhus, the surgeon, Thomas Bell, instantly bled Wells 'from a large orifice' until 'the artery felt like a mere thread under my finger'. When Wells recovered from the bleeding, the surgeon gave him purgative calomel and nutritious salap, followed by senna and salts.[102] Bell bled the boatswain again later that day and sponged his body with vinegar. The surgeon recorded that because the place he was in was so very close and hot, he had Wells 'brought out on deck'. Although the deck was certainly preferable to the man's berth, it still held its own dangers. Bell ordered the crew to put screens up to shelter Wells from any currents of wind. The surgeon continued to draw Wells's blood and administer calomel. By the fourth day of his sickness, Wells began to slowly recover, and he returned to his duty nearly three weeks later.[103]

As a sailor, Wells cut a distinctive figure; this was 'a remarkably athletic and muscular young man', quite different from the pale, sickly-looking convict patients on the *Prince George*. The previous case in the surgeon's journal was of Edwin Hughes, a 16-year-old convict 'of thin make and delicate habit of body'. Had he removed the boatswain to the hospital, rather than to the open air on deck, Bell believed, he would not have recovered from fever. However, when Hughes fell ill, the surgeon did move him from his berth in the prison to the hospital, where, during his illness, Hughes 'barely slept from the heat'. Bell noted that the air temperature between the decks was eighty-nine degrees Fahrenheit.[104] Bell still treated Hughes conscientiously; he paid strict attention to his cleanliness, and frequently changed the man's bed linen and clothing. As it became clear that he had more than one case of fever, the surgeon also took extra measures to purify the whole ship, sprinkling the prison with chloride of lime three or four times a day.

Bell undoubtedly paid attention to what he considered the constitutional requirements of the individual men, but his treatments are striking because they suggest a social geography of health. Wells, an important member of the ship's crew, recovered on deck. Hughes, a convict, remained confined in the hospital below and eventually died. From the ill-ventilated sailor's berth to the airy (but not too draughty) deck, and back to the over-heated hospital, a socio-medical geography of the ship emerges as the surgeon attempted to juggle the internal and external environmental conditions of being at sea with the requirements of his medical duties.

Dividing ship decks into compartments, hospitals, berths, and cabins performed important social, moral, and disciplinary as well as medical functions; on emigrant ships separate spaces housed single men, women, and married couples. The more complicated the requirements for social divisions within ships, the more problematic the process of ventilating these spaces became. On convict ships, carpenters fitted extra bars and stanchions to construct prisons and secure hatches. The physical division of the ship's internal structure had profound implications for the physical as well as the moral well-being of convicts and emigrants.[105] In 1857, for example, a group of intermediate passengers on the *Red Jacket* petitioned the captain directly to request that he put a stop to the Sunday prayer meetings that were being held on their deck, 'as they prevented ventilation'.[106]

When the owners of the *Sir George Seymour* fitted the ship to carry military pensioners and their families to New Zealand, they divided the lower deck into four compartments: a hospital, a cabin for the Sergeant Major, and two further compartments for the single men and women. Although in its dimensions the *Sir George Seymour* was a 'capacious' vessel that 'afforded ample room' to the emigrants, the surgeon of the ship, Harry Goldney, described the partitions as an 'evil' that 'greatly obstructed the air'. The death of the Sergeant Major released the need for one of the compartments. Goldney immediately ordered the ship's carpenter to remove the woodwork and restore a flow of air to the decks below.[107]

Conclusion: steaming ships

The interior spaces of ships created deep unease in theory and in practice. Writers and surgeons alike used metaphors of suffocation and poison, drawn from imperial, domestic, and professional experience, to warn against and explain the ill-effects of confinement. Often, the explanatory power of calculating ship space paled beside evocative comparisons drawn from an earlier age of pest houses, slave ships, Black Holes, and Assize fevers. Sailing ships, governed by the winds and waves, could not be modern spaces, and they absorbed and emanated the steams and sweats of the ocean outside, and of the sick and healthy people within.

To conclude this chapter, it is worth making a brief comment about the advent of steam. The introduction of iron hulls and steam power, we have often assumed, ushered in a spectacular transformation in the nature of shipping during the nineteenth century. Although in the 1850s a particularly fast new sailing vessel known as the clipper made expensive and fire-prone steamers look distinctly unattractive and untrustworthy, the trajectory of steam's triumph is clear in extant accounts.[108] In time, steam vessels certainly did negate some of the most obviously wind-reliant failings of sailing ships, but their internal spaces continued to exert a pathological influence, which mingled with new concerns. In the 1840s, for example, the naval steam vessel *Eclair* seemed to act as a tropical incubator, capable of delivering yellow fever directly into the heart of London.[109] In the 1880s, William Wilson's *The Ocean as a Health Resort* warned potential travellers that although great advances had taken place in the construction of 'large, powerful and commodious steamships', nevertheless some of the objections to steam 'such as the too rapid transition from one kind of climate to another – must always remain'.[110] In 1883, the *British Medical Journal* complained that

> no effort has yet been made to apply to these steamers the more effective systems of tube and fan ventilation, or any of the modern devices for purifying the air, and maintaining an equable and healthy temperature. We hear too of old-fashioned water closets which almost constantly smell, and are frequently neglected throughout the voyage; of foul gases from the bilge being conducted by scupper pipes into the sleeping compartments of passengers; of basins communicating with offensive receiving pipes and water-closets.[111]

Just as they had done for centuries, the leaks, holes, and openings which funnelled the odour of water closets and the gases of the bilge still travelled to and through places where they were not wanted. In the late nineteenth century, engineers struggled to pacify the pathologically generative potential of ship space. These problems of confinement, ventilation, heat, and the steams of bodies took on new significance as Australia-bound vessels headed into the tropics.

Notes

1 United Kingdom, House of Commons. 'The Humble Memorial of the Passengers per Ship *Dirigo*', 15 July 1854, *Emigrant Ship 'Dirigo'* 1854 [492] xlvi, pp. 17–18.

2 Alain Corbin, *The Foul and the Fragrant: Odour and the Social Imagination* (London: Papermac, 1996), p. 106.

3 Robin Haines and Ralph Shlomowitz, 'Explaining the Modern Mortality Decline: What can we learn from sea voyages?' *Social History of Medicine* 11:1 (1998), pp. 15–48, pp. 17–18.

4 Christopher Lawrence, 'Disciplining Disease: Scurvy, the Navy, and imperial expansion, 1750–1825', in David Philip Miller and Peter Hans Reill (eds) *Visions of Empire: Voyages, Botany and Representations of Nature* (Cambridge: Cambridge University Press, 1996), pp. 80–106, p. 85.

5 John Pringle, *Observations on the Nature and Cure of Hospital and Jayl-Fevers* (London: A. Millar & D. Wilson, 1750), p. 8.

6 Pringle, *Observations on the Nature*, p. 8.

7 Guenter Risse, '"Typhus Fever" in Eighteenth Century Hospitals: New approaches to medical treatment', *Bulletin of the History of Medicine* 59:2 (1985), pp. 176–195, p. 181.

8 Felix Driver, 'Moral Geographies: Social science and the urban environment in mid-nineteenth century England', *Transactions of the Institute of British Geographers* 13:3 (1988), pp. 275–287, p. 280.

9 John Howard, *The State of the Prisons in England and Wales with Preliminary Observations, and An Account of Some Foreign Prisons* (Warrington: Cadell, 1777), p. 17.

10 'Act for preserving the Health of prisoners in gaol and preventing the gaol distemper', 14 Geo. 3.c. 59 (1774).

11 For discussions of changing institutional and social spaces see Robin Evans, *The Fabrication of Virtue: English Prison Architecture, 1750–1840* (Cambridge: Cambridge University Press, 1982), pp. 94–95; Jeanne Kisacky, 'Restructuring Isolation: Hospital architecture, medicine and disease prevention', *Bulletin of the History of Medicine* 79:1 (2005), pp. 1–49.

12 Alfred Russel Wallace, *The Wonderful Century: Its Successes and Failures* (Toronto: George N. Morang, 1898), p. 8.

13 Governor Macquarie to the Commissioners of the Transport Board:

[Enclosure] Surgeon Redfern to Governor Macquarie, 30 September 1814, *Historical Records of Australia* (Sydney: Library Committee of the Commonwealth Parliament, 1916) Series 1, Vol. 9, pp. 275–293, p. 288, emphasis in original. (Hereafter Redfern's Report).

14 Redfern's Report, pp. 287–288.

15 Cited in Corri Zoli, 'Black Holes of Calcutta and London: Internal colonies in Vanity Fair', *Victorian Literature and Culture* 35 (2007), pp. 417–449, p. 418.

16 Linda Colley, *Captives* (London: Pimlico, 2002), pp. 255–256.

17 Christopher Hamlin, *Public Health and Social Justice in the Age of Chadwick: Britain, 1800–1854* (Cambridge: Cambridge University Press, 1998), p. 115.

18 Michael Brown, 'From Foetid Air to Filth: The Cultural Transformation of British Epidemiological Thought, c. 1780–1848', *Bulletin of the History of Medicine* 82 (2008), pp. 515–544, p. 526.

19 Gerard O' Brien, 'The New Poor Law in Pre-Famine Ireland', *Irish Economic and Social History* 12 (1985), pp. 33–48, p. 48; Anon. 'The Policy Magistracy', *Sydney Gazette and New South Wales Advertiser*, Thursday 3 August 1837, p. 2.

20 William Henry Duncan, M.D., *On the Physical Causes of the High Rate of Mortality in Liverpool* (Liverpool: J. Walmsley, 1843), p. 19.

21 Evans, *The Fabrication of Virtue*, p. 95.

22 Corbin, *The Foul and the Fragrant*, p. 51.

23 United Kingdom, House of Commons, General Board of Health, *Report on Quarantine* 1849 [1070] xxiv, pp. 86–87, 100.

24 United Kingdom, House of Commons, Copy of a Letter from the Colonial Land and Emigration Commissioners to H. Merivale Esq., 11 February 1853, *Reports Relating to the Mortality on Board Certain Ships* 1852–3 (205), p. 14. For a detailed account of the voyage of the *Ticonderoga* see Robin Haines, *Doctors at Sea: Emigrant Voyages to Colonial Australia* (Basingstoke: Palgrave Macmillan, 2005), pp. 19–31.

25 Robert Rankin, 'Emigrant Ships', Letters to the Editor, *The Times*, 26 January 1853, p. 5.

26 Public Records of Victoria, VPRS 1084, Outwards Letter Book, Governor La Trobe to Secretary of State, 26 Jaunary 1853, cited in Mary Kruithof, *Fever Beach: The Story of the Migrant Clipper 'Ticonderoga' and its Ill-fated Voyage and Historical Impact* (Mount Waverly, Victoria: QI Publishing, 2002), pp. 78–79.

27 Anon. 'Letter to the Editor', *The Argus* (Melbourne), 31 December 1852, p. 3.

28 Olaudah Equiano, *The Interesting Narrative and Other Writings*, first publ. 1789 (London: Penguin, 2003), pp. 56, 58.

29 Editorial, 'The Records of Our Irish Emigration to the North American Colonies', *The Times*, 26 January 1853, p. 4.

30 Anon, 'Letter to the Editor', *Melbourne Argus*, 31 December 1852, p. 2.
31 United Kingdom, House of Commons, CLEC to Merivale, 11 February 1853, *Reports Relating to the Mortality on Board Certain Ships*, pp. 13–15.
32 Mary Poovey, *Making a Social Body: British Cultural Transformation, 1830–1864* (Chicago and London: University of Chicago Press, 1995), p. 25.
33 Chris Garland and Herbert S. Klein, 'The Allotment of Space for Slaves aboard Eighteenth-century British Slave Ships', *The William and Mary Quarterly* 42:2 (1985), pp. 238–248, pp. 239–240.
34 See Peter Dunkley, 'Emigration and the State, 1803–1842: The nineteenth-century revolution in government reconsidered', *Historical Journal* 23:2 (1980), pp. 353–380, p. 355.
35 United Kingdom, House of Commons, CLEC to Merivale, 11 February 1853, *Reports Relating to the Mortality on Board Certain Ships*, pp. 9–10.
36 Robert Rankin, 'Letter to the Editor' *The Times*, 24 January 1853, p. 5.
37 United Kingdom, House of Commons, Report of the Immigration Board at Melbourne upon the 'Wanata', *Reports Relating to the Mortality on Board Certain Ships*, p. 5.
38 United Kingdom, House of Commons, CLEC to Merivale, 11 February 1853, *Reports Relating to the Mortality on Board Certain Ships*, pp. 9–15.
39 'George Gipps to Lord Glenelg', 16 March 1839, *HRA* 1:20, pp. 65–66.
40 TNA, ADM 101/77/2, Journal of surgeon Henry Golding on Emigrant Ship *Garrow* (1838–1839), Remarks.
41 AONSW, Reel 2852: 4/4821, Reports on Conditions of Immigrants and Ships, July 1837–February 1840, *Garrow*.
42 AONSW, Reel 2853: folio 179, 55/37, 'Letter from Agent for Immigration to Colonial Secretary reporting the arrival of the Ship "Constitution" and the disposal of the immigrants by that vessel', 22 August 1855.
43 AONSW, 4/4821, Reports on Conditions of Immigrant Ships, July 1837–February 1840, *Heber*.
44 AONSW, 4/4821, *James Pattison*.
45 AONSW, 4/4821, *Florist* from Gravesend.
46 TNA, ADM 101/76/10, Journal of surgeon J.F. Hampton on emigrant ship *Florist* (1839), General Remarks.
47 TNA, ADM 105/36, *Hashemy* Correspondence, John Ross to Colin Arrott Browning regarding the *Hashemy*, 20 December 1848.
48 TNA, ADM 105/36, *Hashemy* Correspondence, Richard Gamble to Colin Arrott Browning, 2 January 1849.
49 TNA, ADM 101/67/10, Journal of surgeon John Hampton on convict ship *Sir George Seymour* (1844–5).
50 TNA, ADM 101/79/2 Goldney, Journal on *Sir George Seymour*, General Remarks.

51 Stephen Hales, *A Description of Ventilators Whereby Great Quantities of Fresh Air May with Ease be Conveyed into Mines, Gaols, Hospitals, Work-Houses and Ships* (London: W. Innys, 1743), pp. 30–31, 39.

52 Samuel Sutton, *An Historical Account of a New Method for Extracting the Foul Air out of Ships &c* (London: J. Brindley, 1745), pp. 31–32.

53 Arnold Zuckerman, 'Scurvy and the Ventilation of Ships in the Royal Navy: Samuel Sutton's contribution', *Eighteenth Century Studies* 10:2 (1976–77), pp. 222–234, p. 234.

54 Trevor H. Levere, 'Dr Thomas Beddoes (1750–1808): Science and medicine in politics and society', *British Journal of the History of Science* 17:2 (1984), pp. 187–204, p. 197.

55 James Ewell, *The Medical Companion*, 3rd edn (Philadelphia: printed for the author, 1819), p. 313.

56 G.O. Paul, *Observations on the Alarming Progress of the Gaol or Typhus Fever* (Gloucester: D. Walker and Sons, 1817), p. 19.

57 Henry MacCormac, *On the Nature, Treatment and Prevention of Pulmonary Consumption* (London: Longman, Brown Green and Longmans & J. Churchill, 1855), p. 55.

58 James Lind, *An Essay on the Most Effectual Means of Preserving the Health of Seamen, in the Royal Navy*, 2nd edn (London: D. Wilson, 1762), p. 21.

59 William Turnbull, *The Naval Surgeon; Comprising the Entire Duties of Professional Men at Sea.* (London: R. Phillips, 1806), p. 65.

60 Thomas Trotter, *Medicina Nautica: An Essay on the Diseases of Seamen*, Vol. 3, 2nd edn (London: Longman, Hurst, Rees, and Orme, 1804), p. 269.

61 Robert Finlayson, M.D., 'An Essay Addressed to Captains of the Royal Navy, and those of the Merchant's Service; On the Means of Preserving the Health of their Crews: With Directions for the Prevention of Dry Rot in Ships', *Pamphleteer* 26:51 (1825), p. 13.

62 TNA, ADM 101/12/4, Journal of surgeon William McDowell on convict ship *Blenheim* (1839), General Remarks.

63 Francis F. Sankey, M.D., *Familiar Instructions in Medicine and Surgery, with Observations on the Means of Maintaining the Health of Men on Ship Board, or when Employed in Unhealthy Localities* (London: Parker, Furnivall, and Parker, 1846), Appendix, p. 19.

64 TNA, ADM 101/5/10, Journal of surgeon Andrew Sinclair on convict ship *Asia* (1841).

65 TNA, ADM 101/76/7, Journal of surgeon John Patchell on emigrant ship *Crescent* (1839–40), General Remarks.

66 ML, MSS A3234 / mfm CY 1388, Journal of surgeon Niel Campbell on emigrant ship *King William* (1842–1843), General Remarks.

67 TNA, ADM 101/38/4, Journal of surgeon James McTernan, on convict ship *James Barry* (1835–1836). General Remarks.

68 TNA, ADM 101/79/6, Journal of surgeon James Lawrence on Emigrant Ship *Westminster* (1838), General Remarks.

69 TNA, ADM 101/79/6, Lawrence, Journal on *Westminster*, General Remarks.

70 Christopher Hamlin has suggested that Arnott's report on the causes of fever, in particular, illustrated 'how utterly arbitrary was the reasoning on which the sanitary movement was founded'. His 'illustrative facts' ranged from annual cases of disease in a girls' school to grave robbers 'struck down' by the emanations from putrid corpses; Hamlin, *Public Health and Social Justice*, pp. 110–111.

71 Hamlin, *Public Health and Social Justice*, pp. 85–86, 106, 110.

72 Neil Arnott, *On Warming and Ventilating; with Directions for making and using the Thermometer Stove, or Self-Regulating Fire, and other new apparatus* (London: Longman, Orme, Brown, Green, and Longmans, 1838), p. 58.

73 Arnott, *On Warming and Ventilating*, p. 14.

74 Robert A. Bayliss and C. William Ellis, 'Neil Arnott, F.R.S. Reformer, Innovator and Popularizer of Science', *Notes and Records of the Royal Society of London* 36:1 (1981), pp. 103–123, p. 105.

75 Charles Bateson, *The Convict Ships, 1787–1868* (Glasgow: Brown, Son and Ferguson, 1985), p. 393.

76 TNA, ADM 101/3/4, Journal of surgeon Andrew Millar on convict ship *Anson* (1843–4), General Remarks.

77 TNA, ADM 105/27, Reports on experiments with chloride of lime and other innovations (1816–1829), Fred Fincham to Commissioners of the Victualling Board. For a study of the early disinfectant industry, see David McLean, 'Protecting Wood and Killing Germs: "Burnett's Liquid" and the origins of the preservative and disinfectant industries in early Victorian Britain', *Business History* 52:2 (2010), pp. 285–305, p. 286.

78 TNA, ADM 105/27, Reports on experiments with chloride of lime, Copy of letter from Commander P.C. Friend to Fred Fincham (n.d.).

79 Admiralty, *Instructions for the Royal Naval Hospitals at Haslar and Plymouth* (London: William Clowes, 1834), p. 68.

80 TNA, ADM 305/101, Alphabetical List of the Gentlemen attending Lectures at Haslar 1827–1840. Though the reason is unclear, all attendance at lectures abruptly stopped in 1830, and resumed only sporadically between 1832 and 1840.

81 For eighteenth-century medical trials see Erica Charters, '"The Intention is Certainly Noble": The Western Squadron, Medical Trials and the Sick and Hurt Board during the Seven Years War (1756–1763)', in David Boyd Haycock and Sally Archer (eds) *Health and Medicine at Sea, 1700–1900* (Woodbridge: Boydell Press, 2009), pp. 19–37.

82 For the changing relationship of the Navy to eighteenth-century science see Lawrence, 'Disciplining Disease', pp. 90–92, 97.

83 TNA, ADM 101/69/1, Journal of surgeon George Fairfowl on convict ship *Sovereign* (1829), General Remarks.

84 TNA, ADM 101/44/4, Journal of surgeon Obadiah Pineo on convict ship *Lord Lyndoch* (1838), General Remarks.

85 TNA, ADM 101/38/5, Journal of surgeon Campbell France on convict ship *John Barry* (1838), General Remarks; TNA, ADM 101/15/10, Journal of surgeon Henry Kelsall on convict ship *Cape Packet* (1842), General Remarks.

86 ANMM, MS KAT, Diary of Richard Hall on the ship *Kate*, Liverpool to Melbourne (December 1852–April 1853), 29 January 1853.

87 TNA, ADM 105/36, Correspondence regarding sickness on Convict and Emigrant Ships (1836–1851), *Cadet* Correspondence: Letter from J. Nicholas to William Burnett, 28 November 1848.

88 TNA, ADM 105/36, *Cadet* Correspondence, Henry Richardson to William Burnett: Report on *Cadet*, 8 December 1848.

89 TNA, ADM 105/36, *Cadet* Correspondence, Henry Richardson to William Burnett: Report on *Cadet*, 9 December 1848.

90 Quoted in Samuel E. Finer, *The Life and Times of Edwin Chadwick* (London: Methuen, 1980), p. 298.

91 TNA, ADM 101/66/2, Journal of surgeon Samuel Donnelly on female convict ship *St Vincent* (1849–1850): General Remarks.

92 TNA, ADM 101/12/1, Journal of surgeon John Moody on convict ship *Blackfriar* (1851).

93 Lind, *Essay on the Health of Seamen*, p. 96.

94 United Kingdom, House of Commons, *Report from the Select Committee on Transportation* 1812 [341], ii, p. 107.

95 United Kingdom, House of Commons. *Report of the Commissioner of Enquiry into the state of the colony of New South Wales* 1822 [448] xx, p. 6.

96 *Report of the Commissioner of Enquiry*, p. 6.

97 TNA, ADM 101/56/7, David Thomson, Journal of the female convict ship *New Grove* (1835); Bateson, *The Convict Ships*, pp. 351, 361, 363.

98 NMM, MRF/151, Journal of Alfred Fell, Diary on board the Emigrant Ship *Lord Auckland*, 1841–1842.

99 TNA, ADM 101/78/5, Journal of surgeon D.G. Miller, on emigrant ship *North Britain* (1839), General Remarks.

100 TNA, ADM 101/79/7, Journal of surgeon G. Roberts on emigrant ship *William Nicol* (1837), General Remarks.

101 TNA, ADM 101/60/7, Journal of surgeon Thomas Bell on convict ship *Prince George* (1837), Case 6: George Wells.

102 Salap was a powder derived from the root of an orchid, which, when mixed with water, formed a supposedly nutritious jelly.

· 103 TNA, ADM 101/60/7, Bell, Journal on *Prince George*, Case 6: George Wells.

104 TNA, ADM 101/60/7, Bell, Journal on *Prince George*, Case 5: Edwin Hughes.

105 Joy Damousi, *Depraved and Disorderly: Female Convicts, Sexuality and Gender in Colonial Australia* (Cambridge: Cambridge University Press, 1997), p. 12.

106 MMM, D/ECW/1/F4, Diary of William Bower Forwood on *Red Jacket*, 20 November 1857–28 January 1858, 12 December 1857.

107 TNA, ADM 101/79/2, Journal of surgeon Harry Goldney on freight ship *Sir George Seymour* to Auckland (1847).

108 Ben Marsden and Crosbie Smith, *Engineering Empires: A Cultural History of Technology in Nineteenth-Century Britain* (New York: Palgrave Macmillan, 2005), pp. 89, 98.

109 Mark Harrison, 'An "Important and Truly National Subject": The West Africa Service and the health of the Royal Navy in the mid nineteenth century', in David Boyd Haycock and Sally Archer (eds) *Health and Medicine at Sea, 1700–1900* (Woodbridge: Boydell Press, 2009), pp. 108–127.

110 William S. Wilson, *The Ocean as a Health Resort* (London: J. & A. Churchill, 1880), p. v.

111 Anon, 'The Medical and Sanitary Departments of Ocean Steamships', *British Medical Journal*, 13 January 1883, pp. 63–64.

Voyage I:
Eliza Baldwinson (1832)

Some time on Wednesday, 23 March 1832, Eliza Baldwinson crept into Daniel Brice's parlour. Eliza had lodged in London with Brice, his wife, and their daughter, since before the previous Christmas, having told the family that she was a servant out of work.[1] Mrs Brice was in charge of the household domestic affairs, and she had agreed to take Eliza without discussing the terms of Eliza's rent with her husband. Eighteen-year-old Eliza was no orphan; both her mother and father worked at the Olympic Theatre, on nearby Drury Lane, but when Eliza ran out of money, Daniel Brice took pity on her and let her stay on in the house to do needlework. That the Brices trusted Eliza is evident: she had access to the parlour where the wife and child slept.[2]

On that day in the spring of 1832, Eliza opened the wardrobe where Mrs Brice kept her clothes and pulled out a gown and a long, black velvet train dress from among the mistress's evening wear. Perhaps bundling the items hurriedly into a bag, Eliza turned out of the front door of the house and headed for a pawnbroker's on Drury Lane where she met a man named Robert Harris. Giving her name as Ann Bennett of 6 Brownlow St (her own lodgings were next door at 8 Brownlow St), Eliza pawned the black dress. She returned to the shop on Saturday, having told the Brice family that she had taken a room in Oxford Street. Two days later, Mrs Brice realised that a dress was missing, and a further search revealed that the gown, too, had gone astray. Within two weeks Robert Suttle, police constable B97, had apprehended Eliza. On 5 April, at the Old Bailey, she was found guilty of the crime of theft. Eliza's was a case of 'simple larceny', and she was sentenced to transportation to Australia for a period of seven years.[3] From the streets of London, Eliza's world was to expand considerably.

Three months later, as cholera spread across Britain, Eliza boarded the convict ship *Fanny* in the Thames with ninety other women. Eliza had travelled with fifteen other women from the Middlesex Gaol Delivery who had all been convicted at the Old Bailey on the same day. Eliza was part of the largest group, who came from Newgate gaol in London. Other women had been sent from much further away – many on their own – from Plymouth, Monmouth, Lancaster, York and Norfolk.[4]

The night before Eliza's transport sailed for Australia, the sailors spent their last evening on shore drinking in the inns near the Thames. One man, who returned to the ship 'in a complete state of intoxication', caught the eye of surgeon Francis Logan. Three days later he identified the inebriated sailor again 'in a complete state of collapse', and now ill with cholera. In his General Remarks, Logan identified the sailor 'most probably' as the cause of the cholera which first broke out on the ship. The man's messmates explained that 'he had been ill with purging from the moment that he came on board', but when surgeon Logan enquired as to why none of the sailors had informed him of the man's illness, the Chief mate replied that the sailors believed that 'nothing except the effects of the drunkenness was the matter with him'.[5]

Through the heavily studded wooden lattice designed to allow ventilation into the prison, Eliza and her fellow prisoners would have heard (and smelt) all the details and aftermath of the rowdy departure from London. Through these same openings in the ship's wooden structure, Logan explained, cholera 'came amongst the women'. By 30 June, the female convicts began to present themselves to Logan with symptoms of cholera and diarrhoea. Eliza was one of these women. She first saw the naval surgeon on 4 July, even as the ship remained anchored in the old Thames quarantine station at Standgate Creek. On the previous day, the women had witnessed the death of the heavily pregnant Jane Mills within hours of the surgeon's finding her also 'in a complete state of collapse'. In comparison, Eliza's case must have seemed trivial. She soon recovered.

Although the convict ship *Fanny* was at last free of the English coast, the effects of these first few weeks lingered in the health of its company. Surgeon Logan again added Eliza Baldwinson to his sick list as the ship sailed past Madeira. He explained that she 'had suffered much' during the passage, as well as the time spent on the English coast, from 'repeated relapses of cholera and remittent fever'.[6] The following day, Eliza told the surgeon that she felt 'violent pains' in her stomach and bowels. Logan thought that she suffered from a milder 'modified' form of cholera which did not produce the same kind of violent purging that he had witnessed in the earlier cases. Nevertheless, he noted that her hands and feet seemed to spasm under the influence of the disease.[7] Logan bled Eliza's arm, which relieved the young woman's headache. The following day he bled her again. By the morning, Eliza appeared 'considerably better', but she remained very sick as her body purged itself of the cholera. Logan prescribed mercury, and again Eliza improved rapidly. A week later, she was 'greatly better'.

The first two months of Eliza's voyage had been dominated by cholera, but as the *Fanny* reached the tropical latitudes of the Atlantic the character of illness that the women experienced changed; Hannah Besford, another of the convicts, came down with a fever. The master's log confirmed that they sailed only eight degrees of latitude north of the equator. The emergence of these new illnesses, Logan explained, was 'owing to the ship having been so near the coast of Africa'. As the Captain steered to the west and headed for the Brazilian coast, Eliza weakened again. Near the island of Trindade, a small rocky island nearly a thousand miles east of Rio de Janeiro, Eliza was the first of the women to complain of the symptoms of scurvy. Hannah Besford, who had been the first of the fever cases, also re-appeared on the sick list with scurvy.

A nurse, appointed from the convicts, cared for her sick companions in the ship's hospital. Surgeon Logan gave Eliza two ounces of lemon juice daily, as well as 'a proper proportion' of sugar. His dismay increased as Eliza deteriorated. All over her body, sets of small vesicles – fluid-filled blisters – merged into each other until 'nearly the whole body was one continual ulcer'. Logan's attempts to use lemon juice, the fashionable nitrate of potash and preserved meats to cure her scurvy all failed.[8] Finally, the *Fanny* arrived at the Cape of Good Hope, where Logan ordered fresh supplies of meat, fruit, vegetables, and water. Yet, as they continued their journey south, the travellers' bodies still seemed unable to adjust to the constantly changing climate. After leaving the southern tip of Africa, Logan wrote that the 'effects of the cold damp atmosphere' produced more cases of fever among the women. From the middle of December – a full six months after the women had first set foot on the ship – until the end of January, fever dominated the surgeon's sick list, before finally they arrived in Sydney on 19 February 1833.

The number of deaths during the voyage – eight – had been high, but the voyage had been a long one, and moreover, it had begun with cholera. Eliza's experience was visceral indeed, as she suffered from cholera, fever, and then scurvy, and yet, like so many thousands of others, she survived, and began her new life in New South Wales. Through the trail of official papers that followed Eliza from the Old Bailey to Australia, we can piece together a little of her experience of travelling the world. Surgeon Logan's account of her voyage reveals a great deal. We must be wary, however, of substituting Logan's words for Eliza's thoughts. Logan recorded what Eliza said, though not often in her own words; the pain in her stomach is perhaps the most clearly autobiographical of the pieces of information we have. As Hamish Maxwell-Stewart and Lucy Frost remind us: 'every narrative or snippet of life we retrieve is constrained within technologies of penal power and inflected by the colonial politics of the period within which the words were written'.[9]

We cannot fully comprehend the agony of mercury treatment and scurvy in a body already weakened by fever and cholera. Can we understand anything of what the voyage might have meant to Eliza, and to other convict men and women? Did surviving the sea make her believe that she could do anything? Perhaps not, but it must have changed her. Eliza was first a London lodger, then a Newgate convict, then a global voyager, and then a colonist. We have a few more glimpses of her subsequent life in New South Wales. In the colony, she married a man named James Lock and became a nursery woman. In May 1839, almost exactly as her seven years' sentence came to its end, the Superintendent of the New South Wales convict office reported through the *Government Gazette* that Eliza Baldwinson had absconded from her husband.[10]

Notes

1 'Eliza Baldwinson, Theft > simple larceny, 5th April 1832', www.oldbaileyonline.org/browse.jsp?id=t18320405-262&div=t18320405-262 (accessed 1 February 2011).

2 On the freedoms and constraints of London lodgers, see Amanda Vickery, 'An Englishman's Home Is His Castle? Thresholds, boundaries and privacies in the eighteenth-century London house', *Past and Present* 199 (May 2008), pp. 147–173.

3 After 1827 judges no longer distinguished between petty larceny – the theft of an item valued under one shilling – and grand larceny, referring to a theft of over one shilling.

4 TNA, HO 11/8, Convict Registers for *Fanny* (1832), pp. 367–368.

5 TNA, ADM 101/27/3, Francis Logan, surgeon's Journal on female convict ship *Fanny* (1832), General Remarks.

6 TNA, ADM 101/27/3, Logan's Journal on *Fanny*, Case 9: Eliza Baldwinson, 19 September 1832.

7 TNA, ADM 101/27/3, Logan's Journal on *Fanny*, General Remarks.

8 TNA, ADM 101/27/3, Logan's Journal on *Fanny*, Case 9: Eliza Baldwinson, 19 September 1832.

9 Lucy Frost and Hamish Maxwell-Stewart, 'Introduction' to *Chain Letters: Narrating Convict Lives* (Melbourne: Melbourne University Press, 2001), p. 3.

10 *New South Wales Government Gazette*, 8 May 1839, p. 554.

3

Geographies
of the tropical Atlantic

After negotiating the swells of the English Channel or the unpredictable Irish Sea, the captains of Australia-bound ships steered into the Atlantic and headed south-by-south-west through the notoriously heavy seas of the Bay of Biscay. Sailors called out as coasts, islands, and peaks appeared on the horizon. Some vessels skirted close enough to the north-western tip of the Spanish mainland to glimpse the Cape of Finisterre. Sailing further to the west of the Iberian coast took ships past Madeira. As the cool waters of the Canary current welled up from the ocean and aided southerly journeys, the shimmering volcanic peak of Tenerife rose in the distance to a height of two miles.

Lying in their berths, prostrate with seasickness during the early part of the voyage, many migrants might well only have heard only 'the cracking tone of command and the wild hoarse response of the seamen' on the decks above their heads.[1] As they spent more time on deck in the calmer, warmer waters beyond Europe, men and women who had never been to sea before appreciated for the first time the enormous expanse of ocean that would surround them for another three to six months. Although James Backhouse, a missionary, declared himself unable to 'conceive of anything more desolate than the ocean over which we have sailed week after week a circle of blue waters surrounding us', the ocean was much more than a characterless expanse.[2]

Under clear skies and with fair breezes, the sight of islands such as Madeira and Tenerife reassured surgeons and travellers who understood the significance of its healthy Mediterranean climate. The hopes of invalids such as Mrs Bateup lay precisely in the expectation that they would breathe such restorative airs during their Australian voyage. The islands and coasts of the southerly passage through the Atlantic loom large in first-hand accounts; travellers' evaluations of their health at sea drew deeply on a long tradition of colonial medical topography, and accounts of the tropics repeatedly demonstrate the belief that health-fulness could be mapped and navigated. In 1853, the passengers of the

Elizabeth produced a newspaper every week during their voyage from Bristol to Melbourne, and named it *The Tropical Times*. Intended to entertain the passengers 'during a long and tedious voyage', the journal carefully recorded the general state of the weather, air temperature, and pressure in a meteorological table. A 'Statistical Account of the Progress of the Ship' detailed the ship's daily position of longitude and latitude, as well as the daily wind speed. The surgeon also provided a weekly medical report on the health of the passengers, opinion pieces, and observations on the voyage. In such a 'delightful climate' as Madeira, one *Tropical Times* editorial said, 'we are not surprised that invalids should recover under its genial influence'.[3]

New creatures also inhabited the warmer water: whales spouted, porpoises rode the bow wave of ships in full sail, and flying fish leapt through the air, often landing on the deck. With its membrane extended into the air as a sail, the nautilus seemed to navigate the ocean just as humans did. As the *Andromeda* sailed past Palma, the convict women could see that porpoises resembled pigs, but the flying fish 'were something so far beyond their comprehension' that one of the crew members, W. James Gales, wrote that he 'never heard one of [the women] venture to give an opinion'.[4] Sailors and passengers often fished for these, as well as albacore, turtles, and smaller sharks. Their capture and display aroused fascination and allowed impromptu dissection demonstrations on decks, but their unfamiliarity also signalled that as they headed towards the tropics, the maritime environment, the passengers' knowledge of their health, and their relationships with the sailors, would continue to change.

Sailors introduced new ways of interpreting these surroundings as they told migrants that the appearance of sharks around a becalmed ship foretold of disease and death. In 1838 an anonymous diarist described how 'at dark an immense number of [sharks] were about the ship, attributed by the sailors to the number of sick onboard, as the sharks can, as the sailors say, smell the disease from afar'.[5] Another diary, from 1850, contains a similar scenario. 'A lot of sharks kept hovering round the ship for two or three days. I saw one of them very distinctly the water was perfectly clear & the [creature] was quite close to the ship, & the sailors say there will soon be a death on board.'[6]

Measuring air temperature, examining wildlife, and observing the angle of the sun, as the passengers of the *Elizabeth* did, all took on practical significance beyond their obvious function of passing the time. This chapter explores the ways in which passengers used an eclectic range of corporeal, scientific, cultural, medical, and colonial frameworks to evaluate their encounter with the maritime environment.

It shows that understandings of health were not just related to being *at* sea, but also to constant movement *through* the different regions, environments, and climates of the oceans.

Maritime tropicality

Until the opening of the Suez Canal in 1869, most Europeans who sailed to India, Australia, southern Africa, or the Pacific first experienced the tropics from the deck of a ship in the open Atlantic.[7] This was by no means a tropical vision of 'abundant and luxuriant vegetation' in the Humboldtian sense, but the experience of the tropical seas foreshadowed the more prolonged problems that colonists would endure in tropical and colonial lands. What kinds of existing and new knowledge did travellers bring to bear in their evaluation of this 'tropicality'? How did their tropical experiences relate to preconceptions?

In order to understand how medical experience and knowledge evolved over the time and distance of the voyage, it is crucial to appreciate how constant movement through distinct regional maritime climates affected travellers' knowledge of health and illness. Of all these regions, the Atlantic tropics perhaps most define the environmental experience of voyaging to Australia. Intense sun marked itself on travellers' bodies as skin prickled, tanned, burnt, and blistered. Some travellers relished the speed with which their skin went nut brown, but for others, the sun was too strong. It caused sunstroke and headaches, and seemed to be responsible for cases of measles and smallpox.[8] Food rotted as the climate seemed to penetrate and infect bodies, minds, and objects. This could be a visceral experience of heat, sun, and atmosphere, but it was also an interpretative exercise: physical experience mutually reinforced geographical preconceptions.

Forming a belt around the globe, the tropics define the outer limits of the regions where the sun shines directly overhead, from 23.27 degrees north of the equator to 23.27 degrees south. The northern Tropic of Cancer bisects present-day Mexico, Egypt, Saudi Arabia, India, and southern China. The southern Tropic of Capricorn runs through Australia, Brazil, Chile, and southern Africa. Historically, the idea of the tropics as a geographically distinct region lying to the south of Europe was a powerful idea, rooted in the classical belief that the habitable regions of the earth lay between the frigid zone to the north and the torrid zone to the south.[9] The moment of tropical arrival was an important marker of progress during the early stages of the Australian voyage, and diarists marked this moment as exactly as they recorded the weighing of the anchor, the first sight of land, or the arrival in Australia. Robert Espie White separated his diary of the voyage into three chapters, the third of which is entitled 'Tropics'. He recorded exactly the time at which the ship's crew calculated they had crossed the Tropic of Cancer, 'on Thursday 2nd October at 6 pm'.[10] We can also place Henry Curr here, at 4.53 am on 20 July 1856. Later that day, Curr noted his first impressions of the torrid zone. 'The sun is exactly perpendicular,' he wrote. 'No shadow whatever, and the heat most oppressive.'[11] The sailors' calculations of latitude, as well as his own observations of the sun's position, affirmed his sense of bodily discomfort. There had been, he believed, a distinct, uncomfortable change in the climate.

Writers at sea measured the tropics by latitude, but longitude was also important. As vessels passed the entrance to the Mediterranean and the islands between Europe and Africa, the prevailing north-easterly trade winds and the cool waters of the Canary current naturally propelled ships to the south and west, away from the African coast and into the open Atlantic. Using the principle of Vasco de Gama's *volta do mar*, captains effectively embarked on a double crossing of the Atlantic, sailing towards Brazil before turning back to the south-east, to head for the southern tip of Africa. This double crossing enabled ships' crews to take advantage of the north-east trade winds to head to the west (away from the African coast and out to sea), where they would also be more likely to find a favourable wind that would send them back to the east.[12] Just as travellers mapped the relationship between health and climate by the passing of coasts and islands such as Madeira, so they drew on colonial experience that associated the Brazilian coast with recuperation and the African coast with sickness. The *volto do mar* steered ships clear of the notoriously dangerous African west coast, and closer to Brazil.

Although geographically in the tropics, the coast of Brazil benefited from the same north-easterly trade winds that ventilated Madeira. The Anglo-Portuguese treaties of the seventeenth century had secured British ships the right to anchor in Brazilian ports. In the nineteenth century, Rio de Janeiro remained an important outpost providing fresh food and water, and facilities for refitting and repairing European ships.[13] Until the 1820s, visiting ships often included British convict transports. Rio's strategic position as a European outpost providing abundant fruit, fresh meat, and water for ships that had endured the equatorial voyage further confirmed its status as a healthy and restorative land.[14] Nevertheless, these were, above all, voyages to the south, a fact that remained even in the nineteenth century 'no unimportant thing for a European whose world was north', as Greg Dening has observed.[15]

Explanatory frameworks: debility, putridity and astrology

Historians have repeatedly demonstrated the extent to which ideas about the tropics continued to influence knowledge of climate, race, science, and medicine into the modern era.[16] By emphasising the effects of heat, humidity, airs, and locality, the British experience of health and illness abroad reinforced a framework of neo-Hippocratic medicine that persisted throughout the nineteenth century. Before the emergence in the latter part of the nineteenth century of a geographically specific discipline that became known as 'tropical medicine', surgeons treated diseases using standard therapeutic approaches. Some surgeons used the lancet to bleed out and reduce 'congestion' of the sort that 'invariably takes place in natives of the temperate zones on their first appearance between the tropics', whilst others urged frequent bathing and purgatives as both prophylactic and treatment.[17] Diseases such as fevers, diarrhoea, and debility were 'tropical' because of where they occurred, their seriousness, and to some extent the kind of person in which they occurred.[18] Temporally and geographically, sailing voyages emphasised these medical continuities even as they reinforced the correlation between latitude and health.

Surgeons' journals reveal a clear geographical progression in the kinds of illnesses that occurred during voyages south. Influenza, rheumatism, and agues predominated in the first weeks of the voyage, generally improving as ships reached the Mediterranean climate around Madeira. As ships entered the tropics, surgeons described the eruption of furuncles and boils on people's skin. Prickly heat, also known as 'lichen tropicus', caused great discomfort, particularly for young children, as their bodies attempted to excrete acrid fluids through the skin. Bowel complaints – commonly attributed to the change of diet – worsened and included constipation, diarrhoea, and dysentery. Headaches and dizziness signalled the onset of synochus or inflammatory fevers. Surgeons and passengers alike employed remedies suitable to the climate. On the *Almorah* in 1820, the surgeon ensured that every man drank 'a sufficient quantity of salt water to purge him twice a week while within the tropics'.[19] John Martin, an Irish political prisoner who sailed on the *Mountstuart Elphinstone* in 1849, relied on 'plenty of solution of chloride of lime' to try to sweeten the odours from the hospital opposite his cabin and took regular doses of calomel and rhubarb, as the heat made him feel 'uncomfortably full and stupid'.[20] Cleanliness, ventilation, and disinfection of the interior spaces of the ship gained added significance.

Surgeon Niel Campbell found that 'getting into the tropics caused many women to be in a debilitated state and very languid', and believed that all ships should be supplied with stout to support the strength of women and children.[21] Surgeons often repeated common assumptions about women's physiological and psychological fragility and their greater susceptibility to fear, anxiety, and extreme climate. In 1837, the surgeon of the emigrant ship *William Nicol* explained that 'the females felt the change' severely. Particularly for those women nursing young children, 'general debility ensued' and they became subject to frequent faintings and bowel complaints. Although the women gradually recovered on a diet of preserved soup, the children continued to suffer. National character traits seemed, to Roberts, to explain suffering further, as did a rural or an urban background. He described the Scottish emigrants as dirty: only a third of them spoke English, and he could not communicate with them to discover what was wrong with the children. The emigrants seemed unable to adapt to the voyage, 'having inhabited an open country and unaccustomed to the least restraint'.[22]

As the accumulating pressures of the voyage took their toll, ships' surgeons constantly struggled with their desire to allow convicts and emigrants to stay on deck, but at the same time to enforce the rules that separated women from men, particularly at night. Surgeons' instructions advised that the men on emigrant ships 'should agree amongst themselves to keep large Watches on deck at night, so as to leave the sleeping-places below more airy'.[23] While the men thus remained on deck during the evening and long into the night, single female emigrants, children, and convicts were locked into their compartments at nightfall. Surgeons may have believed that these actions were in the interests of morality, but they also reinforced the common belief that women were particularly prone to physical and mental collapse in the tropics.

By the 1830s, surgeons increasingly used a language of debility to explain the effects of heat on those who had previously suffered from, or seemed predisposed to, sickness. On the *Gilmore* in 1831, Robert West told the surgeon that he had suffered from epileptic fits for several years. The surgeon's notes explain that 'since arriving within the tropics he has had frequent and severe attacks after each attack he is left in a langoured and debilitated state unable to move'. Several weeks later, once out of the tropics, the young convict had recovered, and was removed from the sick list.[24]

Historians have argued that, in general, medical writers became increasingly pessimistic during the nineteenth century about Europeans' ability to acclimatise to tropical climates, even as their mortality rates in places such as India, Africa, and northern Australia fell.[25] At sea, however, the physical immediacy and transitory nature of the immersion in the maritime tropical climates tended not to raise the same questions of degeneration, adaptability, and acclimatization that characterised so much tropical comment in this, and later periods. Instead, the sea voyage was an introduction to what might be termed the everyday pathologies of colonial life. As the *Morning Light* sailed through the tropics in 1856, many of the passengers suffered from sunburn. Henry Curr, a priest, described 'the skin shaling off their faces the same as the skin off a new potato just before it comes of age'. The heat and sun affected non-human bodies, too. Curr continued:

> We are all without exception suffering from the effects of extreme heat. Every article of food is so impregnated by it that it is almost impossible to eat. The water is positively warm, the butter is perfect liquid, and even old biscuits one would suppose only just taken out of the oven.[26]

In Australia during the mid-nineteenth century, sunstroke, alongside anxiety and isolation, was diagnosed as one of the primary causes of insanity.[27] Such environmental perils might have signified the disorientation attendant on life in a new land, but it is also true that by the time colonists set foot in Australia the dangers of the sun had already become part of the knowledge 'baggage' they carried with them.[28] On the *Susan*, in 1838, the surgeon attributed several cases of synochus and synocha fever to 'the change of climate and from [the emigrants] exposing themselves to the suns rays'. One woman had been washing her clothes on deck the day before becoming ill.[29] To provide protection from the sun, surgeons insisted that the sailors hoist awnings over the decks. Another surgeon admitted that he did not know the cause of the cases of night-blindness, but he suspected that with so little to do during the daytime, the military guard on the *Lord Lyndoch* had developed eye disorders by passing their time lying on the poop, 'sometimes asleep exposed to the strong rays of a tropical sun'.[30] *The Tropical Times* recorded two cases of 'serious disturbance of the nervous system resembling sunstroke', accompanied in one case by fits. A week later, the journal reported that 'some of the passengers have had their ankles burned with the sun producing extensive vesecation, while it may be noticed that headache is induced almost immediately by exposure to its rays'. As the passengers became accustomed to the heat, however, they became 'more animated'.[31] Sailors employed their own measures to deal with the heat. On the *Kains*, while the surgeon ordered the crew to stay clear of the sun and moon and always wear a broad-brimmed hat, a sailor, Charles Picknell, instead left his shirt and belt off and 'took to chew tobacco and eating garlick'. He reported that he was 'in good health'.[32]

Surgeon Charles Queade's journal from the convict ship *Phoenix* provides important evidence of the way that different kinds of medical knowledge coexisted. As the *Phoenix* passed seven degrees north of the equator, on 1 May 1824, the surgeon, master, officers of the guard and ship's officers were poisoned after eating a 'bonetta' fish. Although commonly eaten by sailors 'with a good relish', the bonetta had been left to hang overnight without being cleaned, and had then been cooked for the Cabin's breakfast. The surgeon became too seriously ill to assist the sick ('my head felt as if struggling to deliver itself of the vast load of fluid that was rushing through it'), and left every other person who had eaten the fish to find their own remedies. While the surgeon 'was bled immediately to the extent of 18 oz', the junior officer took 'large doses of sulphate of magnesia'. By contrast, the first and second mates took 'a sailor's remedy for all complaints a strong glass of grog'. They reported that this too had relieved their illness. After the dose of grog was repeated in the evening the surgeon recalled that he 'heard no more about the Bonetta from them'.

The surgeon believed that the poisonous quality of the fish was due to 'the decomposition that takes place during the rapid putrefaction that occurs in all animals whether land or marine in tropical climates'. The sailors, on the other hand, expressed the 'generally received' opinion 'that fish hung up and exposed to the rays of the moon for a night become poisonous'.[33] Sailors had long believed that exposure to the moon's rays could cause such conditions as paralysis, vertigo, and 'swelling of the face'.[34] Queade believed that the sailors' beliefs about the moon's effects on the bonetta were 'unfounded'. This may seem unsurprising for a man with formal medical training, well versed in theories of acids, alkalis, and putrefaction. It was, after all, over a century since Richard Mead's *Of the Power and Influence of the Sun and Moon on Humane Bodies* (1708) had suggested that the moon had a particularly powerful effect in the tropics, and such overt medical astrology had gone out of fashion amongst metropolitan practitioners by the nineteenth century. Yet, as Mark Harrison has shown, ideas about the moon continued to hold significant explanatory power for the environmentally sensitive practitioners of military and naval medicine.[35] During Australian voyages the dangers of the moon often excited comment, and could be no less crucial than the sun to how travellers developed their first understandings of the tropics. Surgeon Thomas Bell described the 'diversity of pimples, boils, furunculi with deep seated cores, cutaneous efflorescences, excoriations, prickly heat, moon blindness, and ring worm' that occurred in the tropics.[36]

Queade's account of the bonetta poisoning also illustrates that the doctrine of putridity remained as important as ideas about debility for understanding the effects of climate. Processes of putridity were most apparent when in the presence of a dead body. During the voyage of the *Alfred* from Plymouth to Sydney in 1838, an emigrant named Robert Muir recorded that the ship's third mate had died. Caught in the calms north of the equator, the *Alfred* had progressed only two degrees of latitude south in a week, and on the day the man died, there was 'nothing but calm'. Muir declared himself 'astonished at the rapidity with which decomposition goes on in these latitudes. Five hours after Clark's death he was spotted all over, & tainted the air.'[37] Another anonymous diary from the same voyage also recorded the author's shock at the decomposition of the third mate's body. The process of decay 'proceeded so rapidly that he had to be buried at 10 o'clock'. The writer was struck by the death of the sailor, who previously had been in good health, 'this in fact being the only illness he ever had'.[38]

For emigrants, Pat Jalland has argued, the stark reality of these confrontations with death 'anticipated the unforgiving conditions of early colonial settlement'. The swift and unceremonial way in which corpses were launched into the deep seems to symbolise the barbarity and hardship of life and death at sea.[39] Yet, the diary entries referring to the third mate's death make it clear that environmental as much as cultural considerations determined the swiftness with which crews dispatched bodies into their maritime graves. To keep a body for more than a few hours posed a very real threat to the health of the ship's company, particularly in places where the putrefying effects of heat and sun marked the bodies of the living, and caused the tar between the decking planks to bubble and ooze.

Nearly four decades after Queade's experience with the poisonous bonetta, virtually the same story appears again. This time it was the surgeon who insisted on the power of the moon. During a voyage from Auckland to Liverpool in 1860, a doctor warned his passengers to test carefully that the fish they caught were not poisonous.[40] The doctor showed the passengers how to put the fish in the ship's oven with a silver coin in the middle. He explained that 'deep sea fish are sometimes poisonous, said to be caused by the moon's rays shining upon them'. The fish passed the test: 'The silver came out quite bright had they been poisonous it would be green.'[41] It is tempting, in writing histories of medical knowledge, to look for examples that reinforce the idea that, as medical authority became more self-consciously 'scientific', 'superstitions' held by those without formal medical training either died out, or no longer served a useful purpose. These examples remind us that we cannot fix changing ideas about health and medicine into any clear chronological pattern. In different places, and at different times, what counted as useful knowledge also shifted.

'In a bad place': off West Africa

In June 1830, Charles Picknell had finished his apprenticeship and left Hastings for London. He spent three days looking for a ship until, on 14 June, Captain William Goodwin gave Charles and his friend, Edward Hutchings, an order to join the convict ship *Kains*. On 25 June Picknell 'signed articles' for 'Sidney, New Holland, vandemons land [*sic*] to hell or elsewhere'. As was customary, he received his first month's pay in advance of the voyage. Two days later, female prisoners from London boarded the *Kains*, followed by women who had travelled from prisons in Liverpool, Birmingham, and York. With its full company, the transport sailed from Woolwich on 8 July 1831. As the *Kains* sailed along the English south coast on 15 July, guns fired on the shore to mark the burial of King George IV.[42] Picknell's diary is a rare account of the voyage to Australia from the sailor's perspective and vividly illustrates how the changing geography of the ocean moulded understandings of health and illness.

After a month at sea, much of it in stormy and rough weather, Picknell recorded the first sighting of land since leaving England: 'Was island port santo. inhabited with portagues. mountains in the clouds. larbert watch saw it 50 knots befor we got to it.'[43] Continuing south towards the African coast, dolphins and flying fish surrounded the ship in the water, while 'mother carey's chickens' – petrels – fluttered along behind. The captain stopped for three days at 'Tenreef' for fresh beef, vegetables, and water. Here, the prisoners were allowed 'to purchase as much fruit as they pleased' before the *Kains* sailed south once more. 'No land. no ship. all is well,' Picknell wrote.[44]

As the *Kains* crossed the northern 'tropick line' in mid-August, the tone of the journal changed. Picknell had fallen 'verry sick' and now placed himself 'in the doctors hands'. With little for the sailors to do in the calms north of the equator, Picknell's observations of the sea and fauna around him mingle with his notes on his own health. On 27 August they were 'companied with martains and swallos. great many of us afflicted with soar biles all over.' The sun made Picknell 'rather giddy headed', and the whole ship's company suffered from 'the pricklyheat', an intense itching caused by sweat trapped beneath the skin's surface. The *Kains*, he wrote, was 'in a bad place'.[45] For nearly six weeks after the *Kains* first entered the tropics, it had lurched back and forth across the equator without a steady wind. The English sloop *HMS Atholl*, 'in search of pirates and slavers from the isle of sension bound to surleyhoan', bore down on the *Kains*. The same day another sail appeared; as the crew went after it the unidentified ship warned that they were 'too near sickly Africa'.[46] The crew of the *Kains* paid heed, and 'hove about'.

The seas off the coast of Africa were far from empty of European ships, a fact that does, of course, have its own long and violent history.[47] In 1792 the Sierra Leone Company had established Freetown with 1,200 black African-American loyalists from Nova Scotia. The first British attempts at colonisation were disastrous, primarily because of disease. Into the nineteenth century Sierra Leone's reputation was dominated by sickness: between 1819 and 1836, 48 per cent of European troops died, most of disease.[48] The re-establishment of the colony as a British Crown protectorate coincided almost exactly with the abolition of the slave trade, and from 1808 the British Naval West Africa Squadron patrolled three thousand miles of the West African coast between Cape Verde and Benguela (in modern-day Angola) to intercept 'pirate' ships and suppress the traffic in slaves. Between 1807 and 1864, the Royal Navy liberated more than fifty thousand 'recaptives' in Freetown.[49] In 1819, the Navy had also begun to use Ascension Island – Picknell's 'isle of sension' – for sailors who needed shore leave to recover from fever.[50] These contexts shaped Picknell's understanding of the 'bad place' beyond the Cape Verde islands. The voyage of the convict ship *Kains* briefly intersected with this post-abolition naval world off the West African coast, but it was not the only convict ship to encounter *HMS Atholl*. In 1848, as the *Eden* approached the Cape Verde islands, its surgeon, Robert McCrea, operated on the leg of a man. As he did so, McCrea 'received some poisonous matter into his system through a small wound which he had in the point of his right thumb', and soon died. Robert Beith, another naval surgeon, joined the convict ship from the *Atholl*.[51]

The links between the West African patrols and Australian voyages included chance meetings, shouted warnings, and the shimmering glimpses of sails on the horizon, but they also reveal a core aspect of naval medical employment. In the decades after the end of the Napoleonic Wars, British naval surgeons had two clear opportunities for foreign employment: West African patrols or Australian voyages. Many surgeons spent periods in both services. In June 1831, a young Scottish assistant naval surgeon named Alexander Bryson

was made acting surgeon of the *Atholl* as it patrolled the coast of
Africa. During 1831, Bryson was concerned primarily with fevers. A
decade later, Bryson took up a posting as a convict-ship surgeon on
the *Marquis of Hastings*, and we will have cause to meet him again
in the following chapter as he berated his fellow surgeons for their
approach to remedying scurvy. Both postings offered the ambitious
Bryson a chance to theorise, experiment, and publish on some of the
most pressing military medical problems of his time. After his voyage
to Australia with convicts, Bryson returned again to West Africa,
to fevers, and to his publication of *The Climate and Principal Diseases
of the West Africa Station* (1857). Certainly, Bryson was an unusually
driven individual, but other surgeons also interspersed the publication
of contributions to the study of fevers and quinine, based on their
West African experiences, with service as convict-ship surgeons.[52] This
exchange of personnel and ideas connected Australian voyages into a
global naval and imperial network that stretched from Britain, to West
Africa, India, the Caribbean, and into the Pacific.

Nevertheless, Picknell's account of the meeting with the *Atholl*
and the shouted warning from the unnamed ship under its lee also
shows that there was something more broadly meaningful about Sierra
Leone's reputation. Beneath the publications and career opportunities
for naval surgeons who climbed their way through Britain's imperial
projects around the globe, knowledge about Africa was bolstered as
much by the circulation of oral information among groups of people
on ships' decks as it was by surgeons' professional networks and career
trajectories. As the *Mountstuart Elphinstone* passed Africa, John Martin
noted only that the first mate 'is quite entertaining with his stories
about the Hooghly & Sierra Leone & the East'.[53] Records of this kind
of knowledge exchange are of course only fragments, but they attest
to the importance of an accumulating fund of information with which
travellers related their experience of the Australian voyage to a global
geography that included the African coast as a key reference point.

In 1838 one writer – becalmed and surrounded by sharks – lamented
his ship's position at eight degrees north of the equator, and in close
proximity to the African coast: 'The Doctor's list of the sick still
presents a long melancholy number. OH! If we could only get a good
rattling breeze to carry us out of these deadly latitudes.' Preconceptions
about the significance of the ship's position, combined with a growing
tally of sickness to create fear. 'We are now nearly opposite to Sierra
Leone, which must be truly described as "The White Man's Grave",' the
diarist wrote.[54] The climatic reputation of the West African coast had
long been common knowledge. In the eighteenth century, James Lind

warned of the seasonal 'malignant and fatal vapours called harmattans' that infested the West African coast. Sailors chanted "'beware beware the Bight of Benin, for one that come's out, there's forty go in'".[55] By the 1830s, Phillip Curtin has argued, the deadly image of the 'White man's grave' had become somewhat of a cliché: knowledge about West Africa's deadly reputation circulated as an 'unstated assumption' held by colonial officials, a 'common knowledge' that did not need to be written down.[56] Indeed, it was extraordinary, James Johnson declared, that when Africa was the 'grave' of Europeans, 'no work on the diseases of Africa should have emanated from the medical press of this country'.[57]

For travellers, it seems, the pathological idea of West Africa did need to be written down: again and again, throughout this period, the West African coast appeared in traveller's journals and diaries. In late November 1841, William Charles Wills wrote:

> We are now clearing the part off the coast of Africa where the climate is considered so unhealthy – a fact which is borne out not only by the indisposition of two or three of the passengers, but also by the appearance and colour of the sails, which are of a brownish yellow, and assume a jaundiced complexion.[58]

Having long suffered from asthma, Wills was surprised to find himself in such good health in such a 'thick and sultry' atmosphere. The *Louisa* had not even sailed within sight of the African coast, but for two weeks the airs of Sierra Leone had seemed to become part of the material structure of the ship. Medical knowledge derived from colonial experience in West Africa extended easily to sea, but the proximity of the African coast coincided geographically and meteorologically with another potent source of maritime fear. Calms, as one emigrant wrote, made the atmosphere in the ten degrees of latitude north of the equator 'quite suffocating'.[59]

Flows of wind and water, in the Atlantic as around the rest of the world, created natural ocean highways. By encouraging particular routes of human travel – including the Atlantic *volta do mar* – oceans played a material role in shaping the history of European exploration and imperialism and determining the routes taken to transport gold, silver, and slaves.[60] The further to the west that ships sailed south through the Atlantic, the less was their chance of encountering the three bands of calms that stretched across the Atlantic from west to east. Two subtropical bands of high pressure, lying around thirty degrees north and south of the equator, were known as the horse latitudes. All of these regions were variable and unpredictable, shifting north and south with the season. Of the three areas of calm, the doldrums, in the middle, had gained a fearsome reputation for disabling ships, sometimes for weeks at a time. Their position was never certain: the doldrums drifted from roughly five degrees south of the equator in January to fifteen degrees north in July, and it was the uncertainties of this strange region that caught the imagination of travellers.[61] The maritime experience of emigrants and convicts who sailed to Australia were no less shaped by the reliability of the trade winds and currents, but also at times by periods of unreliability, limbo, and a very real sense of being stranded. Ships sailing south through the Atlantic towards the tip of Africa had no choice but to cross these calm regions; dealing with them was at once a navigational, meteorological, and medical concern.

As the *Sarah* crept towards the equator in 1849, Hugh May Wilson's diary illustrates this attention to westerly as well as southerly location. He described how passengers dispensed with the usual greetings and asked each other instead 'How far are we now from the line?' or, 'Any more deaths last night?' Finally, the captain of the *Sarah* altered course to head towards Brazil. 'We ran westward to get clear of the fatal African atmosphere, which seemed to breathe disease among us,' he said.[62] As Wilson interpreted the meaning of the *Sarah*'s place on the sea, longitude gained almost as much concrete significance as latitude. His meditations on West Africa remind us that 'the tropics' were not uniformly pestilential and show how the region of the Atlantic in the ten degrees of latitude north of the equator took on a particularly malign significance. The ill-effects of land and sea blurred as these two sources of danger merged into each other in the conversations that people had on deck. For sailors, calculations of latitude and longitude were a vital aspect of navigation that daily fixed location. For passengers, comparing different calculations provided reassurance, the knowledge that the ship still moved. When the wind died, and the sea became calm, the sense of being stranded in the open ocean induced fear. Some diarists, particularly those who found the tropical heat trying, fretted about what might happen if they should encounter calms ahead. A 'calm of long continuance', Richard Hall wrote in 1853, 'would be disastrous' to the passengers' health.[63] In 1838, the *Alfred* had 'veered round and round' but made no progress whatever 'towards raking us out of this dreadful heat'.[64]

Ships' captains did not worry (as Columbus had done in the fifteenth century) that their vessels and crews would burst into flames as they headed south across the tropics.[65] Nevertheless, before regular systems of emigration to Australia became commonplace, heat and calms inspired a very real fear of the unknown for uninitiated travellers. When Henry Widowson sailed to Van Diemen's Land with horses and cattle in 1825, he witnessed 'lots of thunder and rain accompanied by vivid lightning scarcely without a cessation'. Such 'visitations', he discovered from the sailors, were 'exceedingly common to this atmosphere'. Widowson was unwell. He fainted in the hold and had to be carried back to the deck. As the heat continued, he feared for his cattle, and also that he and his fellow passengers might 'share the same fate as some ships becalmed here for a month or more, and living under the constant dread of having their ships set on fire by the burning sun, their water exhausted and people dying with fever'. Addressing future readers, he wrote: 'You can form no idea of natural heat in England compared with the climate we are now living in'.[66] Widowson later wrote an advice manual for agricultural settlers, in 1829, but made no mention of his own voyage through the tropics, although his experiences clearly influenced his recommendation that settlers should sail from Britain in the early summer, and choose a vessel greater than 350 tons. Smaller vessels, Widowson explained, 'lacking free circulation of air, are also much warmer in crossing the equator'.[67]

By the 1830s, as the Australian colonies became more than a penal colony beyond the seas, emigrants had a variety of advice manuals at their disposal. These guides advised on who should consider emigrating, covered the practicalities of procuring a passage, provided lists of agricultural and mechanical tools to take, and sketched out an idea of the Australian climate, land, and the practicalities of setting up a new life. Yet, while the majority of these manuals explained how and what to pack into cases, clothing required for the voyage, and the scales of rations that an emigrant should expect, they did not usually describe the voyage itself. Peter Cunningham's famous account of early colonial New South Wales urged only that passengers should 'guard equally against giving and taking offence' during the voyage. Although Cunningham had undertaken four voyages to New South Wales, he recounted no more about the voyage than a 'terrible feud' that had occurred among cabin passengers which had 'originated simply in the carving of a batter pudding!'[68]

David Lindsay Waugh's *Three Years' Practical Experience of a Settler in New South Wales*, which ran to at least eight editions in 1837 and 1838 alone, was notably different.[69] Composed of extracts from letters 'written in unrestrained confidential intercourse' to the author's nearest relatives, Waugh wrote first of the experience of being at sea on the *Isabella* in 1833. He recounted the voyage through the English Channel, the seasickness that ensued, and the gales as the ship left Land's End. Now in the tropics, the author reassured his father (and the reader) that he stayed well:

there are threatening symptoms of a calm, however, although we have been going all day at six knots, yet for six hours yesterday and last night, we were barely making one an hour. As for the heat you dreaded so much, here we are 6˚ from the Equator, and the thermometer never yet above 80˚ with a sea breeze all the time. The surgeon has been five times across, and, in a dead calm and no wind, never saw it above 84˚. I sleep on my plain mattress with neither blanket nor sheet, putting on my cotton drawers and my night shirt, I am very comfortable.[70]

Although writers still struggled to convey to their readers the feeling of heat and helplessness, Waugh's manual attempted to reassure emigrants that their experience of the area around West Africa would rarely match the dread of their expectations. The doldrums, and the tropical climate in general, were manageable. Indeed, as the passengers of the *Elizabeth* 'bade adieu to the Torrid Zone' in 1853, their newspaper observed that 'the heat has been often oppressive, and sometimes almost insupportable, but not at any time so intolerable as we had anticipated.'[71]

Nevertheless, even as the increasingly routine nature of Australian voyaging helped to contribute to a growing awareness in the public consciousness that ships in this region were not enveloped in flames, writers still used the common awareness of the doldrums and West Africa to represent the dangers of climatic extremes. In particular, Matthew Fontaine Maury's *Physical Geography of the Sea* (1855) used the example of the Australian voyage to convey to its readers the dangers of calms (and thereby to promote his wind chart project). The doldrums, Maury wrote, are 'one of the most oppressive and disagreeable places on earth. The emigrant ships from Europe for Australia have to cross it. They are often baffled in it for two or three weeks; then the children and the passengers who are of delicate health suffer most. It is a frightful grave-yard on the way-side to that golden land.'[72] Maury's description of the Australian voyage stretched the idea of the graveyard chronologically and geographically beyond the colonial experience of West Africa and out to sea. The familiarity of a common experience that increasingly attested to the tropics' very survivability, paradoxically also helped to keep the idea firmly in the popular imagination that the Australian voyage was associated primarily with death and suffering.

The equator

Beyond the unnerving, unpredictable calms of the doldrums and the airs of the West African coast, European sailors invested crossing

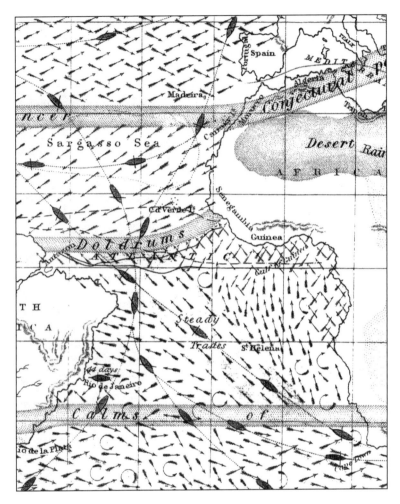

Figure 2 Matthew Maury, detail from 'Winds and Routes', showing tropical winds and calms (1855).

the equator with as much significance and meaning as any point of land. As the northern stars disappeared below the horizon, and the midday sun moved to the north, sailors marked this moment of departure, transition, and the world turning upside down with a theatrical 'crossing the line' ceremony. With an elaborately costumed cast of characters, razors made from iron hoops, and vile 'medical' concoctions, the ceremony was, as Greg Dening has suggested, 'a grotesque satire on institutions and roles of power'.[73]

During the ceremony the ship's captain allowed the usual hierarchies of maritime discipline to be temporarily relaxed, as the most experienced sailors assumed positions of authority in Neptune's court and performed the initiation of sailors and passengers – the 'greenhorns' – who had never previously ventured into the southern hemisphere. Many emigrants' diaries and journals of the Australian voyage contain detailed and remarkably consistent descriptions of these ceremonies. In the evening before the ship crossed the equator, Neptune appeared. He informed the ship's company that he would return the following day to see if there were any strangers on board and to shave them. On the day of the ceremony, Neptune returned with his entourage, which usually included his queen, a barber, several policemen, a baby who represented the 'Royal Belly', a bear, and a doctor. After the novices had been questioned and shaved, they were then 'bathed', and repeatedly held below the water in barrels or in sails slung between the masts.

Wearing the tell-tale spectacles of a learned man, and 'carrying the tools of his profession', the equatorial Doctor might carry pills, smelling bottles, enema syringes, a lancet, or pegs 'to clip on the patient's nose'.[74] On the *Alfred* in 1838, Neptune's doctor appeared as 'a very pompous formidable looking personage, accompanied by six assistants, each carrying a large bottle of medicine, full of all sorts of disagreeable looking materials'.[75] One published diary from 1856 described how Neptune ordered 'the sham doctor' to feel each seaman's pulse:

> upon which this man of physic prescribes for him a more disgusting medicine than is to be found in any druggist's shop in the United Kingdom namely sheep's manure dissolved in water, which is at once forced down the throat of the patient. After squeezing his nose most unmercifully, and satisfying himself that the draft is in the stomach of the unfortunate patient, the doctor then orders the barber to lather his face with the preparation at hand, consisting of tar mixed with a greasy matter, commonly called slush.[76]

In another account, the Doctor played a full part in the violence that accompanied the initiations. If the sailor refused to answer any of his questions, Neptune

> cried out 'poor fellow he has fainted, fetch the Doctor'. The Doctor comes. 'What's the matter, What's the matter? – Oh yes he has fainted; but we'll soon bring him to'. Then the doctor commences operating by taking hold of the patient's nose, to prevent his breathing. This of course compels him to open his mouth to breathe the doctor crying out 'give him air, give him air'. But there before him stands the barber, brush in

hand eyeing intently for the opening mouth; but stubbornly he holds his breath until nature becomes exhausted, he opens his mouth for air and in went the lather brush.[77]

As surgeon-superintendents gained greater authority on naval and government- chartered ships, the satirised figure of the Doctor became one of the most prominent members of Neptune's court, and the ceremony took on the appearance of a bizarre medical carnival. W. James Gales' description of the equatorial ceremony on the *Andromeda* is worth repeating at length for this reason, but also because it is a rare account of the ceremony on a convict ship. The first appearance of Neptune had an 'astonishing' effect on the women of the *Andromeda* as his 'tremendous and sudden bellowing' hailed the ship. Each sailor on Neptune's list of 'strangers' was

> hauled away forward by Neptune's constables blindfolded and questioned one at a time (the sick not allowed to be present) whither he would beg Neptune's mercy for which he is presented with a speaking trumpet and when in the act of opening his mouth to answer, a bucket of water is capsized into the trumpet for which he is sure to receive the benefit of at every word, after this operation he is well soused with as sharp a supply of water as all hands can give him each being furnished with a bucket filled for that purpose ... till Neptune cries enough; all the time this pleasant dose is administering the victim is motionless standing across a line when over he is passed away to the hands of the barber and doctor the former of which seats him on the edge of the bathing tub laying a wet sack on his naked shoulders to wipe his razor with.[78]

Gales' account is filled with the paraphernalia of a warped kind of medical authority. The ceremonial Doctor's face was partially covered 'with a piece of cows hide with a couple of holes cut in it to represent spectacles' and he wore 'a red coat ... that reached down to his heels and a pair of boots with tassels standing with a look that gravity itself might well laugh at'. Operations and doses turned the surgeon's familiar diagnostic descriptions on their head. Now, it is the physician who becomes the 'thin meagre sickly looking fellow'. He felt the sailor's pulse and prescribed 'what medicine his care might require'. The Doctor's mate, 'a painted devil bedaubed from heel to trunk with tar and lampblack or some as foul an ingredient', stood by. Strung around the mate's body were 'pill boxes ... numbered 1, 2, and 3 with bottles of various drugs and washes all calculated to restore the almost drowning patient'. Once the sailor took the medicine, the barber began to tar his face; 'selecting his keenest razor he not very gently scrapes it off till Neptune passes his word.'[79]

After their initial bewilderment, Gales believed that the convict women passed 'a fine night'. Indeed, they had already been partly responsible for dressing Neptune, who was 'rigged in the best attire the convicts could invent'. Several of the women apparently 'declared it was worth while being transported if it was for nothing but being present at such a scene'.[80] After Neptune and his initiates had retired below decks to clean themselves, 'the rest of the day was directed to mirth and revelry'. Towards evening 'the grog went round the song poured forth its melody the gentle murmur of the waves joining in chorus to the favourite strain ... nothing occurred to molest the happiness of the crew who were allowed to carry on their sports without interruption' for four nights.[81]

In 1818, one convict ship surgeon explained that the women of the *Elizabeth* had expressed a wish to see 'the usual ceremony', and he had allowed it to go ahead as a reward for their good behaviour. As the sailors were initiated, the women '[joined] in free sprinkling of water, with much good will and humour. Few of them [escaped] a complete drenching, and in the evening they were indulged with half a pint of wine each', having conducted themselves 'very orderly'.[82] It is of no little significance that both of these accounts refer to female convict ships, on which the possibility of a real mutiny was less than on male convict ships. For some convicts and emigrants who probably appreciated the satirical implications of such an attack on authority, the ceremony appears to have been an exciting release of tension after the heat and calms, and they willingly submitted to the rituals. On the convict ship *Bussorah Merchant*, William Maybury explained that each man was 'blindfolded greased with dirty fat shaved with tar and a long stick called Neptune's Razor while the rest of the crew were throwing wet swabs and buckets of water upon them, the scene was truly laughable, a great deal of mirth was displayed upon this occasion'.[83]

Other passengers found the rituals deeply offensive. On the *Morning Light*, even though the sailors used treacle, having been forbidden from using tar, Henry Curr, a Catholic priest, thought the proceedings 'perfectly disgusting and foolish and I wonder it is tolerated, so much nakedness is displayed'.[84] George Willmer also retreated to his cabin, having observed several of the sailors and passengers undergo their 'operation'. As the sailors came to Willmer's door, he 'immediately took up a sword to intimidate them. This posture of self-defence led to a parley.' When the sailors promised not to handle him roughly, Willmer 'ventured out and was only compelled to taste a little clean water while blindfolded. They did not even dip me in the water.'[85] The crossing of the line ceremony was not a harmless pantomime. Passengers who objected to the festivities fought to protect themselves from being forced into the ritual. George Wilcox described how he and eight other passengers 'took possession of the 'tween decks, pulled down the gangway ladders, and arming ourselves with anything that came to hand, assumed a posture of defence'. After a discussion in which the passengers declared that they 'cared nothing about customs, nor would we be insulted by anyone', the captain 'gave immediate orders to stop it, and Neptune and Co departed about their usual business'.[86]

For surgeons, the crossing of the line ceremony was a real test of their authority. That surgeons rarely mentioned ceremonies is suggestive, but their instructions also reveal growing official anxieties about the potential for disorder that accompanied the crossing of the line. In 1838, surgeons were instructed to allow the convicts to be on deck as much as possible. In so doing, they needed to be on their guard against any attempts at mutiny and to take 'precautions to prevent any surprises'. By 1848, the Admiralty had amended these instructions. They now stated that the surgeon must 'redouble [his] vigilance while within the tropics, instead of, as may have been the case, relaxing the discipline of the ship in those latitudes.' Disorder and climate were closely correlated. In addition, the convict-ship surgeon was 'to issue strict orders forbidding any ceremonies or amusements upon the occasion of passing the Line'.[87]

In contrast to the concern about convict ships, the surgeon's instructions and charter party for emigrant ships stated simply that 'emigrants are not to be molested on crossing the line'.[88] Yet, in 1855 the emigrant ship *Norman* became the subject of an Immigration Board inquiry after emigrants made many complaints, including that they 'had water pumped upon them by the fire-engine on crossing the line; in consequence of which many of them were thoroughly drenched'. Some of the young women 'attributed a long continued illness to that cause'.[89] The Immigration Board withheld the master's gratuity that rewarded a healthy passage, but instructed that because 'the surgeon had watched in silence the master compromising himself and the charter party', the master could still receive his passage-money.

Conclusion

The case of the *Norman* neatly illustrates why crossing the line was such an ordeal for surgeons. Whether the surgeon had authorised the ceremony, or whether he had simply been unable to assert his authority, is unclear. This was a personal failure, but it also represented a medical failure. Sailors' baptisms had often involved ducking into the sea; by the nineteenth century, revelries remained on- rather than overboard. For sailors, hanging huge sails across the deck and filling them with hundreds of gallons of sea water was, of course, far safer than risking a dunking over the side. Surgeons, on the other hand, watched helplessly as the sailors quite literally brought the sea into the ship, in defiance of one of the fundamental foundations of his medical knowledge. The growing prominence of the surgeon as a central figure in the crossing the line ceremony was certainly a satirical comment on his growing disciplinary authority, but the equatorial sousings, dunkings, and pourings also represented a denial of the relentless monotony of the surgeon's medical mantra: ships, at all costs, must be kept dry. It is little wonder that surgeons rarely mentioned the equatorial revelries in their own accounts of Australian voyages. Crossing the line marked a transition between departing and arriving, but as the sailors celebrated with their grog in the warmth of a tropical evening, it must also have reinforced the knowledge that voyages still had a very long way to go.

Notes

1   NMM, JOD 239, Journal kept by William Roberts on the *Sussex* (1854), 16 October.

2   Warwickshire County Record Office, CR 2926/63, Letter from James Backhouse on *Science of Scarborough*, n.d. (c. 1833).

3   Bristol Record Office, 41067/1, *The Tropical Times, printed and published on board the Barque Elizabeth during a voyage from Bristol to Australia, 1853*, Issue III, 19 February 1853, p. 1.

4   NMM, MSS/87/061, 3, Journal of W. James Gales, crew member on the convict ship *Andromeda*, Cork to Sydney (1834), 7 June.

5   ANMM, MS ALF Anonymous diary on *Alfred* (1838–1839), 13 October 1838.

6   PRONI, 1944/9/1, Anon, Logbook from voyage on *Fear Not* (1850).

7   Denis Cosgrove, 'Tropic and Tropicality', in Felix Driver and Luciana Martins (eds), *Tropical Visions in an Age of Empire* (Chicago and London: Chicago University Press, 2005), pp. 197–216, pp. 201–202.

8   ANMM, MS CRE, Diary of George Charles Bannister on ship *Credenda*, from England to Geelong (1853), 27–30 August 1853.

9   Driver and Martins, 'Introduction', in *Tropical Visions in an Age of Empire*, p. 8; David Livingstone, 'Tropical Hermeneutics: Fragments for a historical narrative, an afterword' *Singapore Journal of Tropical Geography* 21:1 (2000), pp. 92–98.

10 ML, M864, Journal of James Espie White, including voyage from

Liverpool to Melbourne on ship *Henry Fernie* (1863), Part 2: 'First Part of the Voyage'.

11 ANMM, MS MOR, Diary of Henry Curr on *Morning Light*, Liverpool to Australia (c. 1856), 20 July.

12 For an explanation of the *volta do mar*, and its role in European exploration from the fifteenth century, see Alfred Crosby, *Ecological Imperialism: The Biological Expansion of Europe* (Cambridge: Cambridge University Press, 1986), pp. 113–118.

13 Luciana Martins, 'Navigating in Tropical Waters: British maritime views of Rio de Janeiro', *Imago Mundi* 50 (1998), pp. 141–155, p. 143.

14 William S. Wilson, *The Ocean as a Health Resort* (London: Presley Blakiston, 1880), p. 16.

15 Greg Dening, *Mr Bligh's Bad Language: Passion, Power and Theatre on the Bounty* (Cambridge: Cambridge University Press, 1992), p. 76.

16 See for example, Warwick Anderson, *Colonial Pathologies: American Tropical Medicine, Race, and Hygiene in the Philippines* (Durham and London: Duke University Press, 2006); David Arnold, *The Tropics and the Traveling Gaze: India, Landscape and Science, 1800–1856* (Seattle and London: University of Washington Press, 2006); Mark Harrison, *Climates and Constitutions: Health, Race, Environment and British Imperialism in India, 1600–1850* (New Delhi and Oxford: Oxford University Press, 2002); Eric T. Jennings, *Curing the Colonizers: Hydrotherapy, Climatology and French Colonial Spas* (Durham and London: Duke University Press, 2006).

17 TNA, ADM 101/56/8, Journal of surgeon Robert Malcolm on convict ship *Nithsdale* (1829–1830), case no. 12: Joseph Worthington.

18 Michael Worboys, 'Germs, Malaria and the Invention of Mansonian Tropical Medicine: From 'diseases in the tropics' to 'tropical diseases', in David Arnold, *Warm Climates and Western Medicine* (Amsterdam: Rodopi, 1996), pp. 181–207, p. 185.

19 TNA, ADM 101/2/1, Journal of surgeon S. Alexander on convict ship *Almorah* (1820–1), 11 September 1820.

20 PRONI, 560/2, John Martin, Journal of voyage from Ireland on the convict ship *Mountstuart Elphinstone* to Australia, 1849–1850, entry for 7 July 1849.

21 ML, MSS A3234 / mfm CY 1388, Journal of surgeon Niel Campbell on emigrant ship *King William* (1842–1843), 4 November 1842.

22 TNA, ADM 101/79/7, Journal of surgeon G. Roberts on emigrant ship *William Nicol* (1837), General Remarks.

23 Admiralty, *Instructions for Surgeons-Superintendents on Board Convict Ships* (London: William Clowes, 1838).

24 TNA, ADM 101/29/8, Journal of surgeon George Roberts on convict ship *Gilmore* (1831–2), case no. 2: Robert West.

25 Mark Harrison, 'Tropical Medicine in Nineteenth-Century India', *British Journal for the History of Science* 25:3 (1992), pp. 299–318.
26 ANMM, MS MOR, Curr, Diary on *Morning Light*, 20 July (c. 1856).
27 Catharine Coleborne, *Madness in the Family: Insanity and Institutions in the Australasian Colonial World, 1860–1914* (Basingstoke: Palgrave Macmillan, 2010), pp. 38, 74.
28 Dane Kennedy, 'The Perils of the Midday Sun: Climatic anxieties in the colonial tropics', in J.M. Mackenzie (ed.) *Imperialism and the Natural World* (Manchester: Manchester University Press, 1990), p. 120.
29 TNA, ADM 101/79/4 Journal of surgeon Charles Kennedy on government emigrant ship *Susan* (1838–1839), General Remarks; Case 7: Margaret Walmsley.
30 TNA, ADM 101/44/3, Journal of surgeon James Lawrence on convict ship *Lord Lyndoch* (1836), case no. 8: Charles Moore.
31 Bristol Record Office, 41067/1, *Tropical Times*, Issue V, 5 March 1853, p. 4.
32 'Charles Picknell's Journal', in Anon, *The Kains: Female Convict Vessel* (Adelaide: Sullivan's Cove, 1989), pp. 19, 22.
33 TNA, ADM 101/59/7, Journal of surgeon Charles Queade on convict ship *Phoenix* (1824), Statement of 'some cases of poisoning'.
34 Karen Ordahl Kupperman, 'Fear of Hot Climates in the Anglo-American Colonial Experience', *William and Mary Quarterly*, 3rd Series 41:2 (1984), pp. 213–240, p. 224; Harrison, *Climates and Constitutions*, pp. 73, 79, 180–181.
35 Mark Harrison, 'From Medical Astronomy to Medical Astrology: Sol-lunar and planetary theories of disease in British medicine, c. 1700–1850', *British Journal for History of Science* 33 (2000), pp. 25–48, p. 26.
36 TNA, ADM 101 60/7, Journal of surgeon Thomas Bell on convict ship *Prince George* (1836–7), General Remarks.
37 ML, Mss B1496, mfm CY 1143, Robert Muir, Diary of voyage from Plymouth to Sydney on *Alfred*, 1838–1839, 21 October 1838.
38 ANMM, MS ALF Anonymous diary on *Alfred*, 21 October 1838.
39 Pat Jalland, *Australian Ways of Death: A social and cultural history 1840–1918* (Oxford: Oxford University Press, 2002), p. 5.
40 Supporting evidence from passenger lists suggests that it is apparently nothing more than a remarkable coincidence that we have two poisonous fish and two ships named *Pheonix*, separated by three decades.
41 MMM, DX/1481 (transcript of MMM. 1994. 157), Diary of Second Cabin Passenger William Hodkinson, on the White Star Line *Phoenix*, Auckland to Liverpool (1860), 30 September 1860.
42 'Charles Picknell's Journal' pp. 10–12.
43 'Charles Picknell's Journal', p. 17.
44 'Charles Picknell's Journal', p. 18.

45 'Charles Picknell's Journal', p. 20.

46 'Charles Picknell's Journal', p. 27.

47 Toby Green, *The Rise of the Trans-Atlantic Slave Trade in Western Africa, 1300–1589* (Cambridge: Cambridge University Press, 2011).

48 Phillip D. Curtin, *The Image of Africa: British ideas and action, 1780–1850* (Madison: University of Wisconsin Press, 1964), p. 362.

49 For the early history of Sierra Leone see 'New Approaches to the Founding of the Sierra Leone Colony, 1786–1808', Special Issue of *Journal of Colonialism and Colonial History* 9:3 (2008). For the involvement of the Navy in the nineteenth century see Raymond Howell, *The Royal Navy and the Slave Trade* (London: Croom Helm, 1987) and Mark Harrison, '"An Important and Truly National Subject": The West Africa Service and the Health of the Royal Navy in the Mid Nineteenth Century', in David Boyd Haycock and Sally Archer (eds) *Health and Medicine at Sea, 1700–1900* (Woodbridge: Boydell Press, 2009), pp. 108–127.

50 Frank Lloyd, *The Navy and the Slave Trade* (London: Frank Cass and Co., 1968), p. 69.

51 TNA, ADM 101/22/5, Journal of surgeon Robert Beith on convict ship *Eden* (1848), General Remarks.

52 J.O. McWilliam, *Medical History of the Expedition to the Niger during the years 1841–2: comprising an account of the fever which led to its abrupt termination* (London: John Churchill, 1843); T.R.H. Thomson, 'On the Value of Quinine in African Remittent Fever', *The Lancet* (28 February 1846), pp. 244–245.

53 PRONI, 560/2, John Martin, Journal of voyage from Ireland, entry for 19 July.

54 ANMM, MS ALF, Anonymous diary written on board *Alfred*, from Plymouth to New South Wales, 16 September 1838–17 January 1839, entry for 20 October 1838.

55 Emma Christopher, 'Steal a Handkerchief, See the World: The trans-oceanic voyaging of Thomas Limpus', in Ann Curthoys and Marilyn Lake (eds), *Connected Worlds: History in Transnational Perspective* (Canberra: ANU Press, 2005), pp. 77–88, p. 81.

56 Curtin, *The Image of Africa*, pp. vi–vii.

57 James Johnson, *The Influence of Tropical Climates on European Constitutions*, 6th edn (London: James Ranald Martin, 1841), p. 4.

58 ML, Mfm M934, Journal of William Charles Wills, Diary on voyage from England to Sidney [*sic*] on the barque *Louisa* (1841–1842), 1 December 1841.

59 NLA, MS 336 Folder 1, Oswald Bloxome, Journal of a Voyage to New South Wales (1838), Sunday 6 May 1838.

60 Richard Drayton, 'Maritime Networks and the Making of Knowledge',

in David Cannadine (ed.) *Empire, the Sea and Global History: Britain's Maritime World, c. 1763–c. 1840* (Basingstoke: Palgrave Macmillan, 2007), pp. 72–82.

61 H. Riehl, *Tropical Meteorology* (London: McGraw Hill, 1954), pp. 1–5.

62 ML, Mss B1535 / CY 1024, Diary of Hugh May Wilson from Deptford and Plymouth on barque *Sarah* (1849) 4 October 1849.

63 ANMM, MS KAT, Diary of Richard Hall on the ship *Kate*, Liverpool to Melbourne (December 1852–April 1853), 22 and 26 January 1853.

64 ANMM, MS ALF, Anonymous diary on *Alfred*, 13 October.

65 For the importance of Columbus' journey south as well as west see Nicolas Wey Gómez, *The Tropics of Empire: Why Columbus sailed South to the Indies* (Cambridge, MA: MIT Press, 2008).

66 ML, Mfm 2116, Henry Widdowson's Diary on *Albion*, transporting cattle and horses to Australia (1825–1826), 9 and 10 January 1826. [The Mitchell Library uses the spelling Widdowson]

67 Henry Widowson, *Present State of Van Diemen's Land* (London: 1829).

68 Peter Cunningham, *Two Years in New South Wales* (London: Henry Colburn, 1827), pp. 19–20.

69 David Lindsay Waugh, *Three Years Practical Experience of a Settler in New South Wales; being extracts from letters to his friends in Edinburgh, from 1834–1837*, 8th edn, with a map (Edinburgh: John Johnstone, 1838), p. iv.

70 Waugh, *Three Years Practical Experience*, p. 11.

71 Bristol Record Office, 41067/1, *Tropical Times*, Issue VI, p. 4.

72 Matthew Fontaine Maury, *Physical Geography of the Sea* (New York: Harper and Brothers, 1855), p. 171.

73 Dening, *Mr Bligh's Bad Language*, p. 77. For other descriptions of the ceremony see Emma Christopher, *Slave Ship Sailors and their Captive Cargoes* (Cambridge: Cambridge University Press, 2006), pp. xiii–xv; Margaret S. Creighton, *Rites and Passages: The Experience of American Whaling, 1830–1870* (Cambridge: Cambridge University Press, 1995), pp. 118–124.

74 Henning Henningsen, *Crossing the Equator: Sailor's Baptisms and Other Initiation Rites* (Copenhagen: Munksgaarde, 1961), pp. 59, 71–81.

75 ANMM, MS ALF, Anonymous diary on *Alfred*, 5 November 1838.

76 George Willmer, *The Draper in Australia* (London: Freeman, 1856), pp. 20–21.

77 ANMM, MS GOL, Diary of Christopher Parrah Gale on *Golden Era* (1855), 12 April.

78 NMM, MSS/87/061, 3, Gales, journal on *Andromeda*, 6 July.

79 NMM, MSS/87/061, 3, Gales, journal on *Andromeda*, 5 July.

80 NMM, MSS/87/061, 3, Gales, journal on *Andromeda*, 5 July.

81 NMM, MSS/87/061, 3, Gales, journal on *Andromeda*, 6 July.

82 TNA, ADM 101/24/1, Journal of surgeon William Hamilton, on convict ship *Elizabeth* (1818), 1 September 1818.

83 NMM, MS87/047, William Maybury, Convict's Log on the *Bussorah Merchant* (27 March–26 July 1828), 30 April.

84 ANMM, MS MOR, Curr, Diary on *Morning Light*, 27 July (c. 1856).

85 Willmer, *The Draper in Australia*, p. 21.

86 ANMM, MS ADE, George Wilcox, Journal of passage to Australia on *Aden* (1849), 5 July.

87 Admiralty, *Instructions for Surgeons-Superintendents on Board Convict Ships* (London: William Clowes, 1838 and 1848).

88 KCL, Special Collections: FCO Collection. Emigration Tracts Vol. XI, 1832–1840. *Instructions for the surgeon's superintendent on board emigrant ships proceeding to New South Wales or Van Diemen's Land* (1838).

89 United Kingdom, House of Commons, Immigration Agent's Report, *Papers relative to Emigration to Australian Colonies* 1857 [144], x, p. 105.

4

'Such concentrated mischief':
scurvy and imprisonment

On 8 December 1841, the convict ship *Barossa* was approximately four hundred miles to the east of the Cape of Good Hope, and eight thousand miles from London. It was summer in the southern hemisphere, but the weather was cold and rainy and the winds boisterous. Having so recently passed the Cape – the last opportunity for procuring fresh meat, vegetables, fruit, and water – the *Barossa*'s surgeon, Henry Mahon, recorded with frustration that ten of the convicts had developed scurvy. 'The sickness seemed', Mahon wrote in his journal, 'as if ushered in simultaneously with our advancement into the high southern latitudes, wherein cold rainy weather predominated with a heavy sea.' Such conditions 'will not fail in producing injurious effects on persons indifferently clad and unprovided for these vicissitudes'. By the time the *Barossa* reached Van Diemen's Land on 9 January 1842, there had been 106 cases of scurvy. Sixty-seven men had appeared to recover during the voyage, but one man had died. As they finally saw land, Mahon wrote that several of the prisoners 'were suddenly seized with sickness and alarming faintness'. The convicts' breakdown, he suggested, was caused by 'the emotions felt on recognising the land of their destiny and brooding on the fate that may await them'.[1] On arrival in Hobart, Mahon sent sixteen of the convicts to the colonial hospital.

Historians have often commented on the detail with which the British government described the physical appearance of convicts in the ships' musters and convict indents. For the purposes of identification, the British government took an extraordinary interest in the distinguishing features of convicts' bodies, including their eye colour, height, and face shape, as well as their scars and tattoos.[2] We know, for example, that Edward Radford, one of the men on the *Barossa*, was transported for stealing twenty yards of lace from a warehouse. Aged 22 years, he stood 5 feet 1½ inches tall. He had a fair complexion, oval face (forehead of medium height) and dark brown hair. His eyebrows were black, his eyes brown, and his nose long. Scars in the corner of his left eye, at the side of his mouth, and over his right eye also distinguished him.[3]

Henry Mahon's journal of the *Barossa*'s voyage contains another remarkably intimate record of Edward Radford's body: his right leg (Figure 3) is the subject of one of eight watercolour studies contained within a thirteen-page report on scurvy.[4] Each picture vividly depicts the swellings, bruising, and eruptions of scurvy in the groin and limbs of several of the *Barossa*'s convicts. Three of the men stand naked from the waist down, two painted from the front, and one from the rear. The remaining five studies depict single legs, each displaying a range of spots and ulcers. The skin covering Edward Radford's shin is covered in dark spots, and dark purple bruising surrounds his knee, but the sketch of Radford's leg is particularly striking for the two trickles of bright blood that ooze from the tumour over his knee cap. In a note next to the sketch, Mahon recorded that this 'bloody discharge continued for some time' after he had made the opening with his lancet.

The painstakingly detailed pictorial representation of this incision in Radford's knee is compelling evidence of Mahon's physical contact with the prisoners on the *Barossa* as he investigated the nature of scurvy. His writing elaborates further: in a section entitled 'Pathological Observations on the Blood and Urine', Mahon described how he bled four of his convict patients to analyse the scorbutic fluids. The blood from Robert Osborne – 'a healthy muscular man' – appeared 'darker and less firm' than that taken from the others. Mahon was able to move the clot 'several times from one vessel to another without [it] breaking up'. When Mahon added a solution of nitrate of potash and muriate of soda to the sample of Osborne's blood, it changed 'from a dark purple to a reddish hue'. As a therapeutic practice, bleeding remained common in the 1840s, particularly for fevers, but Mahon's studies are not just records of disease and its treatment.

Unclothed and unchained, no material effects betray the prisoners' station in life. By recording the physiological details of how scurvy deformed and erupted from within the naked men, Mahon's paintings provide graphic evidence of the examinations, proddings, and incisions undertaken on their bodies. Their prison experience had contributed to the production of disease, and the surgeon took a familiar practice of recording a convict's physical appearance a step further. Mahon's paintings are stark illustrations of the surgeon's power to physically intervene and experiment with the morbid processes that affected prisoners' lives, and they hint at the cumulative effects of imprisonment, transportation, and the sea on prisoners.

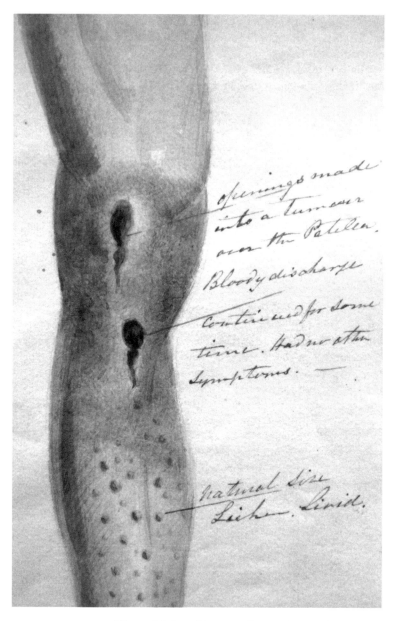

Figure 3 Henry Mahon, Essay on Scurvy (1841–42),
detail of Diagram No. 4: Case 24, Edward Radford.

Mahon's paintings are surprising for a second reason, because they give the lie to great contemporary confidence in scurvy cures. During the early modern period, as European powers expanded their empires into the southern hemisphere, scurvy had inscribed 'maritime' experience on the bodies and minds of sailors. Like tattoos, scurvy distinguished those who bore its inscriptions as seafarers. Thus marked, men became men of the world who were distinguished from landed society.[5] In 1808, Thomas Trotter explained that the ocean bestowed 'a new disposition' on the sailor's morbid state. 'His diseases showed a particular genuis [*sic*] and feature, such as are found only among his own class, and which spring from causes particular to the sea life'. Indeed, Trotter declared, being at sea changed the sailor to 'a different species of being'.[6] Yet, by 1822 Gilbert Blane believed that the 'medical art' had cured scurvy, and thus saved Britain in the Napoleonic Wars. By 1847, J.B. Jukes would suggest that the surgeon on *HMS Fly* had 'never seen scurvy in the Navy before, so completely have modern discoveries and improvements eradicated that naval scourge'.[7] This 'eradication' of scurvy is reflected in the physical arrangement of naval surgeons' medical journals. By the time they began to routinely superintend convict voyages in 1815, surgeons had to write scurvy by hand into the nosological table in which they tallied and ordered cases of disease, as it no longer appeared in the printed list.

For historians too, the story of scurvy has been one of eighteenth-century medical and military triumph. By 1795, the story goes, men such as Thomas Trotter, Gilbert Blane, and James Cook finally forced a corrupt Admiralty establishment to belatedly acknowledge James Lind's discovery of the lemon juice 'cure' and to authorise the regular issue of lemon juice in the Navy in 1795. While the best scholarship acknowledges that scurvy continued to affect merchant ships, polar explorers, and victims of the Scottish and Irish famine throughout the nineteenth century, recent popular studies still describe the eighteenth-century naval 'conquest' of scurvy as 'one of the great socio-military advances of the era'.[8]

Certainly, the issuing of lemon juice on some convict ships in the nineteenth century took on the aspect of a religious ritual. John Martin described George Moxey's 'ceremonious occupations' with the convicts as he took on the persona of 'a deity to be worshipped' on the *Mountstuart Elphinstone*. 'Every man must come round the Capstan, past the lynx eyed Doctor, with his tin in one hand and his cap in the other. Should he venture too close to the Doctor's person, should his foot touch the raised floor surrounding the Capstan, back he goes to try again at the exact performance of his duty.'[9] In 1850, Alexander

Bryson recalled that scurvy had still commanded 'a considerable share of the naval surgeon's attention', in an aggravated form, while 'under the charge of prisoners on the passage to New South Wales'.[10]

The previous chapters have highlighted the ways in which emigrants, particularly those who could only afford to travel in steerage or had their passages paid by the government or Australian colonists, shared with convicts many of the social, environmental, and medical experiences of the early nineteenth-century voyage. Scurvy is one of the most striking exceptions to this theme of shared experience. Scurvy appeared very occasionally on emigrant ships to Australia in the nineteenth century: the surgeon of the *Woodbridge*, for example, recorded that they had put in at the Cape for fresh provisions, including 2,501 pounds of beef and mutton, because the symptoms of scurvy had appeared. The majority of surgeons in charge of emigrants mentioned the disease only in passing, if at all.[11] Yet, for convicts, the disease still figured centrally as part of the transformative experience of time on the high seas. Moreover, it rapidly increased in incidence through the 1830s, so that scurvy became an almost inevitable result of their transportation. This chapter explains why.

Obadiah Pineo and the Cape of Good Hope

Once the captains and crews of ships bound for Australia had negotiated the meteorological uncertainties of the tropical Atlantic, they put the coast of South America behind them and headed south-east, towards the Cape of Good Hope. If surgeons had already experienced the trials of calms, the sudden and severe changes in climate as the trade winds propelled ships south could have equally unsettling consequences for physical and mental health. Temperatures plummeted over a few days, and surgeons recorded the return of the kinds of colds, catarrhs, fevers, and bowel disorders that often occurred in the first few days off Northern Europe. As we have seen in the previous chapter, the African coast played an important role in the geographical and medical imagination of the Australian voyage. In the 'deadly latitudes' of West Africa ships lolled in equatorial calms, sails assumed a jaundiced complexion, and there often appeared to be a clear correlation between maritime latitude, climate, and disease. More subtly, though no less significant for that, the seas around the Cape of Good Hope also played a crucial role in understandings of the medical geography of Australian voyages.

As Jonathan Lamb has shown, Commodore George Anson's disastrous global travels and Captain James Cook's Pacific voyaging had brought the dangers of prolonged voyages to the oceans of the southern hemisphere vividly to the attention of the Admiralty and British public in the eighteenth century. The discursive connection between scurvy and the South Seas, Lamb suggests, was 'extensive and exact'.[12] The further south ships sailed beyond forty degrees of latitude – known as 'Great Circle' sailing – the more likely they were to encounter the roaring westerlies that circled the southern hemisphere and flung ships across the ocean, towards Australia. Captains had to decide whether to take advantage of this time- and distance-saving route and risk scurvy, and the effects of freezing wet weather, or whether to stay further north and accept the prolonged delays, but also the better health, that came with repairing and replenishing with fresh water and provisions.[13]

At the southern tip of the African continent, as the warmth of the Indian Ocean meets the colder waters of the Antarctic and Atlantic, the Cape of Good Hope had been a vital node in European imperial networks since its first permanent settlement by the Dutch in the early seventeenth century.[14] Occupied by the British in 1806, the Cape officially became a British colony in 1814. Some surgeons of vessels bound for Australia struggled to persuade captains who wished not to break their voyage, but others encountered less resistance as they requested to steer for Simon's Bay.[15] Long considered an oasis of health and recuperation, the Cape also came to figure centrally in naval surgeons' reflections and regrets about scurvy.

In 1838, Obadiah Pineo appears to have been happy to let the *Lord Lyndoch*'s crew take full advantage of favourable winds and continue eastwards into the southern Indian Ocean. However, contemplating the voyage as he filled in the 'General Remarks' section of his journal, Pineo lamented that he had not persuaded the captain to steer for the Cape.[16] The surgeon explained that scurvy had appeared in 'a very aggravated form' among the male convicts on the *Lord Lyndoch* after the ship had rounded the southern tip of Africa. Pineo had missed the vital opportunity for replenishment and recuperation. Nevertheless, he still maintained that there had not been sufficient cause at the time to warrant a change in the ship's course. Pineo had 'gone two preceding voyages without calling anywhere & without the loss of a person, of any discomfiture whatever'. He hoped 'to have been equally fortunate in this [voyage], but in that I was deceived. It has been a source of much regret ever since.' Pineo described a typical convict ship regime which addressed all the usual causes of disease:

> the prisons were kept dry, clean and well fumigated with hot vinegar, or sprinkled with cold vinegar and the solution of chloride of lime,

alternatively every day of the week. I have walked through every part of them in the middle of the night, without experiencing the slightest foul smell, not even from the water closets, where a guard was constantly kept that the parts of the prison should not be rendered uncomfortable to any one. The scuttles were kept open most of the time and windsails used at the different hatchway. The ships hold which I examined more than once was in good condition, and her ballast the best and freshest I ever saw. The provisions and comforts for the prisoners were of excellent quality ... I began the general use of lemon juice and sugar shortly after leaving England, and wine some time afterwards.[17]

In his journal, Pineo showed that despite all of his efforts, scurvy nevertheless plagued the *Lord Lyndoch*. The almost uncommonly fresh atmosphere inside the *Lord Lyndoch*, the routines, and medical comforts had failed, and such a widespread occurrence of disease confused Pineo. He considered possible causes that may have aggravated the emergence of scurvy among the *Lord Lyndoch*'s convicts. Perhaps, because the convicts 'were all from the country', the men had 'suffered considerably from the excessive cold of the preceding winter', and he attributed disease to 'a peculiar diathesis, or constitutional temperament of a great portion of these people'. Pineo also suggested that the convicts' change from 'the plentiful exercise and restricted diet' of the English hulks to the 'generous diet and abridged exercise' had triggered underlying disease.[18] Scurvy deceived Pineo. It concealed itself behind an appearance of well-being: 'even when the disease was most general, you could not perceive any symptoms of ill health', he wrote. Scurvy had also fooled the free passengers on board the *Lord Lyndoch*. They too had remarked 'how uncommonly healthy the prisoners appeared'. Pineo begged the Admiralty to obtain an order from the government 'making it imperative on all surgeon superintendents to call at some port, on the voyage to New South Wales', as they had done until the 1820s. Of this necessity, Pineo was now 'quite convinced' to reduce the risk of 'some epidemic arising'.[19]

On arrival in Port Jackson, Pineo sent 113 sick prisoners to the Colonial Hospital. The new Governor, Sir George Gipps (1838–1846), was also busy quarantining emigrant ships for typhus at this period, and he summoned a colonial Medical Board to inquire into the reasons for sickness on the *Lord Lyndoch*. With his journal and professional reputation subjected to scrutiny, Pineo wrote to William Burnett, Physician-General to the Admiralty. As he had done in his journal, Pineo maintained that he had done no wrong. He also re-emphasised his belief that the prisoners' external appearance of health on their embarkation had not allowed him to comprehend the underlying physical state of their bodies. Even as they approached the Cape, the men had seemed healthy, and he 'could not think it possible that any epidemic could reach them after the Cape of Good Hope'.

However, whereas in the journal, which would serve as the official record of his voyage, Pineo had professed himself 'convinced' by the necessity of a stop at the Cape, as he wrote to William Burnett in the Admiralty, he now proffered a very different opinion. 'Nor do I believe at this moment had I touched at the Cape of Good Hope, we should have saved one life ... It could have only *saved appearances* and perhaps prevented the Governor of New South Wales holding a second enquiry on the causes of scurvy which has annoyed me not a little.'[20] Scurvy lurked and then revealed itself, but Pineo's comments also remind us that these medical journals were cards in a constant medical game. In them, surgeons represented a version of the events of the voyage in order to secure their pay. Pineo's letter to Burnett reveals that his 'regret' was less about his failure to prevent scurvy than it was about his failure to protect his professional reputation.

Diet, debility, and a cold climate

James Lind's eighteenth-century trials with lemon juice are famous, but they were not the end of the scurvy story. Like his contemporaries', Lind's writings contained a wealth of ideas about digestion, atmosphere, temperament, and discipline. Sir John Pringle identified putrid bilge water as one of the main causes of scurvy, and advocated that men take antiseptic substances, including lemon juice, vinegar, and tobacco as a cure. In 1764 David MacBride recommended that Captain Cook take sauerkraut and wort on board *Endeavour* because they too contained the acidic 'fixed air' that could restore a healthy state of the blood.[21] Later in the century, scurvy became a key theme in atmospheric explanations of disease, and Thomas Beddoes would argue that too much time in the unwholesome hold of a ship caused scurvy because of a lack of oxygen.[22]

In his influential medical handbook, *Practice of Physic* (1788), William Cullen taught surgeons that scurvy was 'more frequent and more considerable in cold than in warm climates and seasons'. Yet there had been 'no instance of either cold or moisture producing scurvy, without the concurrence of the faulty sea-diet', particularly the eating of meat in a putrescent or salted state.[23] Without a frequent supply of fresh vegetable aliment, he explained, a man's fluids 'would advance further towards putrefaction than is consistent with health'. Alternatively, eating too much salted animal food would carry the 'animal processes' too far, 'evolving a larger proportion of saline matter'. The body's retention of saline matter when, for example, cold wet weather checked the natural processes of perspiration also contributed to the production of scurvy. By emphasising the role of diet, Cullen broke Pringle's link between scurvy and fevers. Cullen and his circle were also instrumental in shifting the focus from putrid to nervous theories of scurvy.[24] Cullen believed that 'weakness, in whatever manner occasioned is favourable to the production of scurvy', while Frederick Thomson also wrote that scurvy appeared to be more 'a gradual subversion of the constitution'.[25] 'In short', Thomas Trotter wrote in 1795, 'whatever can be considered as a debilitating power when applied to the human body, may be justly reckoned among the predisposing causes of scurvy.'[26]

Naval surgeons' ideas about scurvy on convict ships in the nineteenth century reflected the entire range of this conceptual spectrum from diet, through debility, to atmosphere. In 1835 Andrew Henderson concluded that 'diet alone under proper management can prevent scurvy'. He further argued that 'lemon juice or any other acid never was, and never can be either a preventive or cure for scurvy'.[27] By contrast, the surgeon of the *John Barry* described how 'a succession of heavy gales and cold wet weather' prevented the prisoners from being on deck much during the day. 'This confinement below, together with the damp state of the decks, encouraged a tendency towards scurvy and bowel complaints.'[28] Another surgeon traced the causes of scurvy back to the tropics, where 'molecules of animal matter in a state of decay' floated between decks in the vitiated, moist, heated atmosphere of the prison room.[29] In 1850 Alexander Bryson still argued that scurvy had arisen in one convict ship 'in consequence of [the prisoners'] close confinement below, in the damp, vitiated atmosphere of an ill-ventilated [ship's] prison'.[30]

One of the key assumptions that lay behind surgeons' therapeutic approaches to scurvy was that the disease represented a derangement of the blood's chemical state. In scurvy, Dr Elliotson explained in the *Lancet* in 1830, the constitution itself 'is not at all in fault'. Scurvy was a 'purely chemical' disease, and the role of scurvy remedies was simply to restore the diminished state of the sufferer's bodily fluids.[31] When surgeon Francis Logan described the case of the convict Eleanor Hall in 1832 he recorded that she had 'no blotches on her skin nor other symptoms of scorbutus except the extreme debility, yet there being no other disease apparent to produce such debility I put her on the list as a case of scurvy'.[32] Obadiah Pineo was unable to identify any 'excitement' in the sufferers' bodies that explained the outbreak on the *Lord Lyndoch*, and concluded that scurvy was 'a disease of pure debility and great prostration of strength … [that] appeared to have been inherent in the people'.[33]

Emotion and the mutinous passions

Multi-causal explanations remained at the heart of nineteenth-century knowledge about scurvy, just as they had done in the eighteenth century. Too great a reliance on ship's rations, a cold atmosphere, lack of exercise, and fatigue all sped up the progress of disease. In addition, mental causes of scurvy were almost as important as physical causes, and the disease had long been associated with laziness, depressed passions, and homesickness. Thomas Trotter had described the 'groans and weeping, altogether childish', of those afflicted by what he termed 'scorbutic nostalgia'. Such an intense longing for land was both 'the first symptom and the constant attendant of the disease in all its stages'.[34] This relationship between the mental and physical state remained foremost in convict ship surgeons' discussions of scurvy. Henry Mahon described Roland Cameron as being of 'a weak intellect and debilitated frame produced by a former dissipated course of life'. John Edwards, too, was 'feeble and emaciated, of a sallow complexion and anxious countenance'.[35]

Surgeons emphasised the need to elevate convicts' spirits to ward off the depressed 'passions' on which scurvy apparently thrived. On the *Lord Lyndoch*, Pineo ensured that 'we had plenty of musicians and some good instruments. Every day when the weather would allow, we had dancing. Gymnastics and trotting exercise all round the decks & forecastle.'[36] Andrew Henderson was a particularly enthusiastic promoter of mental well-being. In 1833 he encouraged 'every innocent amusement … and a hilarity of mind'.[37] Perhaps realising that hilarity did not sit well with punishment, in his comments on later voyages he became more reserved, but still emphasised the importance of positive mental and physical discipline in slowing the advances of scurvy.[38] When he discovered in 1842 that nearly forty of the convicts on the *Emily* had spongy gums and other signs of scurvy, he 'doubled [his] diligence to stir them up to exert themselves both upon deck and below' through useful work and exercise.[39]

The effect of emotions on the progress of scurvy could be a strange one. As Thrasycles Clarke superintended the women on the convict ship *Kains* in 1830, he described a striking reversal of the causal relationship between ill-discipline and disease. By all accounts, this had been a protracted and frustrating passage through the tropics. By the time the

Kains reached the Cape, so little water remained on board that to pass without restocking, Clarke wrote, would have been 'both improvident and unjustifiable'. In the week preceding their arrival at the Cape in late November, scurvy had appeared amongst some of the female convicts. Many of the women were 'slightly tainted', but Clarke had needed only to confine the two most serious cases to the ship's hospital. In general, Clarke thought, 'if there ever was a hell afloat it must have been in the shape of a female convict ship'. With a 'spirit of devilishness', the women had spent the voyage 'quarrelling, fighting, thieving', and destroying each other's property. And yet, he reluctantly observed a striking reversal of the surgeon's usual association of ill-discipline and disease. The women had seemed to positively affect their own health by engaging in 'conversations with each other most abandoned, – without feeling or shame'. He concluded that the 'absence of depressing feelings' which such conversations engendered had 'probably been in some measure a source of health'.[40]

Joy Damousi has identified convict women's use of bad language, quarrelling, and boisterous behaviour as forms of resistance to authority.[41] Here, on the *Kains*, the women's behaviour resisted disease as their high spirits kept the worst ravages of scurvy at bay. Meanwhile, the crew anxiously awaited a sight of land. 'It is high time we had made land for the scurvy is on board our ship through our bad living and short wauter [*sic*],' Charles Picknell fretted.[42] Finally, the *Kains* reached the Cape. During a month-long stop at Table Bay, the female convicts received fresh meat and vegetables each day, but Clarke believed that the women had already begun to recover at sea, under treatment with lime juice and nitrate of potash, but also under the influence of their own mental strength.

On the *Isabella* in 1840, Henry Mahon suggested that the female constitution in general 'is not so susceptible of being afflicted with scurvy as that of the male'.[43] Ideas about scurvy were gendered, not least because of a long association between scurvy and mutiny. In 1823, surgeon James McTernan reported that the convicts on the *Ocean* had enjoyed a 'tolerable' immunity from disease during the voyage to Australia. However, fifty of the prisoners had suffered from scurvy. McTernan admitted that he would have been 'at a loss to account for the appearance & prevalence of scurvy' had he not been aware of 'a strong predisposing cause': convict mutiny. In the most part, the victims of scurvy on the *Ocean* consisted

of men who by repeated acts of misconduct in their hulks had forfeited every claim to indulgence, had formed a resolution to take whatsoever ship they should be put out in, had actually attempted to possess themselves of the *Ocean* and concerted measures to repeat their attempt.[44]

The convicts' attempts at mutiny failed, and the *Ocean* continued its voyage south, making a quick transition from the heat of the tropics into the temperate climate of the high southern latitudes. These swift climatic changes and decreasing temperatures, McTernan explained, compounded the disappointment and despondency naturally felt by the convicts at the failure of their schemes. McTernan described scurvy as the effect of the changing maritime environment upon the dissatisfied minds and weakened bodies of the desperate men who had twice tried to take the *Ocean*. On arrival in Sydney, McTernan had no qualms about saying that the convicts' 'state of mind' had caused scurvy and invited Governor Brisbane to enquire into the circumstances of the voyage.[45]

Over a decade later, in 1836–37, many of the *Prince George*'s convicts suffered from scurvy during the voyage. Thomas Bell, the surgeon-superintendent, explained that he had examined 120 convicts received from English hulks in preparation for embarkation to the convict transport. Unusually, he had first encountered these convicts in cross irons, 'in consequence of many of them being of desperate character'. The previous month, while they had waited to be transported from the *Fortitude* hulk moored at Chatham, some of the prisoners had attempted to escape. Nineteen men had signed a paper swearing their acceptance only of 'death or liberty'. They had jumped from the *Fortitude*, but found themselves 'anchored to the necks in mud'. Their plot failed, the men were returned to the *Fortitude*. When they embarked the *Prince George* many of the men were 'in a low state of health, such as would arise from long confinement, depressed spirits, want of exercise, despondency and other such debilitating causes'.[46]

As the *Prince George* left the Thames in the middle of December and headed through the English Channel towards the Atlantic, it had immediately met with 'a long continuance of snowy, wet, cold, and blowing weather'. On Christmas night, the ship lost both its anchors in a gale and the whole company 'narrowly escaped with our lives'. The fear, exposure, and seasickness of these first few weeks of the voyage compounded the mental and physical strains of the men's mutinous passions and penal deprivations. For several weeks after their embarkation Bell recorded that most of the men 'could take but little nourishment'. Before they had got far from the English shore a litany of physical and psychological woes 'in a great degree conduced to the disease "scurvy" that has shown itself so early, and with such virulence', Bell wrote.[47]

George Willett

The first of the *Prince George* convicts to develop scurvy was a man named George Willett. A bachelor and farmer's labourer from Essex, Willett was transported to New South Wales for stealing a sheep. He told Bell that he had lived 'very poorly indeed' without any work. 'For the last two winters, being out of employment and provisions high in price, he became very weak for want of food, determined not to die of starvation, [and] stole a sheep for which he was transported.' Bell first suspected that Willett had scurvy on 27 January, when, during the convict's morning ablutions on the deck of the *Prince George*, the surgeon observed 'a number of small petechiae' on Willett's legs. The enforced regular ritual of personal washing was not simply a matter of hygienic discipline, but was also a vital opportunity for the surgeon to observe the physical state of the convicts' bodies. Seeing these small purple spots on Willett's limbs, Bell subjected the man to a further inspection, which revealed that Willett's gums were spongy and tender, the classic symptoms of scurvy.

Bell's regime for scurvy followed a familiar therapeutic pattern; he persuaded Willett to take as much exercise as possible and tried to keep him in the fresh sea air, although he was reluctant to go on deck. As Willett became increasingly languid under the influence of disease, Bell replaced his salt provisions with the preserved meat reserved for invalids, supplemented with wine and sugar. Over the following weeks, the convict's appearance did not improve, although his gums became firmer. Willett complained of headache and tinnitus. When cleaning the convict's ears failed to relieve the headache, Bell applied a blister, which rose well the following day. Although the pain in Willett's head improved, his appetite decreased again and he complained of weakness. In a last attempt to preserve Willett's health, Bell prescribed 'the most generous diet we could afford'. By the time of their arrival in New South Wales, the surgeon recorded a hollow victory: Willett was 'the worst case that did not terminate fatally'.[48] Willett was able to walk the half-mile to the colonial hospital with the assistance of another convict, although colonial accounts record that he died later the same year.[49]

Although his care of Willett was careful and thorough, Bell had made a common association between scurvy, ill-discipline, and laziness; Willett was of 'an indolent and slothful disposition [and] seldom can be got to attend divisions in a clean state'.[50] A causal chain of events – near-starvation, winter exposure, a crime, and then imprisonment – had weakened the man's constitution, and it was not surprising that Willett suffered. In their effects on a person's physical health, little separated the emotions of desperation, homesickness, and exhaustion from laziness, indolence, and failed mutinous desires; so too, these psychological states straddled a porous boundary between cause and effect in scurvy.

New penal discipline

During the eighteenth century there had been some debate as to whether scurvy was in fact two separate diseases: one on land, another at sea. William Cullen's *Practice of Physic* had settled the argument by declaring that scurvy was one disease, wherever it occurred.[51] It is therefore striking, given the strength of Cullen's influence over naval surgeons' medical knowledge in this period, that convict-ship surgeons began again to differentiate between 'land' and 'sea' scurvy during the 1830s. Andrew Henderson explained that sea-scurvy was 'a disease occurring in strong healthy looking subjects, but of a bloated cast or countenance, developing itself in swellings and rigidity of the knee joints chiefly'. On the other hand, land scurvy occurred 'in depraved emaciated habits from scarcity of or pravity of food … showing itself in the sallow anxious countenance, the flabby tongue, an irregular state of the bowels'.[52] Between the 1820s and 1830s the naval surgeons' focus shifted from the maritime to the penal causes of scurvy as prison authorities steadily reduced the dietary scales in Britain and Ireland. If the Admiralty had eradicated the scurvy that attacked the sailor in the hardest-working parts of his body, the scurvy that attacked the depraved, emaciated convict was on the rise.

By 1842, Andrew Henderson was one of the most experienced of the convict-ship surgeons. During the voyage of the *Emily* – his eighth – he described how scurvy emerged unusually quickly before the ship reached the Cape. Scurvy often broke out on ships that had experienced bad weather, particularly those that left in winter, but the circumstances of the *Emily*'s voyage, by contrast, were 'as favourable … as could be wished'.[53] He believed that scurvy had broken out because the *Emily* contained old stores 'of very inferior quality'. Henderson was adamant that men on ships and hulks needed a proper diet, and for a decade had repeatedly written to the Admiralty on the matter of diet and scurvy.[54] And yet, even for Henderson, the inadequacies of the maritime victuals could not fully account for the severity or the early appearance of scurvy. As he looked further into the convicts' history and to their lives on shore, he found a distinct correlation between the convicts' experience of disease and the circumstances of their imprisonment. Where the surgeons of the *Ocean* in 1823 and *Prince George* in 1837 had found mutinous passions, in 1842 Henderson identified the causes of scurvy in the very practice and structure of a changing penal system. Most importantly, the experience of imprisonment itself seemed to Henderson to cause disease.

After receiving his posting to the *Emily*, Henderson had received large groups of convicts from three different prison hulks: the *Justitia* and *Warrior* at Woolwich, and the *Fortitude* at Chatham. The majority of the fourteen cases of scurvy had occurred in convicts from the *Warrior* and *Justitia* hulks and he described how the voyage had taken its toll in different degrees, according to the state in which the convicts had first embarked. 'The 80 prisoners from the *Justitia* and in a less degree the 80 from the *Warrior* were in a very low state of health, bordering upon scurvy when they embarked, otherwise why were the 80 prisoners from the *Fortitude* … not similarly affected?' he asked.[55] In addition, Henderson remarked that the prisoners from the *Fortitude* hulk had been 'much more troublesome to manage' than those from the two Woolwich hulks. This confirmed his belief that the convicts from the *Fortitude* must have been in much better health than those from the two Woolwich hulks. As he contemplated the numbers of cases of scurvy he had witnessed on the *Emily*, Henderson observed that 'no man has much lack [*sic*] or mischief in him, whose spirits are broken from an attenuated state of the blood'. Perhaps, he considered, the convicts' low spirits should have forewarned him of disease, but as others of his colleagues had often done, Henderson pleaded that he could not have realised how sick the convicts were when first he inspected them. 'Men may seem to be enjoying a fair state of health, who are on the very brink of stumbling into maladies of the most fatal character.'[56]

Henderson's conviction that the convicts had been on the verge of scurvy before they embarked the ship mirrored comments by his contemporaries on land. The previous year, Archibald Robertson, the surgeon of the *Wye* hospital ship – the hulk that cared for the sick men of both *Justitia* and *Warrior* – had been not 'in the least surprised at the rate of mortality' during a recent influenza epidemic. 'We now receive prisoners from different gaols who have been subjected to the silent or solitary system, and fed on gruel or bread and water. Their vital powers are injured before they reach us.'[57] In another report, the *Warrior*'s surgeon, Mr Bossy, invited the House of Commons to note the recently introduced 'sources of debility in the health of the prisoners'. The convicts' tendency to scurvy and scrofula had existed only 'since the changes in prison discipline were introduced'. Bossy believed that this state of affairs could be alleviated only by altering 'the diet and forms of discipline to which prisoners were now subjected'.[58] *The Berkshire Chronicle* and *The Times* published a further warning from Bossy:

> When such individuals are subjected to removals that increase the demand upon the power of the constitution, as, to the labour of the hulks or the privations of the voyage to New South Wales, or when exposed to powerful depression from distress of mind, or in unfavourable seasons, serious and destructive effects may be sometimes suddenly developed, the concealed mischief painfully disclosed, and the victims numerous.[59]

On the *Marion* in 1844, Dr Jones also connected six cases of scurvy with prisoners who had come from Millbank. One case proved fatal, the convict 'having brought the disease unquestionably along with him from the penitentiary, as he there laboured under similar symptoms, while a patient in the infirmary, according to his own statement'.[60] Another correspondent, with the pseudonym Medicus, wrote to the *The Times* to condemn the emergence of scurvy. 'It is only to the modern improvements of prison disciplinarians', he wrote, 'that we are indebted for the introduction of this dreadful scourge upon the land.'[61] During the 1830s, systematic deprivations had become an institution-alised characteristic of the nutritional, spatial, and sensory world of the mid-nineteenth-century prison. As these structural disciplinary changes weakened the minds and bodies of convicts, their effects often emerged most visibly on the ships that transported convicts to Australia, in diseases such as cholera and scurvy.

Mr Cameron's nitre remedy

Lemon juice is, of course, key to the therapeutic history of scurvy. Late eighteenth-century writers, most famously James Lind, consistently advocated the acid juices of lemons and oranges, as well as scurvy grasses, water cress, sauerkraut and wort for the widespread treatment of scurvy, because they were 'endowed with peculiarly acrid stimulating juices'.[62] From 1795, naval surgeons issued an ounce of lemon juice per day to troops, crews, passengers, and convicts alike from the fifteenth day of the voyage.[63] These rations had proved very successful on convict ships in the first decades of the nineteenth century: in 1818, David Reid had been able to keep scurvy at bay with 'lemon juice and fresh meat'.[64] In 1823, surgeon Mercer bought fresh beef, vegetables, and six thousand oranges at the Cape. Had he not done so, he believed, 'I strongly suspect my journal would have cost me much more labour for at the time we made Simon's Bay I believe there was not a pound of lemon juice in the ship'.[65] Surgeons willingly used, and believed in the efficacy of, lemon and lime juice. If supplies ran low, or the juice deteriorated on the southerly passage through the Atlantic, ships would call at Tenerife, Rio de Janeiro, or at the Cape of Good Hope to replenish supplies of fresh fruit, vegetables, and meat to ensure continued health until they reached Australia.

Prison authorities were not the only ones experimenting with reduced rations, however. In 1832, the Admiralty reduced by at least a quarter the rations to be supplied to convict ships, including those of lemon juice and sugar. In 1835, the captain of the *George III* sailed through the narrow D'Entrecasteaux channel, only a few miles from Hobart, rather than take the usual passage by Storm Bay, because he had needed 'to reach Hobart-town with the least possible delay, owing to the alarmingly increasing state of the sick list, and the total want of proper nourishment'. The ship hit rocks and sank with the loss of 127 lives. After the wreck of the *George III* in 1835, William Burnett reinstated the old scale of lemon juice.[66]

Even as surgeons knew about, and trusted, the salutary effects of fresh food and juice, chemical remedies seemed to promise better solutions to the problem of scurvy. Volumes in the Admiralty's medical library described Carl Wilhelm Scheele's method, first described in 1784, for making crystalline citric acid from the juice of lemons.[67] In 1795, David Paterson had published *A Treatise on the Scurvy*, in which he introduced his fellow naval surgeons to another potential remedy. During a voyage in 1784 he had tried a solution of nitre and claimed that he had 'restored above eighty seamen from the scurvy' without the use of 'recent vegetable matter'.[68] Paterson did not deny that lemons, limes, and oranges were 'powerful antiscorbutics', but reminded his readers that these could not be depended upon during long voyages. Nitre was cheap to procure and did not decompose with time. Most importantly, a ready supply could be obtained from a ship's regular supplies of gunpowder. Drawing on recent developments in chemistry, his own long experience, and the common belief that poor ventilation caused scurvy and affected the state of the blood, Paterson explained that scurvy was the result of 'contaminated, poisonous or foul air'.[69] Scorbutic sufferers suffered from spongy, ulcerated, and fetid gums and nose, and thus, Paterson reasoned, 'the air, passing through them to the lungs, must, it is presumed, be highly contaminated'. Nitre, he explained, contained 'a very great quantity of dephlogisticated or vital air'.[70] Observing that people with scurvy often exhibited a 'very great desire for acids', Paterson dissolved two ounces of nitre to a quart of ship's vinegar.

Paterson published his treatise in 1795, the same year that the Admiralty began routinely to issue lemon juice to sailors. With hindsight, it is of little surprise that Paterson's treatise on nitre seemingly sank without trace in competition with such a landmark event in the history of scurvy.[71] But it sank only until Charles Cameron remembered the *Fergusson*'s stores of gunpowder, in 1829, at which point nitre made a surprising comeback. The early stages of Cameron's convict voyage followed a familiar narrative. In November 1828, 216 convicts had embarked the convict ship *Fergusson*. Many of the convicts were 'in a low state of health, from deficient nourishment and the depressing passions' during their imprisonment. Bad weather and seasickness early in the voyage further debilitated the convicts' constitutions. Before the *Fergusson* crossed the equator 'the hospital was full of scorbutic patients', and its supplies of lemon juice were exhausted. Cameron explained that when he had remembered Paterson's recipe, he had availed himself of the *Fergusson*'s gunpowder supply and dissolved eight ounces of nitre in vinegar to make sixty-four ounces in total. He also tried mixing the nitre with equal parts of vinegar and lime juice, with a little sugar added. At first Cameron had resorted to the nitre only in desperation, but the remedy's effects, he declared, were 'almost miraculous'; Cameron and the *Fergusson*'s captain subsequently abandoned their plan to divert to Rio de Janeiro, ignored the Cape of Good Hope, and headed straight for New South Wales.[72]

It is worth noting that as he described the effects of Paterson's 'old remedy', Cameron referred to the disease interchangeably as scurvy and 'the Millbank disease'. In 1823, scurvy had broken out in epidemic proportions in the newly opened Millbank prison, after the prison's dietary scale had been criticised as being more luxurious than that of the common labourer. The experiments in Millbank were representative of a prevailing ethos in which prison and the workhouse must not be more attractive than the life of the poorest labourer. The dietary reductions of the early 1820s, Sean McConville has suggested, were 'an extreme but not anomalous experimentation with the outer limits of terror'.[73] By 1825, the disease affected over half of the prison's inmates. Cameron's evocation of Millbank as he dealt with scurvy in the middle of the Atlantic Ocean is significant because it marks the naval surgeons' shifting engagement with scurvy that we discussed above, from a maritime disease of sailors in the southern hemisphere to a penal disease experienced by convicts even before ships passed the equator. As naval surgeons began to encounter scurvy anew in the nineteenth century, Cameron's report also marks the re-invigoration of the naval surgeons' scientific interest in the disease. Cameron's report signals the beginning of nearly two decades of experimentation on convict ships as surgeons returned to the question of how best to prevent and cure their traditional nemesis.

Cameron reported his results with nitre to the Navy Board, and the *London Medical Gazette* published the details in 1831. For the Admiralty, Cameron's mixture was a breakthrough: cheap, durable, and already in abundant supply on ships, nitre seemed to solve ongoing concern about any 'unnecessary expenditure' associated with issuing lemon juice at sea.[74] William Burnett enthusiastically received Cameron's report and proposed that two tons of nitrate of potash should in future be supplied for every hundred men on convict ships.[75] This astonishing remedy, a further letter in the *Medical Gazette* suggested, 'would seem capable not merely of supplying the place, but of superseding the use of vegetable acids altogether in treating the degenerate state of the blood' in various diseases, including scurvy.[76] Burnett provided his convict-ship surgeons with a pamphlet to accompany the nitre, which they referred to throughout the 1830s. Thrasycles Clarke, for example, declared that it was Cameron's remedy (as well as the high spirits of the boisterous female convicts on the *Kains*) that had begun the work of curing cases of scurvy before their arrival at the Cape.[77]

Not everyone approved of the enthusiasm for nitre. In the *London Medical Gazette*, John Elliotson warned that 'some persons now begin to say that the lemon-juice does no good', but he did not believe it wise to dispute the 'authority, so accumulated and so immense as it is, respecting the powers of lemon juice'.[78] On the male convict ship *Bengal Merchant* in 1835, surgeon Ellis tested the remedy and found it wanting. He had divided the sick convicts on his ship into two groups of 'equal number and as near as possible of the same degree of severity and suffering'. To one group Ellis administered the lime juice in doses of 'two ounces, three, four or five times in the day, according to the state of the patient'. To the other group Ellis administered the nitrous vinegar, 'given and prepared as recommended by Mr Cameron'. Ellis concluded that he could not subscribe to the remedy's efficacy. Indeed, he wrote, 'it was well evident that the patients treated by the lime juice alone, improved more rapidly, nor were they so much afflicted with nausea and diarrhoea as those to whom the nitrous vinegar was given'.[79]

Let us return once more to the sheep thief George Willett on the *Prince George* in 1837, because here too the surgeon freely experimented with nitre. In addition to paying careful attention to Willett's diet and making sure he received fresh air on deck, surgeon Bell used nitre as both internal and external remedy. He combined the potash with lime juice and peppermint oil, diffused in a 'small portion of alcohol'. He gave Willett the drink three times a day, mixed with some sugar. Bell also sponged a solution of nitre and vinegar over the lesions on the convict's spotted body. In his general remarks, Bell devoted considerable space to his thoughts on nitre:

> Having been supplied with Mr Cameron's pamphlet on scurvy, which I suppose was intended as a guide to surgeons in this disease, I was determined to give Nitre in solution with lime juice a fair trial. From three to four ounces of the mixture with a little water were given in divided doses from 6am until 8pm increasing or decreasing the dose as circumstances required, seldom in any stage of the disease giving more than eight ounces in the 24 hours and guarding against any irritation that might be produced of stomach or bowels.[80]

Having nearly expended his regular issue of nitre with such liberal use, Bell turned to the ship's supplies of gunpowder. He boiled the gunpowder in water to dissolve the nitre, filtered the liquor, obtained the nitre by crystallisation, and gave some of his patients this freshly made remedy. To others he gave the unadulterated gunpowder. Bell concluded that he could not 'perceive any particular effect produced from the administration of the nitre first given, that obtained from the gunpowder, or the gunpowder itself'.[81]

These experiments that naval surgeons undertook on convict ships in the 1820s and 1830s were only the latest in an ongoing search for a cheap, durable scurvy remedy that demanded relatively little space and would enable ships to remain at sea for months at a time. They also occurred within the context of a broader culture of practical military experimentation in the post-Napoleonic era that we have already encountered in chloride of lime and zinc experiments in Chapter 2 and the enthusiasm for vaccination trials and post-mortem examinations that will come in Chapter 5. Freed from the demands of warfare, and reflecting on its failures and problems, naval surgeons were turning their attention to some of the practical problems that most troubled their eighteenth-century colleagues and their professional status. With their discussions about nitre, lime juice, and citric acid, surgeons added another way to participate in this culture of experimentation, but it is important that these practical investigative impulses of the post-Napoleonic decades also coincided with the busiest years of convict transportation, and with the effects of increasingly severe penal regimes on land. The surgeons' scurvy experiments relied on the weakened bodies of convicts, even as critics of transportation argued that the system 'degraded and brutalised' convicts, and depended upon punishments that were 'irrational and extreme'.[82]

Reflecting on this period, the ambitious naval surgeon Alexander Bryson later summarised that when faced with the impossibility of storing a sufficient portion of fresh vegetables for such long voyages with so many people, his colleagues had begun to substitute 'other articles likely to answer the same purpose [as lemon juice] and which occupy comparatively little space'. To lime juice, vinegar and various pickled vegetables, surgeons had begun to add preserved peas, carrots, and potatoes, nitrate of potash, and crystallised citric acid.[83] By the late 1830s, scurvy developed in the majority of convict ships that arrived in Australia. It had become desirable, Bryson suggested with no little understatement, 'to ascertain, with some degree of certainty, the relative value of these agents, from data which might be subjected to the test of comparison'. In 1840, after a decade of intermittent discussions about nitre, William Burnett officially re-opened investigations into scurvy. Thousands of imprisoned male convict bodies, many of whom, thanks to the circumstances of their imprisonment, would inevitably suffer from scurvy during the voyage to Australia, were to be the source material.

Burnett's experiment

Following the Molesworth Committee reports, the government suspended transportation to New South Wales in 1839. After 1840, nearly all convict ships sailed to Van Diemen's Land, and a few went directly to Norfolk Island. Van Diemen's Land received 2,659 men in 1841, 4,656 in 1842, 3,023 in 1843 and 3,959 in 1844. This was, A.G.L. Shaw has suggested, 'an avalanche', which increased the population of Van Diemen's Land by 40 per cent in just four years.[84] In a period of political and fiscal crisis, the colony also had a new governor, Sir John Franklin (1837–43). Franklin was a Navy man. He had sailed with Matthew Flinders on the *Investigator*, had fought at the battle of Trafalgar on the *Bellerephon*, and searched for the Arctic North-West Passage as second-in-command. As Governor of Van Diemen's Land, he remained an enthusiastic patron of colonial and maritime science, and he would later return to the Navy after his governorship.[85] Franklin's predecessor, Governor George Arthur, had repeatedly complained about the arrival of sick convicts on the Navy's ships. Sir George Gipps in New South Wales had also called Medical Boards to investigate sickness at sea at every opportunity. By contrast, if Franklin was unlikely to openly endorse the effects on prisoners of the Navy's ongoing attempts to investigate scurvy, William Burnett could be confident that he would turn a blind eye.

Against this background, Burnett issued lime juice, citric acid, and 'nitrate of potass' to nearly all of the surgeons in the convict service. Over sixty ships carrying fifteen thousand convicted men from Britain and Ireland to Australia between 1840 and 1844 received the remedies. The formal results of the experiment are contained in a single report in Britain's National Archives, almost hidden in a huge bound volume of miscellaneous letters and correspondence regarding sickness on convict and emigrant ships. In this report, Burnett summarised the results of thirty-nine voyages, but it is also clear that other surgeons, notably the artistic Henry Mahon, submitted other detailed essays and journals.[86]

It is important to note that Burnett made it clear that the surgeons were not to try to *cause* scurvy in order to then cure it; the surgeons were to undertake a trial only '*if* scurvy appeared during the voyage'. On thirty out of the sixty-seven male convict ships that sailed from Britain between 1840 and 1844, the surgeons witnessed no cases of scurvy during the voyage. During a further nineteen voyages, five or fewer cases occurred. The surgeons of several ships did not take part in the experiment. This was a gendered experiment: no female convict vessels were included. Two surgeons were otherwise concerned with the results of very different experiments. John Hampton had received the first prisoners to be transported from Pentonville. On their embarkation they had suffered from convulsions and nausea. Andrew Millar, the surgeon of the *HMS Anson*, was more concerned with finding a suitable method of ventilating a double-decked ship that could transport nearly twice as many convicts as the usual hired vessels.[87] Others simply ignored the experiment altogether. On the *Hydrabad*, which sailed direct to Norfolk Island in 1844, the surgeon appears to have used the voyage primarily as an opportunity for indulging his meteorological interests.[88]

If scurvy appeared during the voyage, the surgeons were to 'place the scorbutic patients, as they presented themselves, in three divisions, each division possessing cases of parallel severity, and presenting, as nearly as possible, similar symptoms'. The prisoners' diet, exercise, and freedom from restraint were to be the same, but each division should receive one of the remedies, and the surgeons would report their results.[89] The surgeons often altered, combined, and varied the doses of the three remedies according to their own personal preference. Moreover, they came to strikingly divergent conclusions about the efficacy of the remedies. Surgeon Deas mixed the nitre with lime juice and citric acid, and felt that both mixtures were useful. George Moxey had little faith in the nitre, while Colin Arrott Browning spoke 'as highly as ever' of Cameron's nitre mixture. On one ship, the sick convicts experienced bad effects with both citric acid and nitre, and consequently the surgeon abandoned both. One surgeon wrote that he had 'limited opportunity' to test the remedies and could not venture a decisive opinion, but professed that he 'had little faith in the Nitrate of Potass'. Surgeon McKecknie on the *Layton* felt that although there was 'little difference' between citric acid and 'nitrate Potass', both were preferable to lime juice. On the *Asia* in 1841, Dr Sinclair reported only four cases of scurvy but believed that 'no benefit appeared to be derived from the use of either of the three articles'. So too, Andrew Henderson reiterated his belief that only dietary management could prevent scurvy, and declared that all three of the articles were 'useless or nearly so'. By contrast, Dr Jones on the *Marion* thought that 'all three of the articles have salutary properties but citric acid most'.[90]

Article no. 17 of the 'Instructions for Surgeon-Superintendents on Convict Ships' (1837) specified that the surgeon was 'to cause lemon-juice and sugar to be issued to the convicts in the proportion of an ounce of each to a man daily'. This should be 'mixed occasionally with the wine allowed to them, or used unmixed as sherbet, unless at any time he should consider it prejudicial to them'.[91] In accordance with these general instructions, as well as the specific orders from Burnett regarding the experiment, the majority of surgeons issued lemon juice as usual during the voyage. However, as Alexander Bryson wrote retrospectively about the experiment for the readers of the *Medical Times*, he revealed that he had been deeply frustrated by the failure of his fellow surgeons to undertake the experiment – in his eyes – 'properly'. Bryson explained that when surgeons issued the lemon juice daily from early in the voyage (as per their instructions), 'like most other remedies, by long continued use' the juice 'would partly, if not entirely, lose its influence on the system'. Thus, the juice would be 'at a great disadvantage, when it came to be used at an advanced period of the voyage in competition with the nitre and citric acid'.

Therefore, Bryson withdrew the convicts' usual allowance of lime juice on the *Marquis of Hastings* 'in order that the effects of each remedy might be more clearly observed' if scurvy appeared on the voyage. Scurvy did indeed appear, 'before the ship had crossed the equator'.[92] Although clearly in defiance of Article 17, Bryson justified his actions by referring to another clause in the surgeons' Instructions. Article 24 stipulated that 'in regulating the diet of the sick', the surgeon 'is not only to employ the articles specially provided for them in the supply of medical comforts, but also *save of their general rations while in health* as may in his judgment be applicable to their respective cases'.[93] In withdrawing the issue of lime juice, Bryson emphasised that he had exercised this discretionary power in accordance with his position of authority. In so doing, he argued, 'whatever proof' he might obtain from the trial 'would be the more conclusive and satisfactory'.

In his journal synopsis, Bryson recorded only eleven cases of scurvy, but his general remarks and his article in the *Medical Times* make it clear that at least sixty of the convicts developed scorbutic symptoms. As scurvy broke out on the *Marquis of Hastings*, Bryson separated the sick convicts into three divisions and gave each group the different remedy 'in a draught of wine and water with sugar'. Aside from the convicts' reluctance to take the nitre remedy, Bryson observed that its first effect was 'to derange the functions of digestion and assimilation already much at fault'.[94] Within two or three days one of the convicts, Jonathan Walker, complained that the nitre 'took away his appetite'. Bryson also observed that the remedy 'excited nausea and vomiting'. Thomas Law said that 'the medicine makes him sick'.[95] In rapid succession, other symptoms of scurvy appeared. Swollen, ulcerated, spongy gums tended to haemorrhage; loose teeth; foetid breath and sweat; livid blotches; indolent boils; rigidity of the tendons; erratic pains of the limbs 'in the bones'; and mental dejection plagued the men. The prisoners sleeping near William Prosser complained about his smell. By contrast, the lemon juice and citric acid had not affected the prisoners' appetites, and scurvy did not 'assume anything like so severe a form' under the treatment with these other remedies. Still, Bryson persisted so that 'no doubt' about the nitre's efficacy should remain in his mind. On 24 September 1842, as the *Marquis of Hastings* reached the Cape of Good Hope, Bryson finally discontinued entirely the use of nitre, and 'procured for the worst cases, particularly for those who had suffered from the Potash plan of treatment, a tolerable supply of oranges'. In conclusion, Bryson declared nitre to be 'objectionable'.[96]

Conclusion

Surgeons consciously made moral decisions about their participation in this experiment; although Bryson withheld the lime juice in order that he could conduct the trial to a particular standard of rigour, he did, in the end, resort 'in humanity' to 'a less equivocal plan of treatment'. As Henry Mahon painted the convicts on the *Barrosa*, with whom this chapter opened, he also made it clear that his 'sole aim was to alleviate the miseries of the unfortunate persons under my charge, prevent illness, and cure disease … With very little assistance and considerable anxiety of mind did I endeavour to avert the fatal blow about to be struck.'[97] Nevertheless, Bryson's apparent willingness to do harm to his prisoners is, to modern sensibilities, deeply disturbing. The occasion of the sea voyage provided a uniquely isolated space and time in which surgeons could experiment with medical remedies. It is not too great a leap of imagination to see how this episode resonates with more recent controversies about the use of prisoners in medical trials.[98]

What did William Burnett make of the varied comments he received from the surgeons? He concluded that the experiment proved the utility of lemon as an antiscorbutic:

> It appears on reading over the journals for 1842 that in 11 ships in which lemon juice was issued daily in the usual manner only 56 cases of scurvy are reported. Whereas in 2 vessels where lemon juice was not issued to the prisoners for reasons specified by the medical officers upwards of 100 cases occurred, many of them of a serious nature before they reached the Cape of Good Hope.[99]

On one level, Burnett's simple conclusion about lemon juice reaffirms the classic history of scurvy's cure. And yet, a century after Lind had carried out his famous clinical trials, William Burnett's deceptively simple conclusion hides so much ongoing uncertainty, and the conjunction of a series of historical trends that made such an experiment possible. Changing penal regimes and reduced ships' rations had a profound effect on prisoners' health at the same time as naval surgeons entered enthusiastically into a period of experimentation. Moreover, from 1840, a redirected system of transportation sent a wave of convicts to Van Diemen's Land, where a sympathetic colonial governor did not open medical enquiries as his predecessors had. Yet, as medical men experimented, scurvy opened up old scars and created new wounds for convicts. The re-emergence and persistence of scurvy on convict ships between the late 1820s and the mid 1840s connects us to larger issues in the history of prisoners' relationship to medicine, and to the histories of social prejudice, intensifying discipline, dietary reduction, and mental stress that accompany the era of disciplinary 'reform'. Cases such as George Willett's reveal a chain of events that took a man from a harsh rural winter to prison, to mutiny, to a surgeon's administration of an experimental mixture thousands of miles away in another hemisphere.

As for nitrate of potash, Paterson's remedy of 1795 may well have finally been consigned to the past by the 1840s. Whether or not nitre had any therapeutic effects it is not within my knowledge or desire to say. However, it is perhaps worth noting that in the twenty-first century, pharmaceutical companies market potassium nitrate as an active ingredient in toothpaste because it is 'clinically proven' to desensitise nerve endings in teeth. The belief of many nineteenth-century surgeons that the same ingredient might reduce the pain of scurvy, a disease so commonly experienced in the mouth and gums, suddenly does not seem so strange.[100]

After Burnett's experiment, scurvy still appeared on convict ships. In 1849, as the *Hashemy* approached the Cape of Good Hope 'the appearance of elevated and spongy gums' and other marks of failing health signalled its appearance. After their experience with cholera at the start of the voyage, guards and convicts suffered alike. The *Hashemy* put in to Simon's Bay at the Cape of Good Hope, and six days later sailed again. With a 'sea stock of fresh meat and live sheep', Browning explained, 'the people soon evinced that they had laid in a stock of health, and they continued to retain their healthy appearance, until we reached Port Jackson.'[101] For Browning it was the *Hashemy*'s visit to the Cape – not the lemon juice – that fortified the minds and bodies of both convicts and sailors for the potentially debilitating passage across the southern Indian Ocean to Australia.

Notes

1 TNA, ADM 101/ 7/8, Journal of surgeon Henry Mahon on convict ship *Barossa* (1841–1842), 'Essay on Scurvy'.

2 Deborah Oxley, *Convict Maids: The Forced Migration of Women to Australia* (Cambridge: Cambridge University Press, 1996), pp. 16–21.

3 AOT, CON 33/1/16, Conduct Record of the *Barossa* (1841–1842), p. 268. While Mahon's medical journal names James Radford, the ship's indent as well as the conduct record names Edward Radford.

4 TNA, ADM 101/ 7/8, Mahon, Journal on *Barossa*, 'Essay on Scurvy'.

5 Marcus Rediker, *Between the Devil and the Deep Blue Sea* (Cambridge: Cambridge University Press, 1989), p. 12.

6 Thomas Trotter, *A View of the Nervous Temperament* (London: Wright, Goodenow, & Stockwell, 1808), pp. 27–28.

7 Gilbert Blane, *Select Dissertations on Several Subjects of Medical Science* (London: T. & G. Underwood, 1822), p. 19; J.B. Jukes, *Narrative of the Surveying Voyage of H.M.S. Fly* (London: T. & W. Boone, 1847), p. 116.

8 The best studies remain C.C. Lloyd, 'The Conquest of Scurvy', *British Journal for the History of Science*, 1 (1962–3), pp. 357–363, p. 357 and Kenneth J. Carpenter, *The History of Scurvy and Vitamin C* (Cambridge: Cambridge University Press, 1986).

9 PRONI 560/2, John Martin, Journal of voyage from Ireland on the convict ship *Mountstuart Elphinstone* to Australia, 1849–1850, entry for 13 July 1849.

10 Alexander Bryson, 'On the Respective Value of Lime Juice, Citric Acid,

and Nitrate of Potash, in the Treatment of Scurvy', *Medical Times* (16 March 1850), pp. 212–214, p. 213.

11 TNA, ADM 101/78/9, Journal of surgeon Alexander Stewart on emigrant ship *Woodbridge* (1839), General Remarks; Robin Haines, *Doctors at Sea: Emigrant Voyages to Colonial Australia* (Basingstoke: Palgrave Macmillan 2005), p. 98.

12 Jonathan Lamb, *Preserving the Self in the South Seas, 1680–1840* (Chicago and London: Chicago University Press, 2001), p. 127.

13 During the 1850s, Emigration Commissioners attempted to ban sailing below 47 degrees south during the southern hemisphere winter, and 53 degrees south during the summer. Robin Haines, *Doctors at Sea*, pp. 104–107.

14 Kerry Ward, *Networks of Empire: Forced Migration in the Dutch East India Company* (Cambridge: Cambridge University Press, 2009), pp. 127–134; Harriet Deacon, 'The Politics of Medical Topography: Seeking healthiness at the Cape during the nineteenth century', in Richard Wrigley and George Revill (eds) *Pathologies of Travel* (Amsterdam: Rodopi, 2000), pp. 279–297.

15 See for example TNA, ADM 101/18/6, Journal of surgeon James Lawrence on convict ship *Cressy* (1843); TNA, ADM 101/46/7, Journal of surgeon Alex McKechnie on convict ship *Mandarin* (1840).

16 TNA, ADM 101/ 44/4, Journal of surgeon Obadiah Pineo on convict ship *Lord Lyndoch* (1838), General Remarks.

17 TNA, ADM 101/ 44/4, Pineo, Journal on *Lord Lyndoch*, General Remarks.

18 TNA, ADM 101/ 44/4, Pineo, Journal on *Lord Lyndoch*, General Remarks.

19 TNA, ADM 101/ 44/4, Pineo, Journal on *Lord Lyndoch*, General Remarks.

20 TNA, ADM 105/36, Correspondence regarding sickness on convict and emigrant ships (1836–1851), Letter from Obadiah Pineo to William Burnett, 15 September 1838 (emphasis in original).

21 For an excellent study of the intertwined medical and political debates that surrounded scurvy in the second half of the eighteenth century, see Christopher Lawrence, 'Disciplining Disease: Scurvy, the Navy, and Imperial Expansion, 1750–1825', in David Philip Miller and Peter Hans Reill (eds) *Visions of Empire: Voyages, Botany and Representations of Nature* (Cambridge: Cambridge University Press, 1996), pp. 80–106.

22 Thomas Beddoes, *Observations on Calculus, Sea Scurvy, Consumption, Catarrh, and Fever* (Philadelphia: T. Dobson, 1797), p. 131.

23 William Cullen, *First Lines of the Practice of Physic, with Practical and Explanatory Notes*, 4 vols (Edinburgh: C. Elliott, 1788), pp. 416, 420.

24 Lawrence, 'Disciplining Disease', p. 95.

25 Frederick Thomson, *An Essay on the Scurvy: Shewing Effectual and Practicable Means for its Prevention at Sea. With some observations on Fevers,*

and proposals for the More Effectual Preservation of the Health of Seamen. (London: G.G.J. & J. Robinson, 1790), p. 41; Cullen, *First Lines*, p. 421.

26 Thomas Trotter, *Observations on the Scurvy* (London: J.S. Jordan, 1795), p. 42.

27 TNA, ADM/101 6/7, Journal of surgeon Andrew Henderson, on convict ship *Aurora* (1835), General Remarks.

28 TNA, ADM 101/38/3, Journal of surgeon John Osborne on convict ship *John Barry* (1834), General Remarks.

29 TNA, ADM 101/21/2, Journal of surgeon William Evans on convict ship *Earl Grey* (1836), General Remarks.

30 Bryson, 'On the Respective Value', p. 213.

31 'Dr Elliotson on Scurvy', *The Lancet*, 2 vols (1830–1831), I, pp. 649–656, p. 653.

32 TNA, ADM 101/27/3, Journal of Francis Logan on female convict ship *Fanny* (1832), Case 15: Eleanor Hall (25 October 1832).

33 TNA, ADM 101/44/4, Pineo, Journal on *Lord Lyndoch*, General Remarks

34 Trotter, *Observations*, p. 44.

35 TNA, ADM 101/ 7/8, Mahon, Journal on *Barossa*, Case 20: Roland Cameron; Case 16: John Edwards.

36 TNA, ADM 101/44/4, Pineo, Journal on *Lord Lyndoch*, General Remarks.

37 TNA, ADM 101/65/2, Journal of surgeon Andrew Henderson on convict ship *Royal Admiral* (1833), General Remarks.

38 For discussion of the role of passions as both positive and detrimental effect on health see Thomas Dixon, 'Patients and Passions: Languages of medicine and emotion, 1789–1850', in Fay Bound Alberti (ed.) *Medicine, Emotion and Disease, 1700–1950* (Basingstoke: Palgrave Macmillan, 2006), pp. 34–35.

39 TNA, ADM 101/25/2, Journal of surgeon Andrew Henderson on the convict ship *Emily* (1842), General Remarks.

40 TNA, ADM, 101/40/1, Journal of surgeon Thrascyles Clarke on female convict ship *Kains* (1830–1831), General Remarks.

41 Joy Damousi, *Depraved and Disorderly: Female Convicts, Sexuality and Gender in Colonial Australia* (Cambridge: Cambridge University Press, 1997), pp. 20–21.

42 Charles Picknell's journal in *The Kains: Female Convict Ship* (Adelaide: Sullivan's Cove, 1989), p. 33.

43 TNA, ADM 101/36/6, Journal of surgeon Henry Mahon on female convict ship *Isabella* (1840), General Remarks.

44 TNA, ADM 101/57/9, Journal of surgeon James McTernan on convict ship *Ocean* (1823), General Remarks. For comparative studies of mutiny see Jane Hathaway (ed.), *Rebellion, Repression, Reinvention: Mutiny in Comparative Perspective* (Westport, CT: Praeger, 2001) and Clare Anderson, '"The Ferringees are Flying – the Ship is ours!": the Convict Middle Passage in

Colonial South and Southeast Asia, 1790–1860', *Indian Economic and Social History Review* 41:3 (2005), pp. 143–186.

45 TNA, ADM 101/57/9, McTernan, Journal on *Ocean*, General Remarks and Summary of All Cases.

46 TNA, ADM 101/60/7, Journal of surgeon Thomas Bell on convict ship *Prince George* (1836–1837), General Remarks.

47 TNA, ADM 101/60/7, Bell, Journal on *Prince George*, General Remarks.

48 TNA, ADM 101/60/7, Bell, Journal on *Prince George*, Case 3: George Willett.

49 AONSW, Convict Deaths and Burials Index 1828–1879, Fiche No. 749–751, 4/4549.

50 TNA, ADM 101/60/7, Bell, Journal on *Prince George*, Case 3: George Willett.

51 Cullen, *First Lines*, p. 414.

52 TNA, ADM/101 6/7, Journal of surgeon Andrew Henderson on convict ship *Aurora* (1835), General Remarks.

53 TNA, ADM 101/25/2, Henderson, Journal on *Emily*, General Remarks.

54 See TNA, ADM 101/65/2, Journal of surgeon Andrew Henderson on convict ship *Royal Admiral* (1833), Report on Scurvy, Preamble.

55 TNA, ADM 101/25/2, Henderson, Journal on *Emily*, General Remarks.

56 TNA, ADM 101/25/2, Henderson, Journal on *Emily*, General Remarks.

57 Archibald Robertson, Medical Report of Wye Hospital (Enclosure G), in United Kingdom House of Commons, *Two Reports from John Henry Capper* 1842 [122] xxxii, p .4.

58 John Bossy, Medical Report of Warrior Convict Hulk (Enclosure I), in United Kingdom House of Commons, *Convicts, Two Reports of John Henry Capper* 1843 [113] xlii, p. 9.

59 'New Prison Dietary (From the Berkshire Chronicle)', *The Times*, 15 May 1843, p. 3.

60 TNA, ADM 101/49/8, Journal of surgeon Dr W.A.B. Jones on convict ship *Marion* (1843–1844), General Remarks.

61 Medicus, 'Prison Discipline', *The Times*, 19 October 1842, p. 5.

62 Francis Milman, *An Enquiry into the source from whence the symptoms of the scurvy and of putrid fevers arise* (London: J. Dodsley, 1782), p. 200.

63 Throughout the first half of the nineteenth century surgeons used the terms lemon and lime interchangeably.

64 TNA, ADM 101/7/4, Journal of surgeon David Reid on convict ship *Baring*, passage to New South Wales 31 October 1818–July 1820.

65 TNA, ADM 101/1/8, Journal of surgeon James A. Mercer on convict ship *Albion* (1823), General Remarks.

66 Michael Roe, *An Imperial Disaster: The Wreck of the George III* (Hobart: Blubberhead Press, 2006), pp. 21, 96.

67 William Henry, *The Elements of Experimental Chemistry* (London: Baldwin, Cradock and Joy, 1826), pp. 210–211.

68 Nitre or nitrate of potash, is better known as saltpetre or potassium nitrate.

69 D. Paterson, *A Treatise on the Scurvy, Containing a New and Effectual Method of Curing That Disease; and the Cause and Indications of Cure, Deduced from Practice; And Observations Connected with the subject* (Edinburgh: Manners & Miller, 1795), p. 7.

70 Paterson, *Treatise*, pp. 10–11.

71 Lawrence, 'Disciplining Disease', p. 105 n. 111.

72 TNA, ADM 101/27/4, Journal of surgeon Charles Cameron on convict ship *Fergusson* (1829); 'Nitre a Remedy for Scurvy', *London Medical Gazette* (13 March 1830), pp. 751–752.

73 Sean McConville, *A History of English Prison Administration*, 2 vols (London: Routledge, 1981), I, pp. 144–145. For discussion of the Millbank scurvy episode see Michael Ignatieff, *A Just Measure of Pain* (New York: Pantheon, 1978), pp. 175–176; William A. Guy, 'On Sufficient and Insufficient Dietaries, with Special Reference to the Dietaries of Prisoners, *Journal of the Statistical Society of London*, 26:3 (1863), pp. 239–280, pp. 251–253; Arthur Griffiths, *Memorials of Millbank* (London: Chapman and Hall, 1884).

74 TNA, ADM 105/7, Medical and Victualling Reports etc to the Victualling Board of the Navy (1829), Committee's Report to the Board.

75 TNA, ADM 105/8, Medical and Victualling Reports etc to the Victualling Board of the Navy (1830), Letter from William Burnett to the Board, 8 May 1830.

76 C. Carlyon, 'Effects of Nitre on the Blood', *London Medical Gazette* (31 August 1831), pp. 626–627.

77 TNA, ADM 101/40/1, Clarke, Journal on *Kains*, General Remarks.

78 Dr Elliotson, 'Universal Diseases-continued. Scurvy', *London Medical Gazette* (25 February 1832), p. 777–781, p. 781.

79 TNA, ADM 101/8/1, Journal of surgeon J. Ellis on convict ship *Bengal Merchant* (1834–1835), General Remarks.

80 TNA, ADM 101/ 60/7, Bell, Journal on *Prince George*, General Remarks.

81 TNA, ADM 101/ 60/7, Bell, Journal on *Prince George*, General Remarks.

82 Kirsty Reid, *Gender, Crime and Empire: Convicts, Settlers and the State in Early Colonial Australia* (Manchester: Manchester University Press), pp. 167–169.

83 Bryson, 'On the Respective Value', p. 213.

84 A.G.L. Shaw, *Convicts and the Colonies* (London: Faber and Faber, 1966), p. 300.

85 In 1839, the Navy despatched HMS *Erebus* and *Terror* to undertake a survey of terrestrial magnetism between the meridians of the Cape of Good Hope and Australia. John Gascoigne, *The Enlightenment and the Origins of*

European Australia (Cambridge: Cambridge University Press, 2002), p. 94; Simon Schaffer, 'Instruments, Surveys and Maritime Empire', in David Cannadine (ed.), *Empire, the Sea and Global History* (Basingstoke: 2007), pp. 83–104, p. 84.

86 TNA, ADM 105/36, Burnett, Report on scurvy.

87 TNA, ADM 101/67/10, Journal of surgeon John S. Hampton on convict ship *Sir George Seymour* (1844–1845), General Remarks; TNA, ADM 101/3/4, Journal of surgeon Andrew Millar on convict ship *HMS Anson* (1843–1844).

88 TNA, ADM 101/35/8, Journal of surgeon J.O. McWilliam on convict ship *Hydrabad*, 11 October 1844–4 March 1845.

89 TNA, ADM 105/36, Letters and Correspondence regarding sickness on convict and emigrant ships (1836–1851), report by William Burnett on scurvy in convict ships (undated, c. 1844).

90 TNA, ADM 105/36, Burnett, Report on scurvy; TNA, ADM 101/21/4, Journal of surgeon Colin Arrott Browning on convict ship *Earl Grey* (1842–1843); TNA, ADM 101/24/11, Journal of surgeon W.H.B. Jones on convict ship *Elphinstone* (1842); TNA, ADM 101/35/8, Journal of surgeon J.O. McWilliam on convict ship *Hydrabad*, 11 October 1844–4 March 1845.

91 United Kingdom, House of Commons, Instructions for Surgeons Superintendent on Board Convict Ships, *Report from the Select Committee on Transportation* 1837 [518] xix, p. 346.

92 Bryson, 'On the Respective Value', p. 213; TNA, ADM 101/50/6, Journal of surgeon Alexander Bryson on convict ship *Marquis of Hastings* (1842).

93 Admiralty, *Instructions for Surgeon-Superintendents on Board Convict Ships* (London: William Clowes, 1838), emphasis added.

94 TNA, ADM 101/50/6, Bryson, Journal on *Marquis of Hastings*, General Remarks.

95 TNA, ADM 101/50/6, Bryson, Journal on *Marquis of Hastings*, Case 22: Jonathan Walker; Case 24: Thomas Law.

96 TNA, ADM 101/50/6, Bryson, Journal on *Marquis of Hastings*, General Remarks.

97 TNA, ADM 101/7/8, Mahon, Journal on *Barossa*, 'Essay on Scurvy'.

98 Susan M. Reverby, '"Normal Exposure" and Inoculation Syphilis: A PHS "Tuskegee" Doctor in Guatemala, 1946–1948', *Journal of Policy History* 23 (2011), pp. 6–28. As a result of Reverby's study, in October 2010 the US government apologised to Guatemala.

99 TNA, ADM 105/36, Burnett, Report on Scurvy.

100 'Why Does Sensitivity Occur?' http://us.sensodyne.com/FAQs.aspx (accessed 23 February 2011).

101 TNA, ADM 101/32/5, Journal of surgeon Colin Arrott Browning on convict ship *Hashemy* (1848–9), General Remarks.

5

Trust and authority below the hatches

In June 1841, John Hood and his son sailed to New South Wales in the government emigrant ship *Lady Kennaway*. Hood's cabin (although 'deficient in comfort') was 'a paradise compared with the other parts of the ship'. Hood had followed the conclusions of the Molesworth Committee about the state of New South Wales society in 1837–38, and the language of the reports coloured his assessment of the *Lady Kennaway*'s emigrants. 'I much fear, that the evidence of Sir F. Forbes and Major Mudie before the committee of the Commons will be verified in this ship before we separate,' he wrote. In the privileged privacy of the cabin's dining room, Hood and his fellow cabin passengers had been told that there 'are many women of the very worst description on board'.[1] Knowledge of disease came to them through 'whispered' intimation and rumour. On 19 June, bad news 'hitherto well concealed has just reached me: we have, it appears, and have had for some days, scarlet fever on board; it was called measles and believed to be such; but truth will out. We are now adopting every precaution to avoid this terrible complaint, and our cabins have been fumigated.' There was 'no running away from it as on land: and in so densely crowded a population, the chances are against us'.[2] To protect themselves from secrecy, inaccuracy, and disease in such close proximity, Hood and his fellow cabin passengers sought refuge in the sulphurous smoke of fumigation.

By the end of August the *Lady Kennaway* had reached its most southerly latitude, where the wind 'blows over the frozen regions, and the icebergs betwixt us and the pole'. Here, the cold was 'very great at night', and rheumatism 'the general ailment of all in this clime'. In his diary entry for 31 August, Hood explained that 'for several days past, the emigrants have been almost continually battened down below the hatches; and the lower region, I am told, is an Augean stable.' The surgeon 'was at work in it'. Hood did not register the implications of the padlocked hatchway and his next sentence betrays his incomprehension at what such a confinement might have meant for those locked below.

'The laziness of some of these emigrants (the women especially) is extraordinary. They lie a-bed for days, and would, I believe, remain so during the entire voyage, were it permitted ... it is with difficulty that the surgeon can expel them from their lairs.'[3]

Three weeks after Hood left England, another male passenger began a diary on a different ship. As the *Lord Auckland*, one of the first emigrant ships for New Zealand, waited to depart the British shore, Alfred Fell described 'a regular clean out below'. The surgeon made all the people take their beds on deck to be 'purified', a routine that they would repeat every week during the voyage. 'Of course', he clarified, 'this only relates to the steerage passengers, where they are so crowded.'[4] Fell experienced the *Lord Auckland* as a roomy and well-ventilated vessel. The surgeon's rules were important, but they did not apply to him. 'Poor creatures', another entry reads, 'it is a horrible place between decks so many people in so small a place I wonder how they live, several of the women told me how glad they should be when it was over.' The closeness below was 'terrible'.[5]

However sparse and uncomfortable their cabins might have seemed, Alfred Fell and John Hood wrote at a great conceptual distance from the experience of being in steerage. In 1957, George Nadel argued that shared ship-board experience and the common dangers of being at sea 'emphasised certain qualities of survival ... it must have been difficult to maintain successfully old world notions of status'.[6] This idea has persisted in popular conceptions of Australian egalitarianism, but diaries such as these two men's show that in fact the opposite was often true. Cabin doors and hatchways between decks reinforced cultural and social distance even as they allowed cabin passengers easy access to comment on the physically proximate world 'below'.

Just as the middle classes of nineteenth-century Britain took it upon themselves to sanitise, moralise, and represent the private spaces of the poor in the name of public health, so writers at sea were repelled, intrigued, and deeply concerned by the habits and habitat of those in the decks below. As surgeons went to work in these threatening spaces, cabin passengers regarded medical men as allies. In Fell's diary the surgeon cleans out; in Hood's he expels. In both accounts the surgeon appears as a figure of authority who imposes sanitary order and reassurance. Socially and politically, surgeons often shared cabin passengers' beliefs, concerns, and their dining table. This relationship was reciprocal: surgeons expected to be able to rely on the cabin passengers to support their interpretation of events and mishaps, and to provide the colonial governor with evidence on their behalf if voyages turned difficult.

The letters and diaries of literate cabin passengers are, of course, important sources for writing the history of nineteenth-century voyages. They wrote of routines, coasts, and ports, storms, equatorial ceremonies, burials, and their fears for those who fell overboard. Some were invalids, intensely aware of the environment around them. But it is important to remember that they still wrote from a privileged vantage point. Gender, class, and social status coloured their experience of voyaging, while deeply held assumptions shaped the way they wrote their accounts. To a lesser extent, people in second-class also considered themselves passengers and not emigrants.

Passengers assumed a freedom of movement that steerage emigrants and convicts could not. If we reverse this vantage point, starting from below the hatchways and looking out, the emphasis of medical relationships shifts. Assumptions about the self-evident benefits of the surgeon's medical authority are replaced by questions about trust, coercion, and the boundaries of privacy. Perhaps more importantly, we see that maritime medical relationships could be much more complex than that of a doctor with his patients. Sailors, messmates, and family members intervened physically, emotionally, and practically. By seeking the counsel of those who shared their living spaces, by caring for those around them, and not least by keeping quiet or choosing to speak out about matters concerning health, convicts and steerage emigrants sought to retain an element of control over their own well-being, as well as that of their children and companions. Questions of consent, trust, and compulsion overlap. Often, and for very good reason, emigrants and convicts remained deeply unconvinced that the surgeons' interests coincided with their own. In this chapter we see how contemporary mistrust of medical authority, so apparent on land among the labouring classes in this period, travelled to sea in respect of practices such as post-mortem examination and vaccination.

Questioning who controlled a person's decisions about health and body illustrates that emigrants and convicts did not share the same experience of voyaging as passengers who could afford to pay for all of their passage to Australia. Closely monitored movement through hatchways was symptomatic of a wider reality: convict transportees and government-assisted emigrants could not assume the right to freedom of movement, or to maintaining control over their bodily integrity. Moreover, surgeons' frustrations with smallpox vaccination, in particular, remind us that voyages hindered, even as they made possible, the larger projects that directly link Britain's social history with that of its colonies.

Hatchways: 'now we let them come up when they choose'

Fanny Davis described the reaction of the single women on the *Conway* to having the hatches closed by the crew while the ship was becalmed in the tropics:

> We got a broomstick and hammered it till they came and opened it for it was so suffocating with the close air; we had it left open all night as it always is. I never saw such an advocate for fresh air as our Doctor is, and I do think that is the secret of all being in such good health. He will not let anyone stop down all day and woe betide anyone who is found in their berth in the daytime.[7]

Davis's account suggests that the women had come to believe in the surgeon's insistence that fresh air preserved health. Why the crew chose to close the hatch on this day, or whether they had openly defied the surgeon in doing so, is unclear. In Davis's account the presence of the sailors is implied, a shadowy 'they' against whom the women appealed to the surgeon for relief from their confinement. Yet, two decades earlier, on the *Lady MacNaghten*, the balance of power between emigrants, surgeon, and sailors had been quite different. In the tropics, the sailors 'drove the women down between decks at the early hour of five in the afternoon'. The women had 'suffered much from suffocation', and frequently fainted, but 'all was useless'.[8]

Sailors appear frequently in discussions about medical authority at sea. Surgeons relied openly on the sailors' physical strength to support their medical authority, and assist with the sick, but the sailor's involvement could have other important consequences. James Gales' account of the voyage of the *Andromeda* in 1834 foregrounds the emergence of a physical relationship between the *Andromeda*'s sailors and the convict women.[9] First-hand voyage accounts from crew members are rare. When compared to the sparsity of the surgeon's account, Gales' diary is even more remarkable. Of the medical occurrences in the tropics, Henry Kelsall, the *Andromeda*'s surgeon, wrote little other than noting that Margaret King 'suffered very much from epileptic fits caused by the heat of the climate – she sometimes had from 10 to 15 in the course of the day'.[10] Gales' account reveals that far more was occurring on the *Andromeda*'s decks.

The *Andromeda* embarked 176 female convicts, thirty free emigrant women and sixteen children for New South Wales in 1834.[11] The free women – wives of previously transported men – shared a compartment that was separate from the convict women's prison, but the surgeon held the key to both rooms. In the early weeks of the voyage, the surgeon locked the prison doors each night at eight o'clock. After leaving Cork on 25 May, the *Andromeda* made good progress, and by the middle of June had passed the Cape Verde islands. In the fine weather the women washed and mended the crew's clothes ('they were very industrious the more work we gave them the better they liked it').[12] Off Madeira, the women had enjoyed watching the porpoises from the deck, but as the heat increased – by mid-June the thermometer on the deck registered 82° in the shade – Gales wrote that 'we had a deal of sickness'. On the night of 15 June the surgeon allowed the free women to bring their beds onto the poop. The next evening, the rules were relaxed further, as the convict women 'could not stand the excessive heat'. The crew 'was oblidged [*sic*] to keep the prison doors open all night and have a great number on deck to attend others fainting and going into violent fits 6 or 7 at a time as if communicated by sympathy'. For the crew, the open doors and the presence of the women on deck at night set a disturbing precedent. The sailors managed to 'get rid of the greater part' of the women by about midnight as the night air cooled, and yet still 'all the poop was occupied by them and their beds the Doctor had a long night of it; bleeding several and using all kinds of restoratives to their fainting'. The next day, the surgeon allowed the women on deck early 'to receive the benefits of the air'. Though the women were all better in the breeze, Gales feared that 'it will be very bad the first calm we get'.[13]

On 18 June, a further relaxation of the rules: a 'great number' of the weaker convicts stayed on the poop for the whole night, albeit without their beds, in case it rained. Gales observed that the women proved 'pleasing company' for some of his crewmates 'such as was amused with dialogue or quaint Irish stories', but he hoped that the situation would not continue long. The women were 'such beggars for tobacco which if given they will next ask for a pipe and then sure tis no use without a light out of the little box'. Although frustrated, Gales admitted that

> I would rather have them here than drag them up while apparently lifeless from their reeking dungeon in nothing but a chemise or struggling in all the agony of something worse than death; this was our task frequently a dozen times a watch during the time of the prison doors being closed but now we let them come up when they choose but generally used to get rid of them about midnight.[14]

While the surgeon was entirely silent on the matter, as the heat continued through the second half of June, the presence of the women on the decks at night dominated Gales' account. On 27 June between thirty and forty of the convicts remained on deck during the night, and soon recognised that they could use the situation to manipulate the sailors' discomfort: 'too hot to stay below several going in fits and others promising to faint if they did not get a smoke of the pipe'. The sailors retaliated:

> a pipe was half filled with gunpowder and filled up with tobacco and laid in a place where it was soon to be catched at, our expectations was soon realised by a loud laugh among the bystanders and the fire and tobacco blowing about the deck it only slightly singed her face but the general laugh that was rained against her with the reprimand from the person that possessed it quite shamed her and I believed deterred a good many from stealing pipes before had been making a constant practice of it.[15]

The crew of the *Andromeda* became intimately involved in the disorder as they shouldered the women from the prison and onto the deck, and later as they tried to re-assert possession of their night-time space. Joy Damousi has argued that women used boisterous behaviour 'in order to be anonymous and to create a space for themselves'.[16] The occurrences on the deck of the *Andromeda* show that these negotiations of space could be intensely physical, and that the mediating role of the sailors was crucial. The women won their space, quite literally, at the expense of the sailors, who then sought to regain the deck. But it was also a geographically specific disorder. As the *Andromeda* left the tropics and sailed into the southern oceans, the women returned below deck. Their physical absence from the sailors' rapidly changing world is reflected in Gales' account; as the crew pumped water and fought to sail the ship through lightning, storms, gales, and squalls, the women recede from view.

This episode tells us a great deal about these women's experience of voyaging, but it is not enough to understand these physical interactions simply as social or sexual intimacies, because we must also appreciate the climatic and medical contexts that first necessitated the breaking of the ship's rigid internal boundaries. The physical interactions between the *Andromeda*'s sailors and the female convicts profoundly affected the relationships that emerged during the voyage. The example of the *Andromeda* is a striking illustration of the ways in which gender, medical necessity, geographical contingency, moral acceptability, and collective responsibility for health played out at the margins of trust, complicity, and coercion.

The heat of the tropics had forced the surgeon to authorise the women's initial transgressions of the ship's internal boundaries. To do so, he had needed the sailors' physical involvement. However, perhaps deeply disturbed by the events he felt unable to record in his official journal, the surgeon had the final word in keeping the men and women apart. When the *Andromeda* arrived in Sydney, Gales' attention returned to the women. The surgeon ensured that all 'the favourites and fancy women' were selected for the 'worst destination'. Gales explained that 'this was truly mortifying a circumstance very unexpected for it was thought by both parties that when on shore they could carry on an intercourse with much less restraint than ever here – this the doctor got credit for'. Throughout his diary Gales had never said whether he had formed any relationship of his own, though it was clear others had, but now the women had gone he felt that the ship was 'lonely and something strange'.[17]

Medical relationships below decks

Charles Cameron had tried to earn the trust of the convicts on the *David Lyon*. Early in the voyage, in mid-April 1830, he had 'been attentive to advise and encourage' the men to 'come to me for laxatives' so that they might avoid the constipation that often accompanied seasickness.[18] Prisoners came to Cameron with ulcers, ringworm, constipation, and venereal ulcers. To these men, Cameron frequently gave medical comforts. By the middle of June, every prisoner also received a gill of wine a day. Two men in particular became used to the finest food that the *David Lyon* could offer. Both William Gibson and James Warboys refused to take the nitre medicine of which Cameron was so fond. Instead, Cameron ensured that they had 'daily something fresh from the Cabin Table'. For these two patients 'everything is cooked that they wish to have … and I even beg for them occasionally from the Captain of the Ship'. When Gibson heard that a sheep had been killed, he 'sent to me that he would like some of the liver'.[19] William Gibson's case dominates Cameron's journal, and it seems extraordinary that the surgeon continually acquiesced to the requests of a man who 'generally has early information of what there is for dinner in the cabin'. Even as he continually tested the limits of the surgeon's generosity, however, Gibson's body became ever more emaciated, and on 29 July he died.

There was another side to Cameron's authority, which he asserted more directly: encouragement was balanced by compulsory weekly inspections. On 23 May he found eight men with 'the itch'. They were 'immediately ordered into hospital and commenced to rub in sulphur ointment twice a day'.[20] Perhaps this, and his liberal distribution of the nitre solution, convinced other convicts to avoid the surgeon's attention and the contents of his medical stores. In the last week of July, Robert

Allen developed a bad headache. Although in pain, he waited four days – by which time he was constantly vomiting – before seeking Cameron's attention. Finally, on 27 July, he spoke to the surgeon. Allen's skin had become cold, his face 'collapsed' and his eyes had 'a wild vacant stare'. When asked why he had not come to Cameron sooner he replied that 'he thought that he would get better soon'.[21]

Cameron was unable to decide what ailed Allen, and he sent for some of the man's messmates, one of whom 'happens to be an old London Apothecary'. The list of convicts on the *David Lyon* reveals that the apothecary was Francis Hartwell. Married, with four children, Hartwell had been convicted of fraud at Middlesex in October 1829, and sentenced to seven years' transportation for dishonestly obtaining two stomach pumps. Previously, he had been in prison for obtaining a hat under false pretences.[22] As a druggist in London, Hartwell would have supplied potions and pills to a varied clientele. At sea, the convicted apothecary could no longer ply his trade, but he could certainly advise a messmate. Cameron's desire to hear the apothecary's version of Allen's illness acknowledged that Hartwell enjoyed the trust of the convicts, but also suggests that the surgeon felt that his authority had been undermined. In 1815, the Apothecary Act required the examination of all future apothecaries, but did not require those already practising to be examined.[23] Cameron's use of the term 'old London apothecary' implied that Hartwell was a shopkeeper, and an unqualified trader of the pre-1815 sort, rather than a modern, learned medical man with certified knowledge of chemistry, anatomy, medicine, physiology, botany, and *materia medica*. Nevertheless, Cameron also realised that at this moment the convict medical man knew significantly more about what ailed his messmate than did the surgeon. Hartwell 'had observed that Allen had been ill for upwards of a week, that he has been during that time extremely irritable and hardly ate anything, but that he would not allow [his messmates] to say that he was ill'.[24] Allen's illness had clearly been trying for those closest to him, but for several days they respected his wishes.

In one sense, Hartwell's relationship with Allen was unusual: not many convicts could have expected to share their voyage with an apothecary. On the other hand, Cameron's regard for the apothecary's version of Allen's illness simply reflected a common method by which surgeons gained information. As Allen's health failed, Cameron again enquired of his messmates whether he had 'got any hurt or blow on the head'. The messmates did not think that he had, and confirmed that Allen had been in the habit of taking his allowance of wine and lime juice.[25]

Emigrants and convicts were often reluctant to seek medical help, even for minor ailments. The surgeon who complained that the emigrants of the *Mandarin* 'threw themselves completely on me, as if they were perfectly incapable of doing anything for their own relief', expressed a frustration that many of his colleagues simply would not have recognised.[26] Peter Cunningham's journal on the *Recovery*, for example, describes how he walked round all the berths morning and evening. He questioned mess captains and examined everyone whom he saw lying down. Many of the convicts attempted to conceal their illnesses, being 'so averse to take medicine that they sometimes permit the disease to make considerable progress before they report themselves.'[27] Some emigrants brought their own trusted remedies onto ships. The surgeon of the *Palmyra* explained how one mother, whose infant was sick with fever and 'lichen tropicus' (heat rash) placed 'great faith' in Morison's pills and 'is in the constant habit of taking a dose every night'. Such self-medication made it 'seem probable' that the mother's milk had affected the health of her child.[28] Yet the surgeon's own remedies for the illnesses of childhood were hardly appealing. During the voyage, parents of children with scarlatina and hydrocephalus refused to let him use bleeding, cupping, or leeches to take the blood from their children's jugular veins.[29]

In the steerage compartments of emigrant vessels, and in the prisons of convict ships, a surgeon had little choice but to trust family members, messmates, and neighbours to take responsibility for those who were or might become sick, or to alert him when someone concealed their illness. For this reason, messmates often found their way into surgeons' case notes. Medical relationships within a mess often revolved around rations, not least because messmates often helped to feed the ill and convalescent. Rations at sea may have been salty, dry, and monotonous, but convicts and emigrants did not refuse food lightly. Andrew Blythe's messmates reported that he had often exchanged his food for tobacco, a habit which, the surgeon concluded, 'no doubt, also had an injurious effect upon his health'.[30] While rejection of food or indifference clearly indicated an ailing companion, an apparently healthy appetite could also conceal underlying sickness. The surgeon of the *Henry Porcher* had kept an eye on Robert Wood since embarkation. He had become 'pale and thin', but his messmates said that he had a 'good appetite'.[31]

Sarah Tainton's 'female companions' said that she had been 'drooping' ever since the *Bussorah Merchant* left the Cape of Good Hope. She had remained on shore during the night, but they firmly denied that she 'was guilty of any excess in drinking, as many of the others were'.[32] Whether welcome or not, intimacies formed in confinement. When Hannah White became 'convulsed' and afterwards 'furiously maniacal', her messmates told the surgeon that the previous night she had complained of 'a noisy hammering in her head'. Hannah talked incoherently and completed only parts of her sentences. Her messmates admitted that she had been scared after being told that the main mast had broken as the spanker-boom jibed violently, but they also explained to the surgeon that Hannah had not menstruated for several months.[33]

Familiarity did not necessarily produce friendship, or even trust, but it did mean that a convict's companions often knew their health intimately. Messmates at sea were often the same men or women with whom prisoners had shared their lives in the prison or hulk. One surgeon described a prisoner 'who always appeared in a low desponding state'. The man 'faltered in his speech and his mental faculties seemed much impaired'. One of the other prisoners who knew him well stated that he had been prone to fits on shore and that 'he has observed a growing aberration of intellect' over the voyage. 'The debility was so great that the exertion necessary to undress him caused him to faint, altho the tenderness displayed by his companions was quite remarkable.'[34] The surgeon tried various medical remedies, included blood-letting, but it is his comments about the convicts' involvement in their companion's illness that reveal something of the social nature of care and medical information that existed beyond the surgeon's own attempts to treat and record illness.

On the other hand, in such close quarters, with little privacy, it is unsurprising that compassion or tenderness often failed. Messmates sometimes took it into their own hands to reveal another's illness to the surgeon, or to take close neighbours to the surgeon against their will, particularly when they smelt bad, when they had lice, or when constant coughing disturbed their own attempts to sleep. James Jee's berthmate and messmates 'made repeated complaints' to the surgeon, 'requesting at the same time to have him removed from among them … one of the principal objections they had to him was his being troubled with vermin'.[35]

Messmates' silences can be as revealing as the occasions when they spoke out. The surgeon of the *Eden*, Gilbert King, objected to the embarkation of William Rogers, who had needed physical support from another man as he arrived at Spithead, but had relented upon hearing that Rogers was anxious to embark. The surgeon of the prison hulk from which Rogers had embarked had assured King that Rogers had never been in hospital. At that moment, the convict's companions kept quiet. They kept quiet too, when they believed that he only had the same seasickness that they all suffered. After he died at sea, Rogers' messmates finally gave a different account of his health: in the hulk he had 'seldom eaten his allowance' and had been 'pensive and melancholy'. He appeared to be 'ever brooding over some deep and secret grief'.[36]

Examining the dead

When the surgeon of the *Bussorah Merchant* unlocked the hatch of the ship's prison on the morning of 18 May 1828, one of the convicts, a 24-year-old man named William Wheally, 'expressed himself much better and wished to go on deck to enjoy the cool air'. For nearly three weeks, Wheally had suffered from intermittent fever and remained in his berth below. Wheally knew his own body, and explained his ailment to the surgeon. 'He says he has been frequently troubled with attacks of intermittent fever while he belonged to the *Dolphin* hulk at Chatham when he had been employed to work in low, marshy and muddy ground & he never perfectly recovered.' Though the tidal stretches of the Thames were long behind him, Wheally recognised this complaint from his life of old. For several days after the illness returned at sea he continued 'low' with little appetite. On 7 May, a week after he had first complained of chills, Wheally reported that he had 'a slight shivering this morning, succeeded by heat, but it was of short duration.' Again, it was the convict, rather than the surgeon, who gave a reason for his relapse: 'He thinks it was occasioned by exposing himself to the cold air. His appetite & strength still bad.'[37]

The *Bussorah Merchant* sailed south through the Atlantic and made a quick transition from the cold air of the English spring to the 'hot sultry weather' of the tropics. The climate became oppressive for the sick and healthy alike, particularly at night 'when the prisoners were locked below'. William Wheally's health failed to improve. The nights of the second week of May were particularly trying. The surgeon's journal entry for 11 May records that he 'had a restless night on account of the heat of the prison & his appetite and strength are completely exhausted'. During another night he again 'slept none because of the heat'. Yet, Wheally apparently recovered on the morning of 18 May. He 'continued on deck about an hour & then went below and layed down on his bed'. Optimism spread to his friends: 'one of his messmates went to call him at eight o clock to know if he would eat any breakfast'. Alas, Wheally 'made no answer'. The messmate sent for the surgeon who 'found him quite dead'. After Wheally had expressed his desire to go on deck, this was unexpected. Dunn wrote that 'he must have died suddenly and without a struggle as several men were sitting close by him from the time he went below till he died & they heard him make no complaint'.[38]

As Dunn wrote about William Wheally's illness on the *Bussorah Merchant*, he blended the effects of Wheally's former life in the hulk, the marsh, and mud of the tidal Thames, the changing Atlantic weather, and the locked prison of the *Bussorah Merchant* into his medical account. The presence of Wheally's messmates was also significant: the surgeon recorded their presence during his illness, when he apparently recovered, and again at the moment of his death. Immediately after Wheally's death, however, the tone of the surgeon's account changed. The close social nature of Wheally's illness disappeared as the surgeon described his post-mortem examination of the convict's body. From the contexts of the ship at sea and the bustle of the prisoner among his messmates, we are thrown suddenly into the silent, anonymous recesses of Wheally's body.

'On opening the body', Dunn continued his account, 'both bags of the pleura were filled with a serious [*sic*: serous] fluid tinged with blood and a small opening was discovered in the pericardium the rupture of which & discharging the contents into the chest might be the cause of his sudden death'. Although Dunn was quickly satisfied that he knew the reason for Wheally's death, as he guided his scalpel from the lungs, through Wheally's abdomen, into his stomach, liver, and enlarged spleen, the surgeon found more and more evidence of disease. 'On exposing the contents of the abdomen the ementum appeared much thickened & diseased. The stomach also was found in a diseased state.' The liver too, was a 'complete mass' of disease. Perhaps the 'enormous quantity' of hydatidi (cysts containing the larvae of tapeworm) finally induced a feeling of revulsion and convinced surgeon Dunn that he had seen enough. Perhaps a shout or a commotion from the deck, or a knock on the door of the ship's hospital, distracted him. Dunn made no reference to where in the ship he performed the post-mortem dissection, or what became of Wheally's remains. Dunn's account removes Wheally's body from the contexts of place, but then, just as suddenly, the entry concludes as Dunn returned to the maritime realities of his work; 'the average height of the thermometer during this month was about 80 on deck', he observed.[39]

The extent to which surgeons who superintended Australian voyages could (or could not) undertake post-mortem examinations provides us with important evidence about their professional motives and the relationships that they forged with the people in their care. Until the Anatomy Act of 1832, surgeons in Britain could only legally dissect the bodies of people who had been hanged as punishment for murder.

With a dearth of suitable teaching material, surgeons often obtained their bodies through body-snatchers. By the early 1830s, long-held fears about these practices erupted into riots and demonstrations around Britain against the Anatomy Act. The subject of anatomical dissection, particularly when combined with the fears surrounding cholera, provoked violent unrest, particularly among the poor.[40]

For surgeons at sea, then, the advantages of maritime isolation were clear; they enjoyed opportunities to undertake post-mortem procedures that few surgeons on land could have imagined. A clause in the 1832 Anatomy Act removed the right of a person's friends to object to an examination. Ruth Richardson has shown how crucial this was for the inmates of workhouses, who were powerless to protect bodies when family members did not arrive within forty-eight hours, but the question of rights over a body was particularly pertinent at sea.[41] Emigrants and soldiers often sailed to Australia with members of their family, and evidence from surgeons' journals suggests that their bodies were less likely to be subjected to post-mortem examination than those of convicts and sailors, who usually went to sea alone. In 1828 the surgeon of the hospital ship *Grampus* already boasted that he could open the bodies of seamen after death 'whenever we wish to do so'.[42] Between March and July 1828, surgeon E. Johnston performed six post-mortem examinations during the voyage of the male convict ship *William Miles*.[43] This is a remarkable tally: in one voyage Johnston had access to more bodies than any surgeon in Britain could imagine. Even as Johnston performed his examinations on the *William Miles*, Burke and Hare were murdering poor people and selling their bodies to an Edinburgh anatomy school.[44] As the public became ever more vigilant against grave-robbery, medical schools faced a severe cadaver shortage, and in 1831, for example, medical men in the whole of London had legal access to a total of only eleven dead bodies.[45]

Naval surgeons had not always been so open about the subject of their examinations. Although surgeons in the West Indies reported dissecting the bodies of soldiers to investigate yellow fever, eighteenth- and early nineteenth-century medical journals rarely included accounts of dissections.[46] While medical men in Britain were under sustained attack, surgeons at sea were gaining greater opportunities to explore and discuss their observations of the dead bodies of convicts, sailors, soldiers, and emigrants. In 1827, the Navy had created its medical library and museum and instructed its librarian 'to receive from all contributors such specimens of Morbid Anatomy, or subjects of Natural History, &c., as may be offered to you'.[47] By the 1850s, naval hospitals in Britain and abroad kept post-mortem registers.

On land, because of the rarity of bodies, anatomical dissections were, quite literally, performances. Surgeons, doctors, artists, students, and assistants crowded around as surgeons demonstrated human anatomy in the auditoriums and dissection rooms of hospitals and medical schools in Britain and its colonies.[48] At sea, things were quite different. Ships were crowded with emigrants, convicts, sailors, and patients, not the students and fellow surgeons trained in the art of clinical detachment. Surgeons had to examine bodies quickly, discreetly, and alone in the cramped confines of the ship's sick bay. Information was disseminated after the fact through written words in the naval surgeons' journals.

That reports of maritime post-mortem procedures became a common requisite, rather than a rare perquisite, aspect of the naval surgeon's role is clear from the number of times surgeons felt it necessary to explain when and why they did *not* perform an adequate examination of a dead body. Colin Arrott Browning professed that he had been determined to perform a post-mortem in a case in which he was 'unable to account for the fatal termination', but the 'circumstances' on the *Earl Grey* in 1842 compelled him to accomplish the examination 'hastily and without any assistance from any one'.[49] Often, the weather intervened. Surgeon Johnston, having already examined six corpses on the *William Miles*, was prevented from opening a seventh 'because of bad weather and inconvenience'.[50] A post-mortem examination demanded great physical control over hands and scalpel, and often proved impossible as ships pitched and rolled in all but the calmest of water. Some surgeons' excuses provide a rare glimpse of their struggles to manage their own health. Henry Brock had 'a great desire to open the body' of John Gooch, but had been unable to do so because he had been afflicted with a feverish attack. He attributed this to his 'exposure in the sun at the Cape of Good Hope where we put in to obtain a supply of medicines and fresh provisions'.[51]

Surgeons' accounts of failure with regard to examining a body reveal more about the communal nature of illness at sea. When James Nohilly, a convict on the *Augusta Jessie*, died in 1839, the surgeon, Thomas Dunn, 'deemed it advisable not to make a postmortem inspection of the body', in order 'to obviate mental depression among the prisoners'.[52] Dunn's decision fitted with an oft-expressed concern about dissection's emotional effects on untrained and susceptible observers and the necessity of keeping people cheerful and usefully occupied during a long voyage in order to ward off other illnesses. Dunn also seems to acknowledge the extent to which James Nohilly's illness had already been particularly troubling for the convicts around him. Dunn had initially objected to Nohilly as he inspected the convicts in Dublin's

Kilmainham gaol, believing him to be unfit for the voyage because of 'apparent mental imbecility'. Dunn recounted the conversation he had with the surgeon and other officers. The Kilmainham officials assured Dunn that Nohilly 'was a man of sound mind, and that the fatuous appearance which I pointed out arose from his total ignorance of the English language'. They had sent for 'an Interpreter of "Native Irish"' who 'in reply to several questions, dictated what appeared to me, on translation, to be rational replies'. Dunn 'reluctantly' sanctioned the man's embarkation but soon realised that James Nohilly was 'a man of infirm health and deranged intellect'.

Rather than chaining or confining Nohilly when his state of mind deteriorated at sea, Dunn put him 'under the immediate charge of a trustworthy fellow prisoner' who had 'no little trouble in managing the unfortunate mania'.[53] From the start, Dunn had carefully managed the convicts on the *Augusta Jessie*. He had formed a constabulary force from military convicts, established volunteer groups for cleaning, and allowed the men to form their own messes. Nevertheless, Dunn's response to Nohilly is noteworthy, not just because he was a convict. Convicts did not routinely travel in chains. Surgeons insisted that physical punishment and restraint should be used only as a last resort for punishment, although many accepted the use of a box for solitary confinement. However, mental disorders had a particularly destabilising effect on crowded ships which had no suitable place to safely hold a patient.

On both convict and emigrant ships, cases of mental illness account for some of the rare occasions when physical restraint was used, albeit with the aim of protecting, rather than punishing. When, on the *Andromeda*, one of the convicts 'went mad', she was confined 'with lashings', for example.[54] Another diary describes how a passenger who had 'gone quite deranged' was first taken down to his berth, 'but a short time afterwards brought upon deck where his hands were put in irons and his legs and body fastened with ropes and a number of buckets of water thrown upon him after which he was allowed to remain for a few hours'.[55] Yet Dunn did not chain Nohilly, and chose instead to entrust him to the care of his fellow prisoners.

Dunn enlisted the help of the *Augusta Jessie*'s 'influential men' to look after Nohilly. He 'assembled the Captains of Messes and all the influential men among the prisoners for the purpose of explaining this man's disease and freely engaging their sympathy and forbearance'. Dunn reported that 'this appeal was not made in vain', an observation that goes some way to explain his reluctance to examine the body, out of sensitivity to the convicts' feelings, when Nohilly died. In the first days of the voyage, as the coast of Ireland receded over the horizon, Dunn had been acutely aware of 'the mental depression consequent upon sea sickness and expatriation', and its medical consequences.[56] Dunn's compassion towards Nohilly and the other convicts on the *Augusta Jessie* is strong evidence that surgeons could treat convicts with a level of humanity rarely associated with medical care in the transportation system.

Other surgeons expressed their reluctance to examine a body in the close proximity of women. One surgeon reported that although one woman was 'a very urgent case for post mortem inspection', it was not practicable on a female convict ship.[57] In 1847 the surgeon of the emigrant ship *Sir George Seymour*, en route to Auckland, explained that 'no post-mortem took place on account of having many sick at the period'. He was also afraid that the procedure 'might produce an ill-effect especially amongst the female emigrants'. The women, he explained, did not share their husbands' desire to emigrate, and 'with whom there existed a great depression of spirits'.[58] The mention of the 'many sick' suggests that the surgeon lacked space, but he also feared the emotional effects of the procedure upon the women.

Opposing dissection

Surgeons did not make these decisions entirely of their own volition. However honourable they professed their sentiments to be, even at sea they could not escape the widespread loathing and fear of dissection. Emigrants, in particular, often collectively made their feelings about post-mortem examinations clear and reminded a surgeon of the limitations of his authority. In the crowded ship, their opposition often forced surgeons to abandon their plans. In 1838 the surgeon of the emigrant ship *Mandarin* explained that in some circumstances 'the surgeon cannot perform post mortem examination on account of the vulgar prejudices of the people'.[59] The phrase 'vulgar prejudice' permeated contemporary medical and political discussions about opposition to anatomical dissection.[60] Leah's contemptuous dismissal certainly conformed to the mood of the era by reducing the emigrants' fears to 'irrational' objections, but it also hints at the uncertainties of his position. The death of an emigrant named Mrs Greer had prompted Leah's exasperation. This was the second death on the *Mandarin*, and two more would follow that week. For a naval surgeon, who needed to ensure that the colonial governor authorised his salary for the voyage, post-mortem examinations were a source of conflict with emigrants, but they also provided a valuable source of medical evidence. A surgeon could use his post-mortem account to argue that the causes of a person's death were internal to their body, rather than a consequence of any fault on his part during his superintendence of the voyage.

Leah's reference to 'the people' implies that he encountered widespread opposition from the emigrants on the *Mandarin*, and it is unclear whether it was this collective dissent, or Mr Greer's assertion of his right to claim his wife's body, that finally prevented the surgeon from performing a dissection. If surgeons did not record the nature of the conversations they had with family members at sea, it is nevertheless often apparent from their journals that the presence of a family member prevented a dissection. When a soldier died of pneumonitis early in the voyage of the convict ship *Lady Raffles*, the surgeon reported that there had been 'no post mortem on account of his wife and the inconvenience of the place'. The entrance to the Thames was certainly not a good place to be disposing of a dismembered body in 1840, but the presence of the soldier's wife also stayed the surgeon's hand.[61] Five years later, the 4-year-old son of another soldier died of what the surgeon diagnosed to be cholera. Here, again, the surgeon explained that he had failed in his attempts to undertake a post mortem because the boy's father was present.[62] Mothers, especially, often refused to allow the examination of their children.

Dissection, Helen MacDonald has written, was 'an activity most likely to be carried out on the bodies of people made vulnerable, through poverty, always, but also through the workings of the law and that particular conjuncture of interests and knowledge called physical anthropology, in which medical men were supreme'.[63] Her study of the culture of dissection in Britain and Australia shows that naval surgeons, notably James Scott, became intimately involved in colonial dissection practices, a culture that was as hungry for the bodies of Aboriginal people, as it was for those of Britain's labouring and destitute poor. Much less well known, and a subject that begs for further historical analysis beyond the scope of this book, is their widespread practice of examining the bodies of sailors.[64] For surgeons, post-mortem examination was both an opportunity to acquire knowledge and a further tool to demonstrate their authority. Nevertheless, the profound mistrust that the subject engendered between Britain's poor and labouring classes and the medical men travelled easily.

Vaccinations

As surgeons complained of intransigence, superstition, and vulgar prejudice they were in fact describing the strategies by which emigrants and convicts sought to retain an element of control over their own and their loved one's bodies. In 1827–28, feelings of mistrust and disrespect between the surgeon of the *Elizabeth* and the female convicts were mutual. Surgeon Joseph Hughes described the women as 'slothful, dirty [and] disposed with a most lamentable recklessness of character unconquerable'. The women threw their clothes and blankets overboard to the 'very faces' of the surgeon and officers.[65] Early in the voyage, Hughes ascertained that all of the convicts had been vaccinated, but he also realised that 'he could never induce them to go through the operation'. He explained that bowel disorders and skin eruptions had further prevented him from vaccinating the children. By the end of November, Hughes admitted that he 'never could vaccinate with satisfaction (that is I never could bring myself to try it under these circumstances)'. As the *Elizabeth* approached its destination, the surgeon abandoned any intention of vaccination. 'I have much prejudice to contend with, but from acting with caution towards them when applying to me, I have secured their esteem and goodwill in their medical capacity.'[66] Nevertheless, in other respects, the women still caused 'considerable trouble'. The subject of vaccination exemplified the precariousness of Hughes's position, as the female convicts of the *Elizabeth* continually found ways to undermine the authority of a man who had not gained their respect.

The practice of vaccination used the lymph of cowpox, or *vaccinia*, to provide protection against the more serious disease of smallpox. After Edward Jenner first reported his findings on cowpox in 1798, the medical profession rapidly adopted the practice, and soon came to see inoculation (the direct transfer of smallpox matter between bodies, also known as variolation) as outmoded and, increasingly, as dangerous. The subsequent career of Jenner's vaccine lymph – like the disease it prevented – is closely tied to that of nineteenth-century imperial travel and communications, and Jenner's vaccine soon arrived in Australia.[67] In 1803, Governor Gidley King requested a supply of the new vaccine matter for New South Wales. The following year the *Coromandel* delivered a supply from the Royal Jennerian Society.[68] By 1806, more than a thousand people had been vaccinated with cowpox in New South Wales and the newly founded colony of Van Diemen's Land. These early attempts at taking vaccine to the antipodes were part of the emergence of a global vaccination network. In 1802, vaccine arrived in Bombay, transported via a relay of children stretching overland from Baghdad.[69] Vaccine also travelled in live cows, in glass vials, and in drops of pus trapped between pieces of glass. In 1803, the Spanish Crown sponsored a Royal Maritime Vaccination Expedition, by which Jenner's vaccine travelled to Puerto Rico, Guatemala, and then on to the Philippines.[70] From 1803, supported by voluntary contributions, the Royal Jennerian Society in London distributed lymph to 'Shipping, the Colonies and every Quarter of the Habitable Globe'.[71] Requiring little formal medical expertise to administer, vials and bottles of vaccine travelled with missionaries, surgeons, traders, and colonial officials.

Naval surgeons were some of the most enthusiastic subscribers to the government-funded National Vaccine Establishment. From 1821, the Commissioners of the Navy routinely sent packages of vaccine virus from the Establishment for convict ships. In 1825, during one of the earliest experiments with government-assisted emigration – a scheme that sent over two thousand Irish labourers to Upper Canada – naval surgeons reported their frustrations, failures, and opinions after attempting to vaccinate the emigrants and their children during these voyages.[72] By 1830, the annual accounts of the Jennerian Society show that the Navy contributed the considerable sum of £1,000 for supplies 'to his Majesty's Forces in the Navy and Settlements abroad'.[73]

Although surgeons and colonists frequently complained about the excessive numbers of children on convict and emigrant ships, they became highly valuable and visible passengers in the context of vaccination. Free from the debilities, constitutional weaknesses, and venereal complaints that plagued adults, previously unvaccinated infants, particularly the healthier children of the military guard, were crucial colonial vaccine carriers. The vaccination of children was also more often successful than that of adults. Before the *John Bull* left Cork in 1821, Dr Trevor vaccinated eight children between the ages of 6 months and 9 years, and two adult women. Initially, the results seemed doubtful, but a week after the operation, the *John Bull*'s surgeon chose 2-year-old Elizabeth Wade, this child 'being the most healthy and free from blemish'. He punctured the pea-sized pustule on her arm, and 'took what lymph I could from it'. Within a month, the scabs on the arms of the vaccinated patients 'had all dried and fallen off', leaving a scar 'sufficient to satisfy me that they had regularly gone through the process'.[74] On the *Mangles* in 1822, the surgeon 'vaccinated Mary Wright's child with matter taken from Sergeant Croft's child, which has had a very fine pock'.[75] In 1842, the surgeon of the female convict ship *Royal Admiral* recorded with obvious satisfaction that 'lymph (decent)' was delivered to Dr Clarke on arrival in Hobart, 'exclusively kept up on the voyage from the children'.[76]

Surgeons could deliver lymph in the form of a person with a pustule or as preserved dry scabs. Alternatively, they could simply give the package of Establishment vaccine (or what remained of it) to the colonial surgeon on arrival, and hope that it was still viable.[77] From the start, it is clear that surgeons juggled two different priorities when they vaccinated at sea. They needed to prevent outbreaks of smallpox during the voyage, but they also needed to deliver lymph for use in the colonies. In 1826, Joseph Hughes's instructions make these two priorities quite explicit when he received for the convict ship *Chapman* 'the usual packet' of Establishment vaccine from the Commissioners of the Navy 'relative to the vaccination of convicts and the preservation of the matter during the voyage'. On journeys to North America, surgeons had complained that the lymph they received from the Navy had been next to useless, and failed in almost every instance. A voyage to Australia took several times longer. Joseph Hughes's attempt to convey vaccine shows how surgeons could use maritime trade circuits and systems of exchange that linked ports and islands including London, Cork, Madeira, Cape Town, Rio de Janeiro, Calcutta, and Sydney. When Hughes arrived in Porto Praya in the Cape Verde islands to replenish the *Chapman*'s water stocks, Hughes gave half of his own vaccine matter to the Chief Physician of St Jago, a gesture which 'was considered a great Boon they having none in the island'.[78] As the *Chapman* crossed the Atlantic, the surgeon attempted to 'inoculate' two soldiers' children with some of the remaining matter. The attempt failed, and Hughes regretted that the lymph would have been of little use to the physician at St Jago either. The *Chapman* then put in at Rio de Janeiro to refit. Hughes's discovery that his vaccine matter was useless forced him to apply to the Principal English surgeon, Dr Dickson, to have the children vaccinated, but he found it impossible to get them to the hospital for the one hour on either Thursday or Sunday morning that it performed the procedure. Hughes learnt from two other English surgeons in Rio that 'several surgeons of convict ships had complained of the same thing' and supposed 'that Damp or some other cause had rendered the virus useless and inert'. They too 'had found the matter they had obtained from several ships to be the same'.[79] The failure of Hughes's attempts to vaccinate, his willingness to share his own precious supply, and his shared frustrations in Rio show how quickly vaccine matter had become an important medical commodity in islands and ports during the first decades of the nineteenth century. Around the Atlantic, surgeons and physicians shared their little parcels of vaccine matter. Yet, these networks of exchange were as frustrating and prone to failure as they were vital.

From the mid-1820s, ships' captains increasingly undertook Australian voyages non-stop, depriving surgeons of these opportunities to distribute, procure, and replenish vaccine matter *en route*. As the *Albion* approached forty degrees of latitude south of the equator in 1828, Thomas Logan vaccinated four of the male convicts with the vaccine he had carried from the beginning of the voyage. Logan hoped to land 'a large supply of recent vaccine virus at Sydney', and had waited four months since the ship left London before he attempted to vaccinate any of the convicts. The day after the procedures, the weather in the southern ocean deteriorated; the ship's motion became violent, the air cold, and the convicts remained below. Logan began to regret vaccinating the prisoners who were confined, crowded together, and 'indisposed by excessive motion, bad air & dismal aspect of the ship'. In Logan's journal, the same meteorological conditions in the southern oceans that so often seemed to cause illness now impeded the action of vaccine. For vaccination to be successful, it required more than a pure body: it required a strong, healthy body. Because of the weather, the bodies of the convicts on the *Albion* were 'in the most unfavourable circumstances to go thro' the disease'.[80]

Surgeons struggled to balance climatic assessment, the risk of smallpox during the voyage, and, not least, their desire to deliver lymph to the colony. As such, there was no consensus among surgeons on convict ships as to when vaccine should be used, and their practices varied widely. Some surgeons vaccinated in the days immediately after embarkation, before the vessel left port. Others waited for seasickness to subside before vaccinating in the first few days at sea. Some waited a month, choosing to vaccinate in the warm air and steady sailing before the tropics. Others still, as Logan did, waited for months in the hope that the matter would be more likely to reach the colony in a useful state. In 1835, one surgeon commented that during the early stages of the voyage the 'extreme irritation of nausea' of seasickness 'may have prevented the vaccine lymph from producing vesicles'. Conditions did not improve; he went on to suggest that 'vaccination can hardly have faced a more severe trial than in a ship with more than three hundred people on board in warm climates'. In the tropics, the heat caused skin irritation, which also prevented vaccination.[81]

Logan's expressions of disappointment contain a rare glimpse of self-criticism. Two days after the attempted vaccinations, his regret about the bad weather had turned to the open admission that 'an error has been committed in delaying the vaccination until the end of the voyage. The matter seems to have become effete. All the prisoners vaccinated on the 18th inst. have resisted the operation of the vaccine matter.' The disappointed Logan admitted that he had 'reserved the process of vaccination for a late period of the voyage' because he 'wished to land a great supply of matter … I wished, in short, to do too much; I have therefore defeated my own object.'[82]

As David Arnold has observed, the practice of vaccination remained 'crude and unreliable' throughout the nineteenth century and the majority of surgeons' attempts to vaccinate at sea were unsuccessful.[83] They commonly blamed 'bad' lymph; matter often 'lost effectiveness', it became 'inert', 'effete', or 'rendered useless by long keeping'. Vaccinations 'totally failed' or were 'unsuccessful in all cases'.[84] In 1840, one surgeon's use of 'decomposed' lymph had very serious consequences. Henry Mahon had received the lymph in December 1839, but the convicts had not embarked in Ireland until the last week of February. By then, the lymph 'must have been decomposed'. Nevertheless, Mahon 'selected twelve healthy children and vaccinated them'. All of the procedures were unsuccessful, but for one of them it had nearly 'proved destructive by being absorbed into the system'. The arm, shoulder, and side of the neck became inflamed and painful, and an abscess formed.[85] Violent reactions of this kind were rare, and usually failure resulted only in the anti-climax of 'slight efflorescences' that receded, and puncture marks that disappeared without producing the tell-tale scarring.[86] Surgeon Logan could afford, therefore, to be candid about his dashed hopes. Vaccine failure was so common that it did not diminish his professional reputation, but his hoped-for success might just have brought him colonial recognition and gratitude, perhaps even an appointment.

Throughout the period, colonial newspapers emphasised the need to maintain a circulation and supply of fresh lymph to and around the Australian colonies. In February 1833, the *Circassian* convict ship arrived in Hobart with a viable supply of lymph. The *Colonial Times* printed a notice that 'Mr Thomas, Surgeon and corresponding vaccinator to the National Vaccine Establishment … will be happy in diffusing its benefits throughout the colony'.[87] Six years later, when the HMS *Pelorus* arrived in Sydney with a supply of 'this invaluable matter', the event demanded formal recognition. For two years, the *Sydney Morning Herald* explained, no ships had arrived in the colony with lymph, although 'various medical gentlemen' had made 'repeated, though unsuccessful attempts' to deliver vaccine matter.[88] By contrast, smallpox *had* arrived in 1828 with the *Bussorah Merchant*, and again in 1835 with the *Canton*. In 1828 the *Morley* had brought whooping cough, and by the late 1830s nearly all convict ships arrived with scurvy. At this time, as we will see in the following chapter, emigrant ships too seemed constantly to deliver contagious fever. The *Herald* observed that 'the circumstances of so many persons having arrived here during the last two years in crowded and sickly ships' threw into sharp relief the difficulties of transporting lymph, and reiterated its urgency. The *Herald* believed it a 'matter of fearful probability that small-pox, one of the most dreadful of all diseases, would have been introduced into this colony' even as lymph would not. A deputation of 'subscribers' presented the surgeon of the *Pelorus*, Dr Reilly, with a 'handsome silver snuffbox'. The engraving explained that this was 'a token of regard for the benefit he has conferred by successfully introducing the vaccine lymph into N.S. Wales'.[89]

How to vaccinate emigrants and convicts

During the 1830s, when the British government began to provide assistance to emigrants who wished to sail to Australia, vaccination practices at sea also changed. The two competing priorities – to vaccinate early to prevent smallpox, and to vaccinate continuously to deliver lymph – became aligned with the two different streams of people: emigrants and convicts. In 1838, the instructions for surgeons of emigrant ships stated that they were to take 'measures … in the course of selecting people, to secure their vaccination; but it will be proper that the Surgeon Superintendent should examine their arms, or see their certificates that the operation has been performed, and that he should perform it anew in any case that may seem to him doubtful'.[90] Emigrant vaccinations occurred before boarding and thereby became another procedure that granted admittance to the ship, besides the tests of eligibility and certificates of character and good health. Emigrants also received instructions clearly stating that 'no family will be allowed to embark unless they furnish previously a certificate from a respectable medical practitioner, that each of their children have either had the smallpox or been previously vaccinated'.[91] David Ross, the surgeon of the *Parland*, complained that despite his instructions, 'I have learnt that several of the children have not been vaccinated'. Two weeks after departing, a child developed smallpox.[92] This policy of vaccinating eligible emigrants at their selection could cause complications when surgeons came to re-inspect the emigrants at the moment of embarkation. On the *Adam Lodge* in 1838, and again on the *Woodbridge* in 1839, emigrants responded to Alexander Stewart's queries about their family's health – and the threat of rejection that such queries implied – by responding that the pustular eruptions on their children's faces had 'taken place after vaccination'.[93] Compulsory child vaccination was introduced in England and Wales in 1853. Historians have identified compulsory vaccination for emigrants from the 1870s, if they travelled from a region with smallpox.[94] It is clear, in fact, that these requirements had existed since the 1830s.

On convict ships, vaccination seems to have served a different function. Rather than being vaccinated before departure, as was the case with emigrants, convicts and their children were routinely used to convey live vaccine matter to the Australian colonies through human chains, as is recorded unequivocally in the journals of naval surgeons.[95] By the 1830s, vaccination also appeared in the convict-ship surgeon's official instructions. He was to 'keep up such a succession of vaccinated cases as may enable him to convey fresh virus to the colony, if the number of Convicts or Passengers on board, who may not have had the Small-Pox nor undergone Vaccination, and who shall consent to be vaccinated, will admit of it'.[96]

These instructions clearly emphasise the colonial importance of delivering vaccine to the colonies, but the wording also contains another crucial detail, in which convicts apparently retained the right to refuse: the surgeon could vaccinate only convicts who consented. The instructions of 1840 removed this clause, but in 1841 William McDowell still reported that 'on inspection of the convicts to ascertain the number requiring vaccination I found that *according to their own declaration*, that they had all been previously vaccinated or had variola'.[97] Other convicts told surgeons that they had been vaccinated, only for it to subsequently become apparent that they had not.[98] Through the 1840s, surgeons' vaccination reports became more routine, and often consisted simply of a list of names. Surgeons received an acknowledgement from the medical officer of the colony 'stating whether he had delivered to him any recent virus', with the date and result of the vaccinations. A great many of the vaccinations failed, and still some convicts refused vaccinations for themselves and their children. In 1848, another surgeon could vaccinate only 'all the infants whose mothers would permit it'.[99]

There was no clear break between the ending of inoculation with smallpox and the introduction of vaccination with cowpox. Surgeons also slipped between the language of inoculation and vaccination well into the 1830s.[100] In 1818, William McDowell 'innoculated with vaccine virus in both arms'. The surgeon on the *Grenada* also 'inoculated ... with vaccine virus'. As late as 1836, another surgeon described inoculating eighteen convicts.[101] For emigrants and convicts, the distinction between inoculation and the new vaccination procedure must often have been unclear – perhaps even irrelevant – and the terminology confusing. It is likely that many poor people did not know if they had undergone vaccination. Many others might have undergone the procedure of vaccination without it having being successful – should they, or should they not, say they had been vaccinated? On the *Bardaster*, the mother of one child said that her son had been 'inoculated', but the surgeon concluded from the appearance of the marks on the child's arm and 'from the operation having been performed by the Medical Officer of the Regt there is no doubt of its having been cowpox', i.e. vaccination. Normally the feverish child's pimples 'would not attract attention', but as cases of smallpox broke out through the *Bardaster*, the distinction between smallpox and cowpox took on urgent importance.[102]

Aside from those who refused, surgeons frequently explained that there were not enough suitable convicts on each ship to ensure a supply of vaccine for the colony. From the first decade of the nineteenth century, English parishes had organised vaccination campaigns aimed at the poor. 'Economy and convenience', one historian has argued, led some parishes to adopt compulsory vaccination, as in Hungerford from 1811.[103] Compulsory vaccination also occurred in prisons: during the 1820s, surgeons reported that when cases of smallpox occurred, they vaccinated all the prisoners who had never had smallpox or who could not show a scar.[104] Charitable organisations provided vaccinations, and from 1840 free vaccination came under the remit of the New Poor Law. Guardians had to provide vaccination 'for all persons who may come to them for that purpose', for which contracted surgeons often received extra payment. The frustration of surgeons who lacked suitable bodies thus provides important evidence about the extent to which poor people were being vaccinated before the Act of 1853 made the procedure compulsory.[105] This is a murky, grey area between consent and coercion and it raises important questions about medical knowledge, trust, compulsion, and informed consent, which are equally pertinent on land and at sea. If, as Nadja Durbach has shown, there was a sense among anti-vaccinators in 1869 that some British mothers were 'too poor to object', then evidence from Australian convict and emigrant voyages suggests that the blurred boundaries of compulsion and consent have a more extensive history than we currently know about.[106]

Throughout the 1820s and 1830s, there is little sense that convict lymph generated the sense of distaste among colonists that would come later as people questioned the race and class of its carriers.[107] In 1844 the convict ship *Tasmania* stopped at Madeira. For the surgeon, Thomas Seaton, this delay offered a rare opportunity to both vaccinate the convicts and save his precious package of pure matter from 'home' for the colony. He procured some vaccine matter in Madeira (he did not say from whom) and vaccinated four of the adult female convicts. This allowed him to keep the package from 'Dr Black' for delivery to the hospital at Hobart Town 'as he had strictly charged me to do'.[108]

Seaton's packet from England was worth considerably more than lymph that had travelled through the bodies of convicts. For them, the unidentified Madeiran lymph had sufficed. In Seaton's actions we glimpse the emerging importance of provenance, an idea that would become crucial to imperial vaccination debates later in the century.

Conclusion

Travelling with vaccine lymph brought naval surgeons into a prestigious global network of medical exchange. Yet, far from being a story of professional triumph, any attempt to trace naval surgeons' efforts to supply live vaccine lymph to the Australian colonies in the mid-nineteenth century reveals a continuing story of messy failure and thwarted hopes. Precisely *because* voyages of several months were a deeply unreliable method of conveying lymph matter to the Australian colonies, success became a matter of professional pride and could make the surgeons important men in colonies increasingly obsessed by the arrival of disease.

For surgeons, voyages provided a space to experiment with remedies, vaccinations, and anatomical examinations. However, these practices also exemplify the questions about compulsion, consent, trust, and medical intervention with which this chapter began. It becomes clear why emigrants and convicts did not necessarily see medical authority as a resource for which they ought to be grateful; nor, often, did they come to share the surgeon's opinions. On an everyday level, many remained reluctant to seek medical help, even for minor ailments. Examples of post-mortem examination at sea also make it clear that if a surgeon was to gain access to the bodies of those under his care, the question of trust was key to his relationship with emigrants and convicts. While the surgeons' official instructions codified his authority, they could not account for the more intangible elements of medical relationships. Put simply, if a surgeon could not gain the trust of those in his care, he did not have authority. If he did not have authority, it was more difficult to perform the experiments and procedures that brought recognition. Through threads such as these, Australian voyages bind together the histories of medicine, social power, colonialism, and migration across national borders and geographical space.

Notes

1 John Hood, *Australia and the East* (London: John Murray, 1843), pp. 4, 20.
2 Hood, *Australia and the East*, p. 13.
3 Hood, *Australia and the East*, p. 57.

4 NMM, MRF/151, Journal of Alfred Fell on Emigrant Ship *Lord Auckland*, London to New Zealand (1841–2), 30 September 1841.

5 NMM, MRF/151, Journal of Alfred Fell, 21 January 1842.

6 George Nadel, *Australia's Colonial Culture* (Cambridge MA: Harvard University Press, 1957), p. 52.

7 ANMM, MS CON, Diary of Fanny Davis, Voyage to Melbourne on *Conway* (1858), 21 July 1858.

8 'The Lady McNaughten – The Sick Female Emigrant Ship', *Sydney Monitor*, 20 March 1837, p. 3.

9 NMM, MSS/87/061, 3, Journal of W. James Gales, crew member on the convict ship *Aurelia* Cork to Sydney (1834). The NMM catalogue incorrectly lists the ship as the *Aurelia*; there were no convict ships named *Aurelia* and this was certainly the *Andromeda*. See Charles Bateson, *The Convict Ships, 1787–1868* (Glasgow: Brown, Son and Ferguson, 1985), p. 353 and TNA, ADM 101/2/8, Journal of surgeon Henry Kelsall on female convict ship *Andromeda* (1834). The Captain of the *Andromeda* was Ben Gales, making it likely that the sailor who wrote this journal was a close relation.

10 TNA, ADM 101/2/8, Kelsall's journal on *Andromeda*. Case 1: Margaret King, and General Remarks.

11 NMM, MSS/87/061, 3, Gales Journal, p. 1; TNA, ADM 101/2/8, Kelsall's journal on *Andromeda*, General Remarks.

12 NMM, MSS/87/061, 3, Gales Journal, 29 May 1834.

13 NMM, MSS/87/061, 3, Gales Journal, 17 June 1834.

14 NMM, MSS/87/061, 3, Gales Journal, 18 June 1834.

15 NMM, MSS/87/061, 3, Gales Journal, 27 June 1834.

16 Joy Damousi, *Depraved and Disorderly: Female Convicts, Sexuality and Gender in Colonial Australia* (Cambridge: Cambridge University Press, 1997), pp. 20–22.

17 NMM, MSS/87/061, 3, Gales Journal, 16 September 1834.

18 TNA, ADM 101/19/3, Journal of surgeon Charles Cameron on convict ship *David Lyon* (1830), 5 May 1830.

19 TNA, ADM 101/19/3, Cameron, Journal on *David Lyon*. 9, 14, 19, 26 June 1830.

20 TNA, ADM 101/19/3, Cameron, Journal on *David Lyon*, 23 May 1830.

21 TNA, ADM 101/19/3, Cameron, Journal on *David Lyon*, Case 17: Robert Allen, 27–29 July 1830.

22 AOT, CON 31/1/20, Francis Hartwell per *David Lyon*, http://search.archives.tas.gov.au/ImageViewer/image_viewer.htm?CON31-1-20,228,28, L,80 (accessed 15 February 2011).

23 Hilary Marland, *Medicine and Society in Wakefield and Huddersfield, 1780–1870* (Cambridge: Cambridge University Press, 1987), pp. 235, 272.

24 TNA, ADM 101/19/3, Cameron, Journal on *David Lyon*, Case 17: Robert Allen, 28 July 1830.

25 TNA, ADM 101/19/3, Cameron, Journal on *David Lyon*, Case 17: Robert Allen, 30 July 1830.

26 TNA, ADM 101/78/2, Journal of surgeon Edward Leah on emigrant ship *Mandarin* (1838), General Remarks.

27 TNA, ADM 101/63/6, Journal of surgeon Peter Cunningham on *Recovery* (1823), General Remarks.

28 TNA, ADM 101/78/7, Journal of surgeon Charles Carter on emigrant ship *Palmyra* (1838–9), Case 6: Sarah Douste.

29 TNA, ADM 101/78/7, Carter, journal on *Palmyra*, General Remarks.

30 TNA, ADM 101/38/5, Journal of surgeon Campbell France on convict ship *John Barry* (1838–9), General Remarks.

31 TNA, ADM 101/33/5, Journal of surgeon Thomas Galloway on *Henry Porcher* (1834–5), Case 20: Thomas Wood.

32 TNA, ADM 101/76/5, Journal of surgeon James Scott, M.D. on emigrant ship *Bussorah Merchant* (1839), Case 17: Sarah Tainton.

33 TNA, ADM 101/48/8, Journal of surgeon John Arnold on female convict ship *Margaret* (1843), Case 7: Hannah White.

34 ML, MAV/FM4/1543, The diary of John Campbell, 1850, surgeon on convict ship *William Jardine* (1850), General Remarks (12th page).

35 TNA, ADM 101/41/1, Journal of surgeon William McDowell, on convict ship *Lady East* (1824–1825), Case of James Jee. See also, e.g., TNA, ADM 101/35/6, Journal of surgeon L.T. Cunningham on convict ship *Hyderabad* (1849), Case 9: Charles Oakes.

36 TNA, ADM 101/22/2, Journal of surgeon Gilbert King on convict ship *Eden* (1836–7), Case 2: William Rogers.

37 TNA, ADM 101/14/4, Journal of surgeon Robert Dunn on convict ship *Bussorah Merchant* (1828), Case 5: William Wheally and General Remarks.

38 TNA, ADM 101/14/4, R. Dunn, Journal on *Bussorah Merchant*, Case 5: William Wheally and General Remarks.

39 TNA, ADM 101/14/4, R. Dunn, Journal on *Bussorah Merchant*, Case 5: William Wheally, 18 April 1828.

40 Ruth Richardson, *Death, Dissection and the Destitute* (London: Penguin Books, 1989), p. 222; Sean Burrell and Geoffrey Gill, 'The Liverpool Cholera Epidemic of 1832 and Anatomical Dissection – Medical Mistrust and Civil Unrest', *Journal of the History of Medicine and Allied Sciences* 60:4 (2005), pp. 478–498.

41 Richardson, *Death, Dissection and the Destitute*, pp. 205–207.

42 United Kingdom, House of Commons, *Report and Evidence of the Select Committee on Anatomy* 1828 [568] vii, p. 75.

43 TNA, ADM 101/75/1, Journal of surgeon E. Johnston on the male convict ship *William Miles* (1828); General Remarks.

44 Richardson, *Death, Dissection and the Destitute*, pp. 132–141.

45 Richardson, *Death, Dissection and the Destitute*, p. 101; Helen MacDonald, *Human Remains: Dissection and Its Histories* (New Haven and London, Yale University Press, 2006), p. 11.

46 Mark Harrison, *Medicine in an Age of Commerce and Empire: Britain and its Tropical Colonies, 1660–1830* (Oxford: Oxford University Press, 2010), p. 68.

47 The Army opened a parallel establishment in 1827, and the staff of the two libraries often exchanged books of anatomical studies. *Instructions for the Royal Naval Hospitals at Haslar and Plymouth* (London: William Clowes, 1834), p. 68.

48 MacDonald, *Human Remains*, p. 50.

49 TNA, ADM 101/21/4, Journal of surgeon Colin A Browning on convict ship *Earl Grey* (1842–3), General Remarks.

50 TNA, ADM 101/75/1, Johnston, Journal on *William Miles*, General Remarks.

51 TNA, ADM 101/50/1, Journal of surgeon Henry Brock, on male convict ship *Marmion* (1827–8), General Remarks.

52 TNA, ADM 101/6/6, Journal of surgeon Thomas R. Dunn on convict ship *Augusta Jessie* (1839–40), Case 10: James Nohilly.

53 TNA, ADM 101/6/6, T. Dunn, Journal on *Augusta Jessie*, Case 10: James Nohilly and General Remarks.

54 NMM, MSS/87/061, 3, Gales Journal, 29 June 1834.

55 ANMM, MS KAT, Diary of Richard Hall on the ship *Kate*, Liverpool to Melbourne, December 1852–April 1853, 5 February 1853.

56 TNA, ADM 101/6/6, T. Dunn, Journal on *Augusta Jessie*, Abstract of the daily journal.

57 TNA, ADM 101/25/6, Journal of surgeon John Wilson on female convict ship *Emma Eugenia* (1846), Case 3: Caroline Gardner.

58 TNA, ADM 101/79/2, Journal of surgeon Harry Goldney on Freight Ship *Sir George Seymour* (1847), General Remarks.

59 TNA, ADM 101/78/2, Journal of surgeon Edward Leah on the emigrant ship *Mandarin* (1838), Case 3: Nancy Greer.

60 Richardson, *Death, Dissection and the Destitute*, p. 151.

61 TNA, ADM 101/42/1, Journal of surgeon Robert Wylie on convict ship *Lady Raffles* (1840–1), Case 3: William Collins.

62 TNA, ADM 101/68/3, Journal of surgeon J.A. Mould on convict ship *Sir Robert Peel* (1844–5), Case 4: John Coyle.

63 MacDonald, *Human Remains*, p. 4.

64 MacDonald, *Human Remains*, pp. 47–48.

65 TNA, ADM 101/24/3, Journal of surgeon Joseph Hughes on female convict ship *Elizabeth* (1827–1828), 31 October.

66 TNA, ADM 101/24/3, Hughes, journal on *Elizabeth*, Comments for end of November.

67 Alison Bashford, *Imperial Hygiene. A Critical History of Colonialism, Nationalism and Public Health* (Basingstoke: Palgrave, 2004), pp. 15, 25.

68 Michael J. Bennett, 'Smallpox and Cowpox under the Southern Cross: The smallpox epidemic of 1789 and the advent of vaccination in colonial Australia', *Bulletin of the History of Medicine* 83:1 (2009), pp. 37–62, p. 51.

69 David Arnold, *Colonizing the Body* (London, Berkeley and Los Angeles: California University Press, 1993), pp. 139–140.

70 Martha Few, 'Circulating Smallpox Knowledge: Guatemalan doctors, Maya Indians and designing Spain's smallpox vaccination expedition', *British Journal for the History of Science* 43 (2010), pp. 1–19.

71 Royal Jennerian Society, *Yearly Report* (London: John Westley and Co., 1830), p. 31.

72 Nine emigrant ships sailed from Cork to Quebec. For the surgeons' different approaches to vaccination during the voyages see, e.g., TNA, ADM 101/76/2, Journal of surgeon John Thomson on emigrant ship *Albion* (1825) and TNA, ADM 101/77/1, Journal of surgeon Francis Connin on emigrant ship *Fortitude* (1825).

73 Jennerian Society, *Yearly Report*, p. 41.

74 TNA, ADM 101/38/7, Journal of surgeon William Elyard on convict ship *John Bull* (1821–2), entries for 17 July, 24 July, 14 August 1821.

75 TNA, ADM 101/47/2, Journal of surgeon Matthew Anderson on convict ship *Mangles* (1822), General Remarks.

76 TNA, ADM 101 65/3, Journal of surgeon J.R. Roberts on female convict ship *Royal Admiral* (1842), General Remarks.

77 For the first two methods, see TNA, ADM 101/38/7, Journal of surgeon William Elyard on female convict ship *John Bull* (1821) and for the third, see TNA, ADM 101/12/8, Journal of Oliver Sproule on convict ship *Borneo* (1828), 13 June 1828.

78 TNA, ADM 101/16/9, Journal of surgeon Joseph H. Hughes on convict ship *Chapman* (1826), Entry for 31 May and General Remarks.

79 TNA, ADM 101/16/9, Journal of surgeon Joseph H. Hughes on convict ship *Chapman* (1826), Note on vaccination, after entry for 11 October.

80 TNA, ADM 101/1/9, Journal of surgeon Thomas Logan on convict ship *Albion* (1828–9), Remarks for 18–21 October.

81 TNA, ADM 101/7/3, Journal of surgeon Joseph Steret on convict ship *Bardaster* (1835–6). In India, vaccination had a season, as surgeons recognised that vaccine lymph often failed or produced 'sloughing sores' in intense heat. Arnold, *Colonizing the Body*, p. 140.

82 TNA, ADM 101/1/9, Logan, Journal on *Albion*, General Remarks.

83 Arnold, *Colonizing the Body*, p. 139.

84 TNA, ADM 101/24/1, Hamilton, journal on *Elizabeth*; TNA, ADM 101/22/3, Journal of surgeon William Rae on convict ship *Eliza* (1822), General Remarks; TNA, ADM 101/33/3, Journal of surgeon William Carlyle on convict ship *Henry* (1824–5), General Remarks.

85 TNA, ADM 101/36/6, Journal of surgeon Henry Mahon on convict ship *Isabella* (1839–1840), General Remarks.

86 TNA, ADM 101/38/2, Journal of surgeon Daniel MacNamara on convict ship *John Barry* (1821), General Remarks.

87 'Notice', *Colonial Times* (Hobart), 12 March 1833, p. 4.

88 'P. Reilly, Esq. R.N.', *The Sydney Herald*, Monday 8 July 1839, p. 2.

89 'P. Reilly, Esq. R.N.', p. 2.

90 Admiralty, *Instructions for Surgeons-Superintendents on Board Convict Ships* (London: William Clowes, 1838), Instruction 30.

91 United Kingdom, House of Commons. *Emigration* 1839 [536–1] [536 II] xxxix, p. 15.

92 TNA, ADM 101/78/8, Journal of surgeon David Ross on emigrant ship *Parland* (1838), Case 1: Collins.

93 TNA, ADM 101/76/1, Journal of surgeon Alexander Stewart on emigrant ship *Adam Lodge* (1838), General Remarks; TNA, ADM 101/79/8, Journal of surgeon Alexander Stewart on emigrant ship *Woodbridge* (1839), General Remarks.

94 Bashford, *Imperial Hygiene*, p. 36.

95 Historians have previously assumed that there is no evidence for this process. See Bennett, 'Smallpox and Cowpox', p. 61.

96 Admiralty, *Instructions for Surgeons-Superintendents on Board Convict Ships* (London: William Clowes, 1838), Instruction 18 (emphasis added).

97 TNA, ADM 101/20/5, Journal of surgeon William McDowell on convict ship *Duncan* (1840–1), General Remarks (emphasis added).

98 TNA, ADM 101/7/3, Steret, journal on *Bardaster*, General Remarks.

99 TNA, ADM 101/15/3, Journal of surgeon John G. Bowman on female convict ship *Cadet* (1848), General Remarks.

100 In 1840, the Vaccination Extension Act made inoculation illegal.

101 TNA, ADM 101/30/5, Journal of surgeon Peter Cunningham on convict ship *Grenada* (1821), 11 June 1821; TNA, ADM 101/44/10, Journal of surgeon Robert Espie on convict ship *Lord Sidmouth* (1822–3), 11 October 1822; TNA, ADM 101/8/2, Journal of surgeon John Tarn on convict ship *Bengal Merchant* (1836), General Remarks.

102 TNA, ADM 101/7/3, Steret, journal on *Bardaster*, Case 15: Richard Clarke and General Remarks.

103 E.G. Thomas, 'The Old Poor Law and Medicine', *Medical History* 24 (1980), pp. 1–19, pp. 12–14.

104 For example, United Kingdom, House of Commons, *Gaols* 1825 [5] xxiii, p. 270.

105 Dorothy and Roy Porter, 'The Politics of Prevention: Anti-vaccinationism and public health in nineteenth-century England', *Medical History* 32 (1988), pp. 231–252.

106 Nadja Durbach, 'They Might As Well Brand Us: Working class resistance to compulsory vaccination in Victorian England', *Social History of Medicine* 13:1 (2000), pp. 45–62, p. 52.

107 Alison Bashford, 'Foreign Bodies: Vaccination, contagion and colonialism in the nineteenth century', in Alison Bashford and Claire Hooker (eds) *Contagion: Historical and Cultural Studies* (London and New York: Routledge, 2001), pp. 39–60, p. 41.

108 TNA, ADM 101/71/1, Journal of surgeon Thomas Seaton on female convict ship *Tasmania* (1844), General Remarks.

Voyage II:
Henry Wellings (1858)

Henry Wellings, a 29-year-old painter from Manchester, arrived in Liverpool with his wife, Elizabeth, and two sons, Harry (age 6) and Willie (age 2) on Thursday 27 May 1858.[1] The waterfront would have been crowded with sailors, labourers, Irish migrants, runners, beggars. By boat, the family carried their luggage across the Mersey, through what Henry Melville described as the 'tangled thicket of masts', to the Government Emigrant Depot in Birkenhead, a huge warehouse on the edge of the dock on the opposite bank of the estuary.[2] As the Wellings family showed their papers and certificates, and were allowed to enter the depot, the officer warned that they would have 'any little luxuries' that they had brought taken from them. Henry sent the family's eggs back to Manchester.[3]

Conscious that his family had entered a new chapter in their lives, Wellings had decided to keep a journal in a Manchester and Salford Committee on Education notebook, originally designed to collect signatures in support of the Manchester and Salford Education Bill of 1851–52. On the first blank page Wellings neatly ruled three vertical lines to create columns for Date, Weather, Health and General remarks. His first entry records that this was a 'fine' spring day and his family were 'tolerably well'. Every day without fail, for the next four months, Henry would make an entry in his notebook.

Although they were told that once inside the depot they 'could not get out again', the family found the Birkenhead depot a 'very comfortable, clean and convenient' place, and the officials very civil. Inside the depot, pillars ran the entire length of a dining room able to accommodate six hundred emigrants at long wooden benches. In the evening of 28 May, Henry preached to an impromptu congregation of fellow emigrants and wrote a letter to his mother. As it happened, the family spent less than two days in Birkenhead. At noon the following day, the Wellings boarded the *David McIvor*, with nearly four hundred other men, women, and children from all over Britain and Ireland.[4] The weather was fine and Henry was confident that he and his family were 'all well' in health. Although everything was 'very comfortable and clean', surrounded by the strange environment and unfamiliar sounds of the now crowded steerage quarters of the emigrants' ship, Wellings was, perhaps, only able to sleep fitfully on this first night. The following morning he rose early and went on deck, where he watched and listened as the crew of the *David McIvor* manoeuvred the vessel away from the dock and into the Mersey estuary. Henry took the opportunity to write a last letter to his mother, and preached again. Perhaps it was this preaching that made Henry stand out among the crowd of emigrants. Before the ship had left the river, the surgeon appointed him 'Constable Superintendent of Water Closets'.

Apart from the forfeiting of the eggs, the transition from land to sea had been uneventful. However, the tone of Wellings' diary entries soon changed. Three days after weighing anchor in the dock it was clear that adverse weather prevented the *David McIvor* from leaving the estuary. This, Wellings declared, was 'the most monstrous state of things I ever experienced'. His wife, Lizzie, was heavily pregnant and felt ill. As if to reflect his mood, Wellings wrote that 3 June was 'a dull miserable day everything damp and uncomfortable'. Lizzie was 'still very poorly'. Although Harry, the elder of his two sons, was 'all right', Willie was 'not as well' and Henry himself felt 'rather poorly'. The unhealthy airs of the estuary were having an effect; that night, Henry had 'a very severe attack of ague'. Finally, in the early dawn of 4 June, the *David McIvor* sailed. Although he still felt ill and the weather was rough and cold, Henry left his berth to go on deck, from where he saw the coast of North Wales, with the peak of Snowdon behind. As the emigrants reached the open Irish Sea on the following day, the familiar agues they had experienced in the estuary blended into seasickness. Many on board were 'too ill to get out of their berths: such heaving vomiting crying and groaning', Wellings wrote. Over the following weeks, amidst his comments about rations, cleaning routines, and his own responsibilities at the water pumps, Wellings' voyage diary charted the declining health of his youngest son, Willie, and his concerns for Lizzie, his pregnant wife.

In the strange environment of the open ocean, moments of joy and curiosity relieved a growing sense of monotony. On 10 June, the ship 'fell in with a shoal of porpoises', two of which the sailors caught, cooked, and ate. Below decks, there were also moments of social tension, of fights and arguments, but from the very first days in the Mersey estuary Henry Wellings' narrative binds the health of the family to the accumulating strains of the voyage. As the weather remained cold and dull, with a stiff breeze, in the second week, sickness still prevailed through the ship. 'Think it will never end', Wellings wrote of the weather, the nausea, perhaps even of the sea. The next day, the breeze had become a gale. The passengers remained confined below and most of the people were 'fearfully sick'.

As the *David McIvor* passed Spain, it reached the fine weather and the light breezes of the trade winds. Lizzie improved, but her husband found little else of interest to report. 'Routine', Wellings wrote in large underlined letters on 19 June, although he had managed to get a gill of wine and a book to read from the doctor. The frustrating monotony of these early days was interrupted during the following week by 'a fearful riot in the single men's cabin'. The following night, the second mate caught two of the sailors in the hold. Was it their 'naked light' or that they were 'nearly drunk' that caused such 'a great disturbance' the following morning? From the fine spring days in Birkenhead, the *David McIvor* propelled the family into a scorching summer. Only a month after they had first arrived at the depot, they were now in the tropics. Throughout the last week of June the wind dropped, until on 26 June they were 'becalmed and scorching'. Wellings' attention returned to the health of his son, who had become 'fearfully ill'. 'Expect to lose him', Henry added. As the ship languished in the calm, he stayed up all night with Willie. Within a few days, Lizzie had weakened again. After crossing the equator on July 11, and in the fine weather and trade winds of the southern Atlantic, Willie appeared to improve slightly, but 'somehow he gets thinner every day he is a living skeleton'. Henry confided in his journal that he wished that 'we had a little wine for Willie', but the ship's doctor refused. On 12 July he managed to get Willie a tin of boiled mutton.

A month later, in the middle of a Southern Ocean gale, Willie finally went to the ship's hospital. Wellings invested his hopes in higher powers; 'I pray God will restore him'. Willie 'still continues to breathe and that is all'. Despite Wellings' worry for his son, 14 August was notable: he 'got a glass of grog'. Two days later, another entry, similarly understated and to the point: 'Lizzie delivered of a son at 2.50 a.m. going on favourably.' After the birth, and as Willie continued to linger, Wellings' relationship with the surgeon had improved from his early struggles to obtain medical comforts. 'I cannot but feel very grateful to think how kind the Doctor is to Lizzie and Willie.' Wellings' diary suggests that the health of his family was a deeply personal and private matter. Pride and dignity mingled with his religious faith. Nevertheless, after the family had entrusted Willie to the care of the ship's hospital, and the contact with other people that this necessitated, Wellings seemed to take a new interest in those around him and felt the need to comment on the health of another of the adult passengers for the first time. On 23 August, 'Mrs Isac went into the hospital to day with the itch.'

From spring to summer, the seasons changed within days. By 28 August, as the *David McIvor* sailed fast and deep into the southern hemisphere, 'it is winter with a vengeance'. 'Great sameness' alternated with rough weather and snow as the ship headed eastwards, beyond the southern tip of Africa. Wellings, always sparing with his words, wrote little. On 7 September, in rough, squally, and cold weather, Willie died. That morning they 'could see the hand of death was upon him'. At 2.30 p.m. 'his spirit winged its flight to Jesus'. Framed by a black box, the entry records that Willie's death occurred at about 'Long 104.0 E, Lat. 43.59 S'. Just two weeks from Australia, the family committed the body to the deep, and for the first time Wellings ran out of space on the page for the words he wanted to write.

Closing his account of the voyage, Wellings traced the line of his family's voyage in a hand-drawn map of the world. The map is one of the most revealing and thoughtful sources that we have as evidence for an ordinary working man's understanding of the imperial and maritime globe around which he found himself sailing. Wellings drew his map over the major lines of longitude and latitude and included the tropical lines of Cancer and Capricorn. The coasts and islands that located his understanding of his voyage are the same coasts and islands that populate the contemporary framework of colonial and maritime topography and medical understanding that frames so many Australian voyages. He labelled the Cape Verde islands, St Helena, and the Cape of Good Hope. The outline of the South American continent is erased, redrawn smaller, and the outline of its western coast is unsure. Perhaps also drawing on his own and the sailors' knowledge of important places, he marked England, Asia, China, Spain, France, Borneo, and New York.

Most striking of all, Wellings used an 'X' to mark the exact position of Willie's burial. Fixing the longitude and latitude of his son's final resting place afforded Wellings little immediate comfort. As he reported the *David McIvor*'s 'dreadful rocking' during the night after his son's death, Wellings found that he could not help 'fretting for poor Willie'.

This modest notebook is a rare and moving example of a steerage emigrant's diary.[5] At a first glance, the short, spare entries in Henry Wellings' diary seem to add up to little more than a repetitive tale of woe, in short untidy entries. Addressed to no one in particular, there is little sense of the wonder and weirdness of the tropics, the sailors'

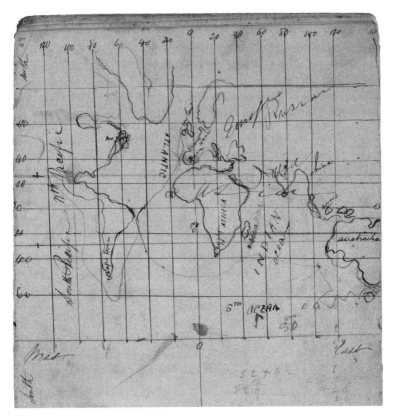

Figure 4 Journal of Henry Wellings on *David McIvor*, Birkenhead to Sydney (1857). Map of the Voyage, page facing entry for 24 September.

stories and beliefs, or the self-conscious literary flourish of the journals that travelling Victorians often wrote and re-wrote. Wellings' columns record terrifying gales and the birth of a son in as matter-of-fact a manner as scorching heat, a glass of grog, or a simple note that the weather was 'fine'. And yet, sometimes it is precisely 'the exhaustive repetitive dailiness' of the sparsest of personal records that can reveal the most.[6] We must take this diary, and its map, as important evidence of how one man 'named the world' of his own journey and began to imagine this world beyond Manchester and into the Australian space that he and his family would come to inhabit.[7]

The maritime environment and the geography of the voyage beyond the ship profoundly shaped Wellings' experience and understanding of the voyage, but through the diary we can also see that the *David McIvor* was much more than a vessel that conveyed a human cargo. This insight is particularly important in the case of the *David McIvor* because, throughout its history as an emigrant ship, the Agent for Immigration's reports had consistently labelled the ship as well as the emigrants on it as sick. In 1856, when the Health Officer quarantined the *David McIvor* in Sydney for the third time, the Immigration Agent wrote:

> The *David McIvor* has now so frequently brought emigrants to this colony that no remarks are necessary as to her eligibility for carrying emigrants, it is however right to remark that however eligible she may be for such a purpose she has always been most particularly unfortunate in contracting some cutaneous or eruptive disease amongst the children during the passage and thus has been subjected each voyage to the annoyance and inconvenience of being placed in quarantine.[8]

For the officials in Sydney, the *David McIvor*'s sickness was repeatedly revealed in the children's varied illnesses. Alleyne's use of the term 'eligibility' echoed the language of the workhouses to imply the worthiness of the *David McIvor*. Again and again, the *David McIvor* had proved an inherently unhealthy vessel. We could argue that the death of Willie Wellings provides further evidence to support the official view, but, as his father's diary ends, it gives us a very different sense of what travelling in the *David McIvor* meant to those in its steerage berths:

> Whoever you are or whatever may be your position (unless you have plenty of money at your command and can well afford pay your passage as a first class cabin passenger in a first class ship or steamer) endeavour to obtain a passage in a government ship … you will be better treated & better fed & cared for you will find yourself more comfortable & clean than in any private ship … parties who take my advice will I am sure feel thankful for these few hints, by a man who has experienced what he is constrained to write having been an Emigrant from Birkenhead to Sydney N.S.W in the Ship David McIver May 27th /58.

Notes

1 Passengers on the *David McIvor*, 24 September 1858, p. 5. http://srwww.records.nsw.gov.au/ebook/list.asp?series=NRS5316&item=4_4795&ship=David%20McIvor (accessed 20 June 2011). Harry is listed as Thomas H.

2 Henry Melville, *Redburn: His First Voyage* (New York: Harper and Brothers, 1850), p. 204.

3 ML, Mss 1963, Journal of Henry Wellings on *David McIvor*, Birkenhead to Sydney, 1857, 26 June 1857.

4 State Records of New South Wales: Shipping Master's Office; Passengers Arriving 1855–1922; NRS13278, [X96–100] reel 406 transcribed by Barbara Farquharson (2005), http://mariners.records.nsw.gov.au/1858/09/038dav.htm (accessed 1 February 2011).

5 Andrew Hassam has estimated that of 1.3 million free immigrants to nineteenth-century Australia, only 300 steerage diaries are known to remain. Andrew Hassam, *No Privacy for Writing: Shipboard Diaries 1852–1879* (Melbourne: Melbourne University Press, 1995), p. xvii.

6 Laurel Thatcher Ulrich, *A Midwife's Tale: The Life of Martha Ballard, Based on Her Diary, 1785–1812* (New York: Vintage Books, 1991), p. 9.

7 Paul Carter, *The Road to Botany Bay* (London and Boston: Faber and Faber, 1987), p. 69.

8 AONSW, Reel 2853, 56/7, Agent for Immigration to Colonial Secretary re *David McIvor*, 31 March 1856.

6

From emigrants to immigrants: quarantine and the colony

After the long, six-thousand-mile passage east from the Cape of Good Hope, the westerly winds that roared around the southern hemisphere's oceans delivered ships finally to the coast of the Australian continent. For many, the first sight of land for several months was Cape Otway, the tip of land that stretched towards Van Diemen's Land (from 1852, Tasmania), around a hundred miles to the south-west of Melbourne. Passing King Island brought vessels into Bass Strait, the channel which separated Van Diemen's Land from the mainland. Beyond Melbourne, captains navigated further through the Strait, past a string of islands. Crews who could not catch a favourable wind into the Strait, or who were headed for Hobart, sailed around the south of Van Diemen's Land. By the 1840s, the majority of ships bound for Sydney also chose this southern route.

Depending on the winds, it took around one or two weeks to sail the final seven hundred miles from Cape Otway to Sydney. The sight of Mount Dromedary (Mount Gulaga) rising above the New South Wales coast marked the beginning of the end of a voyage. Onward, past the vertical cliffs of Jervis Bay, convicts, passengers, and crew alike began to watch for the two headlands that dominated and protected the entrance to the huge natural harbour of Port Jackson, with Sydney within. From the first decade of the colony, a fire had been lit each night on the Southern Headland. By 1818, the architect Francis Greenway had overseen the construction of Australia's first lighthouse. A year later, the surgeon of the *Bencoolen* recorded his first sight of the 'revolving light' of 'Macquarie's Tower'.[1]

Sydney had grown rapidly during the first decades of the nineteenth century, particularly under Governor Lachlan Macquarie (1810–21). From a distant penal settlement known colloquially as 'Botany Bay', designed to strike fear into the heart of potential wrongdoers, it had become an established colonial port town, an important node in global and imperial maritime networks of trade and communication. Ships from India, the United States, and the Cape of Good Hope brought livestock, rum, sugar, meat, and material goods. By the 1820s, the streets of the town had become more ordered, genteel, and dominated by imposing public buildings, grand houses, and carefully landscaped leisure places. Imitating the fashionable British towns of Bath, Bristol, Cheltenham, and Edinburgh, Sydney boasted an 'architecture of social distinction and exclusion'. It was also an architecture that reflected a town beginning to assume a role of importance in the maritime world.[2]

As their vessels sailed into Port Jackson, accompanied by the pilot boat, convicts and emigrants first saw the walled-off grounds around Government House, and the windmills that dominated the skyline behind Sydney's coves, wharves, and buildings. Some emigrants expressed their mixed feelings about going ashore at the wharf. One emigrant had 'many conflicting thoughts, very sorry that the voyage was over, and having to part with so many passenger friends ... and at the same time glad that I had reached the Land of my adoption, ready to begin the "Battle of Life".'[3] Others, in groups, presented memorials to surgeons to thank them for their care. The emigrants of the *Aliquis* also asked the surgeon to pass on 'their humble but sincere thanks for the several kind and judicious arrangements made on their behalf, and for a free passage to the colony'.[4] When convict vessels anchored in the harbour, officials came on board and took down every person's details for their indents, the documents that would follow the convicts through their lives in Australia. This was a process that could take two or three days. The vast majority of vessels entered Port Jackson and disembarked the new arrivals with few concerns about health.

In the first decades of the nineteenth century, quarantine procedures had been informal and ad hoc. In 1814 the governor quarantined the *Surrey*, and in 1828 sent the guards and convicts of the *Bussorah Merchant* to 'a remote part on the North Shore'.[5] A convict named William Maybury arrived at the quarantine ground from the *Bussorah Merchant*. In a letter to Mary, his wife, in England, he explained that 'we are on an Highland called Spring Cove about 8 miles from Sydney Town'. 'We have about 20 tents erected close to the sea where thank God I never enjoyed better health since I was born. I frequently bathe and our living is pretty good.' In his 'small book', which contained the journal of his voyage to Australia, Maybury's feelings about the quarantine ground stand in for his first impressions of the colony as a whole:

> [M]ost on board expected to anticipate a barren and uncultivated country but I am happy to inform you that it is nothing but a paradise or the garden of the world. The surrounding scenery no picture could

excel for beauty the rocks, the water and the situation of the town in general is really grand.[6]

Maybury explained to his wife that this had been 'a very fine voyage' which had improved his health; 'I am much stouter than when I last saw you'. William's head was filled with possibilities. He and his friend 'Polly' would try to remain in Sydney. As soon as he could procure a certificate of leave, Maybury would 'lose no time' in sending for Mary. She should then arrange matters with Mrs Polly – 'you will find her a most agreeable companion' – and go to Henry Capper, the superintendent of the ships that transported convicts. '[H]e will instruct you how to act,' Maybury assured his wife.[7] Quarantine had delayed him from sending news to Mary and all his 'best friends', but it had given Maybury the time to daydream about his prospects for his future life.

As Sydney's population and global contacts continued to expand, it is easy to see why colonial officials believed that the colony needed a formal quarantine station. Dysentery was rife, but it appeared that contagious diseases such as typhus, smallpox, and measles would arrive only by ship.[8] As news of the cholera outbreaks in Britain reached New South Wales, the colonial government passed its own quarantine legislation in 1832.[9] Although Earl Grey's government accepted that quarantine was a subject on which each community 'must to a great extent be permitted to decide for itself', Colonial Secretary Viscount Goderich impressed upon the Governor of New South Wales, Sir Richard Bourke, 'the importance of not aggravating embarrassment by unnecessarily quarantining British vessels'.[10] As the medical professions and governments of Europe began to reject outmoded quarantine procedures, the colonial government of New South Wales embraced them.

North Head, opposite the lighthouse at the entrance to Port Jackson, was ideal for a quarantine station. The seaward cliffs presented towering faces of wave-sculpted limestone, but inside the harbour, the gently sloping beaches of Spring Cove provided a sheltered landing area and a large, open space for airing goods, clothing, and bedding.[11] Most importantly, the headland lay some eight miles off by boat, and on the opposite shore from the town of Sydney. In 1835 Governor Bourke quarantined the emigrant ship *Canton* for smallpox and used a military guard armed with guns to protect the outer boundary of the quarantine station. In the earliest quarantines, the inhabitants lived in tents on shore, while the sick remained on board their ship, anchored in Spring Cove. On 19 July 1837 Bourke formally proclaimed the whole of North Head to be an official quarantine ground.[12]

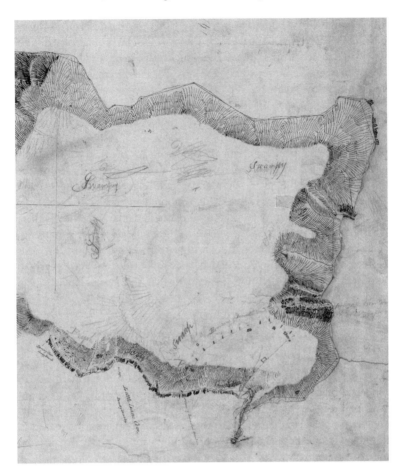

Figure 5 Detail of T.H. Nutt, 'Plan of the Quarantine Ground, North Head, Sydney' (undated).

The colonial government employed convicts in the construction of thirteen whitewashed stone cairns. Clearly delineating the quarantine boundary, these boundary stones would serve as physical reminders of the headland's purpose to separate the sick from the healthy, backed up by the prowling figures of armed guards. The cairns, one of which still stands today, figured prominently in contemporary maps of the quarantine station. T.H. Nutt, a colonial surveyor for New South Wales, drew the cairns out of all proportion to their actual size (Figure 5). Significantly, Nutt also scrawled the word 'swamp' several times across his map of the land outside the quarantine boundary.

Contemporaries would have recognised in this the description of an unhealthy environment that exuded miasma.[13] Nutt's map contributed to a particular colonial representation of the headland; beyond the clearly defined 'healthy ground', the surveyor tried to make the physical environment of North Head collude in the purpose of quarantine.

In 1838 convicts built the first quarantine structures: a wharf, a hospital, and four wooden huts to provide accommodation. From 1838, also, Port Jackson had a health officer. By 1841 he could order a provisional quarantine and employ the necessary medical staff (usually naval surgeons) without requiring any further authority from the governor. From the 1850s, permanent buildings housed the healthy and convalescent and a hospital hulk moored in the bay received the sick.[14] In total, eleven other islands and headlands around the coast of Australia have been used as quarantine stations since the nineteenth century, including Moreton Bay in Queensland, Impression Bay near Hobart and Port Phillip outside Melbourne, but none played nearly so important a part in defining the meaning of the Australian national border.[15]

Defining immigrant status

In 1828, William Maybury and the other convicts of the *Bussorah Merchant* underwent quarantine in Port Jackson for smallpox. In Hobart, the same year, the *Borneo* was placed in quarantine for eight days because of whooping cough.[16] Significantly, these were the last convicts to perform quarantine; formal Australian quarantine measures now began to reflect the politics of immigration, not penal transportation. Between 1837 and 1841, fifteen British emigrant ships – about one in ten of the total – performed quarantine outside Sydney, all for typhus fever.[17] During the same five years, fifty convict ships sailed into Port Jackson. While many of these surgeons also reported multiple cases of typhus, none of the ships was quarantined. There is little medical difference to suggest why immigrants and not convicts should have been quarantined at this point; bowel disorders, skin and eye complaints, consumption, and fevers appear throughout emigrant and convict surgeons' journals. The British government hired the same vessels for emigrants as for convicts; in the late 1830s ships including the *John Barry*, *Maitland*, and *Lady MacNaghten* all sailed to Australia with convicts, before repeating the voyage with emigrants, or vice versa. Convicts and emigrants sailed the same route around the Cape of Good Hope and stopped at the same places. They encountered the same maritime environments and, moreover, they were superintended by the same naval surgeons with comparable authority and instructions.

Amy Fairchild's history of immigration procedures at New York's Ellis Island, *Science at the Border* (2003), helps to explain what this inconsistent treatment means. She describes New York's Ellis Island in the late nineteenth and early twentieth centuries as a processing tool which placed and sorted immigrants and taught them the rules of the nation.[18] This insight is important because it reconceptualises the role of maritime quarantine. Rather than it being a door that prevented the importation of disease, Fairchild describes a modern system of immigration control, making the deceptively simple observation that quarantine officials very rarely turned people back after a long voyage; inspections and quarantines were important not so much because they excluded people with contagious diseases but because they included and initiated immigrants. This inclusion was not unconditional, however. It worked by showing immigrants their place in the hierarchy of the society into which they were attempting to gain entry. 'The assembly line of flesh and bone developed to defend the nation from diseased immigrants served as the inaugural event in the life of the new working class,' she writes. The event impressed upon the immigrant 'the national hierarchy and his or her low place in it'.[19] Quarantines and inspections defined the conditions of admittance to a new society.

In the late 1830s Sydney was growing in size, but its politics were also changing. The problems of unfree labour were intimately related to the politics of immigration as New South Wales made the transition from penal to free colonial society in this decade. Yet for convicts, it was not necessary to define conditions of admittance. Voyages of convict transportation were not discrete events; they were links in a chain that stretched from British and Irish hulks and prisons, on to ships and then through the colonial penal system. From land, to sea, and back to land, convicts remained within a coherent governmental system that channelled, controlled, and paid for their migration. At the border between land and sea, convicts did not change status; they remained convicts. 'Free' immigration was different; even the voyages that occurred under government supervision were less tightly controlled, questions about welfare and responsibility less certain. In contrast to convicts, at the edge of Australia emigrants did change status; they became immigrants.

The 1830s were a decade of intense political, social, and moral debate in New South Wales about immigration and settler relations with indigenous people.[20] Acutely conscious of status and a colonial discourse of respectability, the new Sydney elite were obsessed with morality and with delineating the boundaries of their society. Throughout the 1830s, colonial newspapers and *The Times* in London published letters objecting to the 'culpable negligence' of the British Emigration Committees who had begun assisting emigration, to John Marshall (a ship-owner contractor and agent who dominated the practical implementation of the early schemes), and to the immigrants themselves, particularly single women.[21] Influential colonists such as John Dunmore Lang objected that their money funded the immigration of ineligible British paupers, although only a very few ever migrated under the provisions of the Poor Law itself.

Between 1831 and 1835, 38 per cent of emigrants arriving in New South Wales were government assisted. Between 1836 and 1840, this percentage rose dramatically. Of the 28,985 immigrants arriving in New South Wales from Britain, 22,642 (85 per cent) did so under the auspices of formal schemes of government assistance and bounty schemes whereby colonists specified the kinds of immigrants they required and paid for their passage on arrival, if the new arrivals were deemed acceptable. Immigration was three times transportation in 1839, and by 1840 immigrants outnumbered convict arrivals by four to one.[22] The construction of a formal quarantine station, and the establishment of a permanent Health Officer in Port Jackson, coincided exactly with this period, and must be understood in this context. This colonial society, as one historian has put it, was decidedly 'prickly'.[23] By explicitly identifying certain groups of people with particular kinds of medical and moral failings, quarantine slowed down the emigrants' transition to immigrants, and made it highly visible.

Typhus

On 4 November 1836, the *Lady MacNaghten* sailed from Cork with 412 emigrants on board. The ship's company largely consisted of families selected by the British government's Emigration Committee. The surgeon's journal of the voyage presents a constant battle with fevers, measles, dysentery, and whooping cough during the three months' voyage. Surgeon Hawkins lamented that so many families and young children, apparently entirely unsuitable as settlers, had been allowed to embark on such a long voyage with few spare clothes and inadequate quantities of medical comforts.[24] When the *Lady MacNaghten* sailed into Sydney Harbour on 26 February 1837, ten adults and forty-four children had died during the voyage.[25] By now, Hawkins was dangerously ill – he later died – and the Colonial Assistant Surgeon reported that ninety persons on the *Lady MacNaghten* were sick;

seventy 'in a state of total helplessness' with a contagious fever, the others 'weakly convalescent'.[26]

The Sydney newspapers reacted immediately to the arrival of the *Lady MacNaghten*. On 27 February, the *Sydney Herald* declared the arrival of a 'fever ship' and pointedly remarked that it hoped 'that the strictest attention will be paid to the Quarantine Regulations to prevent so dreadful a malady spreading to Sydney'.[27] The *Sydney Monitor* was more sympathetic, but also condemned the 'deplorable state' of the 'ill-fated' passengers of the *Lady MacNaghten*.[28] The following day, the Colonial Secretary ordered that the ship be quarantined at the newly established station on North Head. Immigrants who remained 'immediately free of disease' would land and lodge in tents and sheds on shore, 'leaving all those who are really infected' on the *Lady MacNaghten*, which would become a hospital ship.[29] The Colonial Secretary employed an experienced naval surgeon at the quarantine station, while Dr Bowler, the Governor's surgeon who had first encountered the vessel offshore while on the *Rattlesnake*, remained with the sick, having joined the ship before it entered the harbour.[30] On 1 March, the *Government Gazette* publicly announced the quarantine. It lasted for forty-five days.[31]

Compared to diseases such as cholera, smallpox, and yellow fever, typhus has played a minor role in the history of modern quarantine.[32] In 1830s Sydney, however, it became crucial to the establishment of a permanent quarantine station. As we saw in Chapter 2, names such as camp, ship, nervous, malignant, and putrid fever had long described a disease that thrived in gaols, prisons hospitals, and, of course, ships. From about 1780, British descriptions of fever had also begun to develop a political edge. Reflecting the degeneration of the social body and produced in the poverty of the 'fever nest', the disease designated as typhus seemed to correspond with institutionalisation, urbanisation, and dislocation.[33] By 1846, David McConnell Reed would describe typhus as the disease of 'filthy, ill-fed, intemperate subjects'.[34] In short, typhus had become a particularly powerful signifier within a broad category of febrile disease. Typhus – and, by implication, the term fever – had become a politically loaded disease of the weak, redundant, and undeserving poor. In the 1830s Thomas Southwood Smith and Edwin Chadwick placed typhus at the heart of their debates about the sanitary condition of England and the workings of the Poor Law.[35] This conceptual framework was not restricted to urbanising Britain. Ideas about poverty, eligibility, and exclusion circulated around the British colonies in the first half of the nineteenth century and contributed to diverse discussions about respectability, status, and exclusion.[36]

In Sydney, typhus became an important part of these discussions as colonists carved out the boundaries of their society.

Five months after the *Lady MacNaghten*, the *John Barry* reached Port Jackson. Fifty cases of fever and nine deaths had occurred on the voyage. Alexander Neill, a naval surgeon who had recently arrived in Sydney on a convict ship, took medical charge of the quarantine station, the *John Barry*, and its immigrants. Neill described how eight of the passengers

> were labouring under typhus, in its most severe form … the disease became highly contagious attacking indiscriminately members of families of all ages but being most fatal in the robust … I was unfortunately seized with the disease, and had a very narrow escape … That the disease originates in the filthy habits of the people there cannot be a doubt, and from the state I found the 'between decks' of the *John Barry* I am only astonished that the fever did not sooner show itself.[37]

Slipping between the terms 'fever' and 'typhus', but clearly indicating that the disease at some point had *become* contagious, Neill pinpointed the disease's origin to the people's 'filthy habits'. Quarantine pitted surgeons against each other. Neill's judgment, ostensibly about the emigrants, also implicitly criticised his fellow surgeon, who had failed to ensure cleanliness during the voyage. Nevertheless, Neill's report also seemed to suggest that it was only *after* the *John Barry* had landed at Spring Cove that the fever became 'highly contagious, attacking indiscriminately'.[38] The *John Barry*'s experienced surgeon, David Thomson, conceded that a lack of cleanliness might have caused sickness to develop during the voyage, but he emphasised that the ship's diet was responsible for the children's illness. He argued that disease had originated *before* the beginning of the voyage, identifying four cases of scarlet fever that occurred about the time of leaving Dundee.[39]

When surgeons such as Neill and Thomson constructed disease aetiologies, they also constructed time-frames. In the case of the *John Barry*, three separate but equally plausible time-frames for disease are apparent. Thomson identified cases of scarlet fever before embarkation; both surgeons talked of general fever (not contagious) during the voyage; Neill discussed contagious fever in quarantine. By emphasising disease in terms of different times and places during the emigration process, Neill and Thomson placed and displaced the blame for the cause of contagion. The when, where, and why of contagion, and who had the authority to decide, were crucial, both for the performance of quarantine and for the professional position of the two medical men.

In 1839 the colonial assistant surgeon, James Stuart, gave evidence to a Parliamentary Committee about his experiences with emigrant ships. Stuart explained that in 1837 and 1838 he had 'frequently received instructions to attend professionally on the passengers and crew of emigrant ships having contagious diseases onboard'. Using William Cullen's term *gravior* to denote a violent or malignant typhus, Stuart explained that a common sickness on the *Lady MacNaghten*, *Amelia Thompson*, *John Barry* and *Minerva* had made quarantine measures necessary. During their voyages, these ships had displayed 'all the forms of continued inflammatory fever, and wherever there were children, hooping-cough and scarlatina, with diarrhoea, dysentery and measles'. Stuart unhesitatingly attributed all these ailments to the same cause: 'the over-crowding of the ships, and want of due ventilation and cleanliness, which must dispose the constitution to inflammatory disease'. Any spaces in the *Lady MacNaghten* and *Minerva* between the luggage and bulkheads, or below the decks, he noted, were 'filled with every sort of filth, broken biscuit, bones, rags and refuse of every description, putrifying [*sic*] and filled with maggots'. In addition, the water closets confined between decks created an 'impure, heavy and almost insufferable' atmosphere.[40]

Surgeons who had superintended voyages had their own explanations of disease. In 1839, the *North Britain* spent forty-one days in quarantine in Sydney. Surgeon Miller carefully avoided using the word contagion, but did describe typhus as 'the most formidable and fatal' of the fevers he encountered during the voyage. Typhus caused twenty deaths on board, and a further six in quarantine. Miller himself suffered a 'very severe attack', which prevented him from assisting the sick for the final seventeen days of the voyage. The first case of typhus, Miller thought, must have been 'imported from the shore'. The second case of typhus was Laurence Rice, a ploughman of 'indolent and dirty habits'. The third patient was John Loyd, of a 'broken constitution'. Loyd had embarked in 'a nervous and debilitated frame of body and mind, from intemperance and drinking'. Loyd died of typhus, and two weeks later so did his wife. Such a family coincidence did not necessarily indicate contagion. After the death of John, the surgeon explained that Elizabeth Loyd had been 'in great lowness of spirits'. Another man who developed typhus should have recovered, 'but he got up and went on deck in wet cold weather' and suffered a relapse. Another man who relapsed 'abandoned all hopes of recovery' and died.[41] In the surgeon's explanation, the environmental circumstances of the voyage aggravated emigrants' individual constitutional weaknesses and created disease. Miller took care to point out other factors beyond his control: the ship's hospital was dark and ill-ventilated and bad weather necessitated keeping the people below 'when it would have been very desirable to have them on deck'.[42]

While Stuart and Miller both proposed arguments about disease that were essentially defensive, these served different purposes. Stuart was justifying his extensive use of quarantine to parliamentary inquiry; he cared little for nuances, he needed generalised, big-picture medical diagnosis: voyages caused disease because the people were filthy, and he drew on the common knowledge that fevers held the potential to become intractable and contagious in dirty, ill-ventilated, crowded conditions. Ships such as the *North Britain*, he argued, were 'one great exciting cause of disease'.[43] Miller's detailed description was more environmentally and constitutionally sensitive. Miller was responsible for one particular voyage, and risked losing his pay if his medical care was found wanting. He focused on individuals and pin-pointed precise turning-points. For Miller, disease was the result of the constant interaction between environmental circumstance and constitutional predisposition, and he did what he could. As he built his narrative of the voyage, Miller played the part of the heroic naval surgeon well; he was adamant that his 'unsparing' use of bloodletting had subdued the cases of inflammatory and rheumatic fevers, and thus prevented more cases of typhus occurring.[44] Despite their differences, both surgeons believed that voyages were pathological processes demanding constant vigilance, and not a little luck with the weather. Both surgeons also relied on the fluidity of febrile identity, and the capacity of ailments to evolve as voyage conditions changed. Although they gave very different accounts, it is clear from both that contagious diseases were not simply 'brought' from Britain.

When the *William Roger* arrived on 26 September 1838, the colonial government had recently appointed a Health Officer and constructed permanent buildings on the quarantine site to house the sick as well as the healthy.[45] It was a busy period for Sydney's Medical Board: only the month before it had investigated Obadiah Pineo's superintendence of the scurvy-stricken convict ship *Lord Lyndoch*. In regard to the *William Roger*, the Health Officer and the Board decided that the cases of disease did not appear 'to exhibit any peculiar malignancy' and it 'did not seem necessary to land the emigrants'. Another ship, the *Palmyra*, arrived the same day, and its situation seemed much more urgent. The surgeon reported that forty cases of scarlet fever had occurred during the voyage. The immigrants of the *William Roger* stayed on board and watched as their counterparts from the *Palmyra* landed at the quarantine station.[46] Within a few days, the new Governor, George Gipps, had released both ships from quarantine. However, as the *William Roger* anchored in Darling Harbour, ready to disembark its immigrants, fever broke out 'with renewed violence'. The Water Police (established in 1832) prevented all communication with the shore until a steamer towed the ship back through the harbour to the quarantine station. This time, the *William Roger*'s immigrants did land and occupied the four new buildings on the quarantine site. Over the following six weeks, fever became typhus 'of the most malignant kind'. Of the 140 persons who were attacked, 25 died.[47]

The *William Roger*'s surgeon, John Reid, was furious. In his report (entitled a 'Correct Statement of Deaths') he proposed a range of causes to explain the fever. First, more attention should have been paid in Britain to the selection of the emigrants; several of those who died 'had their constitutions entirely destroyed by intemperance previous to their embarkation'. Second, the sudden transition from hot to cold climate after crossing the equator had caused the initial cases of fever. His third point was more daring. Reid declared that the fever had only become contagious *after* the emigrants had been put in quarantine. If the Sydney physicians had removed the emigrants from the unhealthy ship immediately, the fever would not have become contagious and endangered the whole ship's company.[48]

Reid penned his report while in quarantine, and he warned of dire consequences; the emigrants' spirits 'are getting depressed after the long voyage and the thought of being detained any time on board with those that are sick'. He had 'no doubt the sooner they are set at liberty the better'.[49] James Lawrence, another naval surgeon who had recently arrived with the emigrants of the *Westminster* (and complained bitterly about the impossibility of ventilating his own ship), supported Reid: 'if the emigrants had been landed immediately on their arrival, instead of being kept as they were a fortnight on board the ship, few cases of fever would have occurred'.[50] Governor Gipps acknowledged that 'it will be scarcely ever possible to prove misconduct or inefficiency against a surgeon', but he nonetheless withheld the pay of the captain and crew of the *William Roger*, as well as surgeon Reid's gratuity.[51] Reid's loss was considerable; surgeons could expect to receive £200 for their superintendence of a voyage.[52]

Even as the immigrants of the *William Roger* remained in quarantine, the *Maitland* arrived in Sydney in November 1838. Whereas Reid had openly criticised the Health Officer and Medical Board, the surgeon of the *Maitland* was more circumspect, even calculating, in his response to quarantine. He 'determined to err on the right side … and not afford an opportunity for my moral character to be impeached'. Smith was unsure about two of his cases. He believed that they might have been hydrocephalus, but the cases displayed prominent 'typhoid symptoms'. Smith was well aware that a 'typhoid fever' had made 'great ravages' on the *William Roger*, and noted the 'dreadful apprehensions' that 'existed in the mind of the Health Officer' when the *Maitland* arrived. John Dobie, the first Health Officer for Port Jackson, was, Smith knew, a 'strong advocate for contagion'. After some deliberation, Smith confirmed the cases as typhus, and the *Maitland* remained in quarantine for fifty-six days.

Smith knew that by choosing the term typhus he might succeed in diverting attention away from his own 'moral character' and towards that of the immigrants. Reid's recent experience on the *William Roger* must have reminded Smith that naval surgeons whose ships ended up in quarantine were in a vulnerable position. Aware that he was under intense scrutiny, Smith offered a full range of causes. Early cases of scarlatina 'must have been imported onto the ship'.[53] Seasickness, anxiety, and fatigue early in the voyage had predisposed other emigrants to disease. Moving further into the voyage, Smith described the aggravated form of disease in the warm latitudes, the great number of emigrants in the ship, and the failures of the parents to feed their children properly.[54] The *Maitland* brought parish-assisted immigrants to New South Wales under the provisions of the Poor Law Amendment Act. Disease, Smith said, 'prevailed nearly in all those families which were in the greatest destitution and who were parochial paupers'. In both health and disease these 'were a very intractable and dissatisfied description of persons'.[55]

Smith had used the powerful language of pauperism to blur the medical events of the voyage into a contemporary discourse of eligibility, worth, and respectability that linked social and political debate in Britain and its colonies. The newly incumbent Governor Gipps confessed that he did not know whether the filthy and diseased state of the *Maitland*'s emigrants resulted from Smith's failure to assert control, their poor state of health when they embarked, or because they came from a poorer class of society.[56] Having set a precedent with surgeon Reid from the *William Roger*, Gipps decided that he would not pay Smith either. Gipps was still frustrated, and set up a colonial Medical Board to discover why ships with government emigrants seemed to suffer so much disease, even after naval surgeons had been made responsible for the selection of government emigrants in 1837. The Board reported that neither the surgeon of the *Maitland* nor that of the *William Roger* had in fact seen their emigrants until the day of embarkation.[57] Colonial accounts suggest that Gipps relented a little; the careful surgeon Smith did receive his money in the end.[58] However, as Gipps pondered the problem of immigrant ships and fever at the end of 1838, he observed that 'a talent for managing men [...] is no less necessary in a surgeon selected to bring out emigrants than medical skill'.[59] John Reid seemed unable to manage either the emigrants on his ship or his professional relationships with the colonial officers. After his angry outbursts about quarantine causing contagion, Reid did not receive his pay.[60]

The modern conception that diseases like typhus are specific biomedical entities, unchanged by time and distance, simply did not exist in the first half of the nineteenth century. When surgeons explained typhus, they did not refer to epidemic typhus in Britain and Ireland.[61] Similarly, although lice and 'vermin' were a constant problem at sea, they were not part of typhus' explanatory framework, as they are now.[62] In 1999 Peter Baldwin proposed that states responded to epidemic disease in the nineteenth century on 'a geo-epidemiological learning curve', in which 'sheer distance from the source and pathways of epidemic advance gave nations thus blessed a sense of security and room to manoeuvre that those closer to the front lines found hard to emulate'.[63] Because both Baldwin's geographical models and, indeed, historians' criticisms of such models rely on the idea of a time and distance barrier, they have failed to take into account the extent to which contemporaries understood voyages themselves as a productive physical and temporal event.[64] Voyages were not simply a vector for pathogens that could be calculated in terms of distance from a fount of disease. In effect, they filled that space in. Voyages were assemblages of people's life histories, the problems of ships, prolonged maritime confinement, and constantly changing environments. During this process, fevers continually evolved.

In addition, as surgeons attempted to deflect attention away from their own authority, they looked for disease before and after the voyage. Some surgeons indignantly suggested that quarantine processes created contagion where none had existed before; others argued that individual emigrants embarked in a sick state, and used the language of pauperism as both a medical and a social diagnosis. Discussions that focus on time and distance, or on how states construct policy, obscure the fact that quarantine has always been a practice ordered by certain people, in a certain place, at a certain time, against certain outsiders.[65] So what did quarantine *mean* in 1830s Sydney?

Newspapers

In a politicised and factious atmosphere, the significance of quarantined immigrants reverberated beyond the medical debates of the quarantine station. Colonists were concerned about typhus, but they objected even more strongly to the immigrants who suffered from it. They readily seized on the moral and political significance of typhus and contagious fever as a marker of poverty. Caught in the middle, immigrants – who considered themselves hard working and respectable – understood quarantine as a slur, a judgment on their capacity as colonists at the moment when they were least secure, when they, quite literally, did not yet have any solid ground on which to stand. Newspapers played a determining role in the discussions that ensued.

When the *Lady MacNaghten* arrived in Sydney, soon after the end of a female emigration scheme to which colonists had violently objected, the *Sydney Monitor* quickly condemned the British Whig government and the 'weak imbecile head' of the Emigration Committee who had selected the emigrants in Ireland. The newspaper accused John Marshall, the Committee's agent as well as the *Lady MacNaghten*'s owner and contractor, of being a 'murderer of the poor Girls', and condemned his 'avaricious packing' of emigrants on the ship.[66]

Throughout March, the language of contagious fever took centre stage in the commentary about the *Lady MacNaghten*'s quarantine. While the *Monitor* retained some sympathy for the immigrants, and suggested that the sickness was 'not of that virulent character which has been represented', the *Sydney Herald* cried contagion, and descriptions of the 'fever ship' were integral to its critique.[67] The *Herald* repeated its hope that the fatal and contagious effects of overcrowding on the *Lady MacNaghten* would be the 'death-blow' to the 'abominable system' of British government-assisted emigration.[68] These were immigrants selected from 'the lowest of the low' and who had embarked in a filthy state, the *Herald* claimed.[69] On 17 April, as most of the passengers from the *Lady MacNaghten* finally left quarantine, the *Herald* scoffed that the colonists would be plundered to the 'delightful tune' of £8,000 to fund the quarantine. Three days later, the *Herald* grudgingly printed a 'ridiculous puff' from the *Lady MacNaghten*'s immigrants, who wished to thank the Colonial Secretary for the care they had received in quarantine. The *Herald* objected that these 'officials' had spent the money of colonists who 'must not continue to be robbed, in order to import useless persons and deadly diseases'.[70]

Certainly, the *Herald* attempted to use the immigrants' letter to its own advantage, but it did print it. Newspapers were more than the mouthpiece for the colonists' vitriol; they were a public forum which immigrants, even as they remained in quarantine, could use to vigorously defend their respectability. As they put forward their own understandings of disease, immigrants attempted to counteract the effect of the colonists' opinions on their future prospects. As early as 1837, the steerage passengers of the *Lady MacNaghten* realised this and used the newspapers to contradict the 'aspersions' that the colonial settlers and officials had 'thrown upon' them.

On 20 March 1837, almost a month before the *Herald* printed their letter of thanks, the *Monitor* had reprinted in full a letter from the *Lady MacNaghten* immigrants. This letter, filling nearly two columns of a broadsheet page, refuted the *Herald*'s initial 'lies'. The steerage passengers described themselves principally as mechanics who had left their homes 'to better our condition'. They reminded the colonists that in this respect they were no different from 'men of rank and property' who 'daily undertook these actions'. As we saw in the previous chapter, the steerage emigrants of the *Lady MacNaghten* believed that the crew's treatment of the women – forcing them below decks early in the afternoon during the heat of the tropics so that they fainted and nearly suffocated – went a long way towards explaining why the entire ship had suffered from fever during the voyage. The crew had also thrown their boxes of belongings overboard and broken their valuables 'to atoms'. Regarding sickness, the letter stated that the first two children had died through 'want of proper sustenance', and men and women had also pined away. The immigrants denied as 'a direct falsehood' the *Herald*'s accusation that they were 'the lowest of the low'.[71]

In part, the official Medical Board inquiry into the circumstances of the voyage was a direct response to this letter alleging ill-treatment from the moment of embarkation. Despite hearing further evidence from steerage and cabin passengers alike, the Board concluded that there was little to support the immigrants' claims of ill-treatment.[72] Six months after the ship had arrived in Sydney, the *Herald* published carefully selected extracts from the Board's report to renew its condemnation of the immigrants and the Emigration Committee. In particular, the *Herald* seized upon the words of the deceased surgeon, who had written that the emigrants 'disregard anything save animal enjoyment, they will be found a useless burden instead of a benefit to the colony'.[73]

For the colonists, the question of quarantine must have seemed a continuous saga in 1837 and 1838. On 14 August 1837 – the same day as it reported the results of the *Lady MacNaghten* inquiry – the *Herald* published a letter from the quarantined steerage passengers of the *John Barry* which emphasised the ship's poor ventilation and crowded state. The cabin passengers had taken up the space of the hospital with their baggage, the letter alleged, and fever had first appeared not in the steerage quarters, but among the wealthier passengers in the ship's cabin. The authors had been 'astonished when the surgeon reported typhus fever', believing that disease had been 'trifling at the time we reached the shore'.[74]

While the letters from the *Lady MacNaghten* represented the immigrants as a united body, the correspondence from the *John Barry* reveals that deep divisions had emerged in steerage during the voyage. The following day, 15 August 1837, the *Sydney Gazette* explained that the first letter was only 'the sole production of an individual who rendered himself conspicuous by his grumbling, discontented spirit on the voyage'.[75] Over the following weeks, the newspapers printed a series of exchanges containing differing opinions from the *John Barry*. A letter to the *Herald* from a 'considerable portion of the steerage passengers, or rather emigrants', denied having anything to do with 'such calumnious stuff'. The surgeon's conduct was 'more like an indulgent parent than one in authority over us', the hospital had been 'the best ventilated part of the vessel', and the disease first appeared 'in a family that had never set foot' in the first-class quarters.[76] The surgeon, David Thomson, was determined that his view of the situation would prevail, and he closed the argument in a letter dated 31 August:

> I was constantly urging the necessity of greater cleanliness, and often predicted that fever or even the plague would certainly break out … Painful as it is to me to hurt the feelings of many respectable men among the emigrants, I must declare that Typhus Fever on board the *John Barry* … was the legitimate offspring of DIRT; and that had my advice been attended to, that disease would never have appeared.[77]

As far as the colonists were concerned, however, the *John Barry* immigrants had provided proof of their worth. They had passed the time in quarantine by constructing a beacon – which had been 'for some time contemplated' – on North Head.[78] The *Herald* decided that, as mechanics or agriculturalists who had been specified by colonists through a bounty scheme, rather than selected by the British government, they were 'not only likely to be of great benefit to the colony, but also, to do credit to the country they have left'.[79] Immigrants were intensely conscious of the social ramifications of quarantine, and a further letter from the *John Barry* signed 'A Steerage Passenger' perfectly encapsulates these fears:

> We did not expect to engage in contributing to the columns of a newspaper…. We have been reluctantly dragged before the public,

while many of us are placed in sorrowful circumstances, and all in a disagreeable situation, but we think it our bounden duty to reply, when the most malicious falsehoods are palmed upon us.[80]

Ships such as the *Lady MacNaghten*, *John Barry*, *Minerva*, and *Maitland* provoked political condemnations, objections to immigrants, passionate defences, medical disagreements, and formal representations which all played out in the colonial newspapers. The threat of contagious fever struck at the heart of broader discussions about honesty, eligibility, class, and labour that circulated in the colony. Surgeons chose their words carefully as they reported to the Health Officer on arrival. Those who objected too loudly to quarantine risked losing their pay. These quarantines were about voyages, at the same time as they reflected and fed on colonial anxieties.

Yet quarantine did not often come as a complete surprise for emigrants; the possibility often loomed long before ships came within sight of land. Arriving in Sydney on 16 January 1839, 'after the number of deaths that had occurred on board', a writer on board the *Alfred* was relieved yet surprised that the immigration officer cleared the ship to enter the colony. During the voyage there were 'great fears entertained at one time that we should be sent to the quarantine ground'.[81] As surgeons compiled their case notes, and considered the wording of their reports in the last days at sea, crew and emigrants cleaned, scrubbed, tarred, and whitewashed, and extracted their best clothes from the stored luggage. By making a good impression in this way, many believed that they had 'nothing to fear from the Health Officer in the way of quarantine'.[82] These efforts often paid off. When the *Florist* arrived in Sydney its company was healthier than when it left Gravesend in June.[83] The Agent for Immigration noted that its immigrants were of 'a good class' and the colonists engaged them all in employment within two days of landing. The Agent commended the surgeon for fostering a 'spirit of healthy competition' in cleaning the berths and deck of the ship.[84] Colonists' advertisements for labourers emphasised exactly these qualities: immigrants 'must be of *good health and character*'; those of 'industrious and steady character, are certain of immediate and constant employment', one notice said.[85] The voyage provided evidence, and colonists responded to immigrants who had displayed qualities of resourcefulness, competition, and pride and, crucially, arrived free of disease. Clean, healthy ships demonstrated immigrants' mental and moral suitability for the colony, by explicitly reinforcing the pervasive association of moral value with physical cleanliness.

'*A lovely spot*'

As the colonial economy of New South Wales entered the depression of the 1840s, the British government suspended its schemes of emigrant assistance. Convict transportation to New South Wales had come to an end by 1840. After the Sydney authorities had so frequently used quarantine between 1837 and 1841, the new Health Officer for Port Jackson used the legislation only once between 1842 and 1848. Neither news of the Irish famine and the 'fever ships' that sailed to North America in 1847 nor the cholera epidemic of 1848–49 provoked any great fear.[86] The *Sarah* left Britain in the midst of the second cholera epidemic. Although cases of cholera continued during the voyage, the ship did not have to enter quarantine.[87]

During the 1840s, when the quarantine station was rarely used, the isolation of North Head drew writers and artists who emphasised its associations with disease and death. Louise Ann Meredith's *Notes and Sketches of New South Wales* (1844) described the quarantine ground as a burial place for 'those unhappy exiles who die during the time of ordeal, and those whose golden dreams of the far-sought land of promise lead but to a lone and desolate grave on its storm-beaten shore'.[88] In 1847, George French Angas came upon the quarantine ground 'unexpectedly in a joyous and merry mood, but instantly felt the influence of the scene'. Describing the 'tombstones of spectral whiteness', Angas declared that he had

> seen no spot where the dead repose which is more melancholy or more exquisitely picturesque than this lonely burial place in the wilderness, where the howling of the storm and the muffled beat of the surge sound a requiem to the dead – those hapless dead, who voyaged so many thousand miles, hopeful and expectant, and perished at the very entrance of the looked for harbour.[89]

In Angas' representations North Head was a wilderness and a place of exile where hopes died, and people perished 'unknelled, uncoffined, and unknown'.[90] These romanticised representations of quarantine are alluring, but also deceptive. The vast majority of emigrants who arrived in Australia did so in good health, even on ships that were quarantined. Healthy people did not automatically associate the physical environments of these lonely headlands with disease and death. Quarantine was as much a social construction as it was an environmental or medical experience. For immigrants it was as much the newspaper correspondence, the cairns, armed soldiers, and medical judgements that made quarantine awful, rather than the place itself.[91]

For example, black crosses had peppered the margins of Charles Scott's diary on the *Annie Wilson*. After the ship had passed the equator, death continued 'making its harvest'. On their arrival in Sydney, Scott explained that 'the Government officials came alongside of us and said on account of sickness that we had on board we must go into Quarantine for a few days'.[92] At sea, Scott had written of his belief that 'I shall not enjoy good health until I land'. Within hours of arrival, he found his health 'greatly improving'. Scott soon forgot sickness as the passengers ate fresh meat, broth, potatoes, and bread. 'It is a lovely day and a lovely spot that we are upon, I should like to live and pass the remainder of my life upon this spot,' he declared. Scott spent his quarantine days 'rambling upon the sea shore, picking oysters, periwinkles, cockles, Limpets [*sic*], crabbs or rambling over the craggs of rocks'.[93] Nevertheless, if after months at sea the physical place of quarantine often appeared as a natural paradise as for Scott, other newly arrived migrants remained more sensitive to its real purpose.

'Watched like felons'

As the second half of the nineteenth century began, Australian colonial society had changed beyond all recognition. Prospectors' discovery of gold further transformed the appeal of the Australian colonies as a destination for migrants. As well as from Britain and Ireland, more ships came from other European countries, California, and China. Health officers continued to quarantine for typhus, but increasingly for other infectious diseases, including measles, smallpox, and scarlet fever. In 1854 the Health Officer at Sydney quarantined a ship for cholera for the first time; this unfortunate vessel was the *David McIvor*, the vessel that would gain such a bad reputation over the following years.[94]

In January 1853 the *Beejapore* arrived in Sydney from Liverpool with 929 emigrants. At the time, this was the largest number of colonists ever taken in one vessel. When the *Beejapore* arrived after a voyage of only eighty-five days (three days faster than the previous record), no other ships had arrived with news from Britain for several weeks; the *Beejapore* had also arrived earlier than two screw steamers that had set off before her.[95] The rapidity of the voyage had 'astonished everyone', Osborne Johnson, one of the *Beejapore*'s two surgeons wrote, a fact which had 'no doubt induced the health officer to visit us so soon'.[96] The size of the *Beejapore*, the number of immigrants, the speed with which it had reached Sydney, the number of sick, not to mention that fifty-six deaths had occurred during the voyage, worried the Sydney officials. The Health Officer, Haynes Gibbes Alleyne, quarantined the

Beejapore as the surgeon reported that cases of measles and scarlet fever remained.

Watching for ships was one of the longest-standing pastimes in the colony of Sydney. Until the 1840s, the sight of sails arriving in Port Jackson was signalled by the raising of a flag on Flagstaff Hill (now the site of the Sydney Observatory).[97] Men from the newspapers raced each other in rowing boats to be the first to handle the precious news from Britain in newspapers and letters. As voyages got faster and more frequent, these habits persisted. William Usherwood, a cabin passenger, described the first visits of the colonists to the *Beejapore* – and noted their particular interest in the newspapers it carried – as it anchored in Port Jackson:

> The reporter from the *Sydney Morning Herald* also came alongside but was not allowed to communicate with us except at a distance by word of mouth. After we were brought up we were visited by the Quarantine Master who took our despatches from us with a pair of tongs & deposited them in a tin case. [N]ot so however the newspapers which we gave them they were received with open hands, opened, and the dates examined immediately, he in return gave us a 'Sydney Empire' which was very acceptable.[98]

Consistent with ideas that contagion could stick to clothes, fabric, bedding, and material goods, the disinfection of mail and despatches was a regular – if deeply frustrating – aspect of the quarantine ritual. Each envelope or package would be pricked with holes or slit open and the papers within treated with a sulphurous smoke, before being sent onwards. In the excitement about the *Beejapore*'s record voyage and the recent newspapers it carried, however, even the Quarantine Master apparently forgot his concerns about contagion; newspapers were too important, too exciting, for further delay.

The quarantine station's distance from Sydney was designed to effect isolation, but the early history of Australian quarantine is dominated by the newspapers (and letters written to them) that continually travelled back and forth through Port Jackson. Despite its apparent spatial rigidity, quarantine was a decidedly porous rhetorical space. Newspapers are a recurring motif in Usherwood's diary, and he often referred to the newspapers that frequently arrived from Sydney. As they kept up with the local news, the *Beejapore*'s cabin passengers felt the need to write to the *Herald* in reply to the article that had announced their quarantine two weeks earlier:

> We are convinced that from the paragraph announcing the arrival of

the ship, how much alarm has been needlessly created in the minds of the resident colonists. That, by this time, the sanatory condition of the emigrants must have been held as truly deplorable to themselves, and extremely dangerous to the future health of the colonial population. Our object in the present communication is, therefore, to disabuse the minds of the population of New South Wales, through the columns of your journal, & have our case brought directly under the consideration of the colonial authorities.[99]

The *Beejapore* passengers emphasised that the thirteen patients currently in the Doctor's hands were all children. As the emigrants of the *Lady MacNaghten* had done eighteen years earlier, the *Beejapore*'s passengers used letters to dissociate themselves from disease. But there are also significant differences in the two letters. The wealthy cabin passengers of the *Beejapore* did not fear that their whole future was at stake, and they did not need to convince colonists that they were not the 'lowest of the low'. Cabin passengers could assume their place in colonial society; they did not need to fight for it, as the immigrants of the *Lady MacNaghten* had done. The *Beejapore* passengers requested that someone in the colony send them a copy of the quarantine regulations 'for perusal', in order to understand on what grounds the authorities had detained the ship. The sense of desperation apparent in the earlier quarantine correspondence from steerage passengers is absent here. This was more a matter of correcting a misunderstanding. Nevertheless, there is a whiff of indignation in the passengers' request. The passengers of the *Beejapore* accepted that quarantine was governed by rules. However, wealthy passengers understood travel in general as a process in which they were free to define how and when they moved through social space, in a way that steerage passengers were not. William Usherwood accepted that such a strict quarantine could be justified, even necessitated, by the 'immense tide of immigration now flowing to these colonies', but also described the troops that patrolled the boundaries of the quarantine station, who had orders 'to shoot anyone going beyond this boundary line, more especially the sick coming into the healthy people's ground'.[100]

Two years later, Charles Moore declared Sydney's quarantine headland 'a most beautiful place to look at' after a voyage in which he had been able to focus on little except smallpox on the *Constitution*.[101] As Moore got to know the landscape of North Head better, his enthusiasm subsided. The natural beauty of the headland jarred with the physical demarcation of space defined by ideas about disease and outsiders. Moore explained that he dared not go beyond the cairns:

'there are sentry boxes for solgers in case of a queer lot and we don't want them to come if we can help it for it is a nasty slur on us the disease as been quite enough'.[102] Like other steerage passengers before him, Moore interpreted quarantine as a judgement.

Similar sentiments were expressed beyond Sydney. On 16 August 1854 a pilot boat from Melbourne greeted the SS *Great Britain*. When the Medical Inspector boarded, he ordered a boat to take three men who suffered from smallpox to the quarantine ground. One passenger, William Bray, recorded with satisfaction that he successfully passed by the inspector. 'I was only asked by him if I had been vaccinated, to which having well remembered being told by mother that I was I said "yes".' As the *Great Britain* anchored, it 'thundered forth a round of 12 guns in triumph and let go her anchor for the good'. The passengers were afforded a 'pleasant view of the city of Melbourne'. With a flourish, Bray signed off, believing that his voyage account ended here. His excitement and feeling of triumph soon ebbed. The following day he began a new notebook entitled 'Lying Quarantine in the Great Britain'. 'To day has been a very long and tedious day,' he wrote. As the Health Officer detained the passengers of the SS *Great Britain*, Bray wrote that they had 'unfortunately subjected ourselves' to the severity of the quarantine laws 'from our having had some 3 or 4 cases of smallpox'. The Medical Inspector's questions seem to have provoked a twinge of uncertainty and doubt in Bray, a nagging feeling of collective responsibility for their situation. On 13 August 1854 – just three days before arrival – one of the *Great Britain*'s sailors had died of smallpox. There had been no public committal of the body to the sea and William Bray supposed that the body of the sailor had been 'thrown overboard in the night' so that the man's death might 'be kept as secret as long as possible from a fear that we shall be obleiged [*sic*] in consequence to lie in quarantine, which would be far from pleasant to us'.[103]

As in Sydney, quarantine facilities in Port Phillip had been constructed in response to the first waves of immigrants over a decade earlier. The first assisted emigrants to boost the squatter population of Port Phillip District had arrived from Sydney in 1839. In June of that year the first immigrants to sail directly from Britain arrived on the *David Clarke*. Between 1840 and 1842 another eleven thousand immigrants, mainly families, arrived under a bounty scheme. Lieutenant Governor La Trobe established a quarantine station near the Port Phillip lighthouse, a 'desolate and forsaken' place, also the base of the Water Police.[104] Throughout the 1840s Port Phillip suffered a chronic labour shortage, but the scheme to send Britain's reformed and rebranded 'exiles' from the new prison at Pentonville attracted growing resentment during the second half of the decade, and was abandoned by 1849.[105]

From a stream, immigration to Port Phillip became a flood during the 1850s. With the discovery of gold, Melbourne 'grew from a small and unknown pioneer settlement into a proud metropolis'.[106] From 1852 to 1855 between thirty and forty-eight thousand immigrants sailed to Victoria each year.[107] The British government chartered double-decked ships, including the *Ticonderoga*, *Wanata*, and *Bourneouf*, to meet demand. The *SS Great Britain*, launched in 1843, was the first large ship to have a hull built with iron, and combined sails with steam. By the 1850s, it regularly sailed the Liverpool–Melbourne route.

Confined within the quarantine rail in 1854, William Bray was at liberty to roam, but words such as 'bondage', 'incarceration', and 'imprisonment' pepper his account. If found beyond the quarantine ground he, and his fellow passengers from the *SS Great Britain*, 'would subject ourselves to being *then and there shot dead immediately* by the Horse Guards and mounted police keeping sentry over us'. If they escaped, Bray believed they would be taken, imprisoned for six months, and made to pay a fine of £300. 'If unable to pay', Bray continued, they would be 'ironed and put to work on the roads *for 7 years*'.[108] Although he had anticipated a spell in quarantine before reaching the land, Bray soon developed a sense that the quarantine was an unjust infringement of his liberty. It was, he wrote, 'a most dreadful affair' that 'six or seven hundred souls all healthy and strong in our own colonial port' could be obliged to submit 'to this awful incarceration' and 'watched like felons'. Bray's writing suggests a sense of colonial possession – this was 'our' port – and it directly plays on references to Australia's penal beginnings. In quarantine, 'we are cast out from all society and not allowed to correspond or exchange words with any of God's creatures in this lower world'. To make matters worse, the captain of the *SS Great Britain* had refused to obey initial orders to return to the entrance to Port Phillip some forty miles from Melbourne. On the second day of the quarantine, the *HMS Fantome* 'sent us a message in the shape of a cannon ball … which fully satisfied the Captain that he must obey the orders'.[109]

As Bray's days in quarantine became a second week, the colonial doctor requested that 'all those not having had the smallpox' were to be vaccinated. A week later again, the request became an order; all of the passengers must be vaccinated, before being permitted to enter Melbourne.[110] We saw in Chapter 5 that vaccination at sea performed two functions: it protected voyages from outbreaks of smallpox, and it enabled surgeons to transmit live lymph to the colonies. Here, in quarantine, the vaccination and revaccination of passengers at the boundaries of the colony became part of the process of admittance. By infecting disease matter directly into the body, vaccination worked, as Alison Bashford has put it, 'rather more through a logic of contagion, than a logic of quarantine'.[111] The two processes here overlapped. As an element of Australian quarantine practice, vaccination worked as a form of medical bargaining: if you allow us to vaccinate you, the health officers could say, we will release you from quarantine. Because vaccination was not reliable it coexisted with, rather than displaced, ongoing strategies of isolation and chemical practices of fumigation. After three weeks of camping at the Port Phillip quarantine ground, and submission to a second vaccination, William Bray landed in Melbourne. He deeply resented his 'incarceration' but also acknowledged that his days in quarantine had given him an opportunity to exercise after so many weeks at sea. Quarantine had given him 'a good appetite' and 'much additional strength'. Bray believed that the time he spent in quarantine had improved his health as he prepared for his new life working on the gold diggings.

Conclusion: carving the rocks of North Head

In a period that lasted 150 years, from 1832 to 1984, thirteen thousand people were quarantined at Sydney's North Head for diseases including typhus, smallpox, plague, cholera, and measles.[112] These quarantines lasted from two to ninety-six days. During that time, the headland became, quite literally, a slate onto which immigrants carved and etched an enduring record of their voyaging, as well as the fact of their arrival. On the rock faces of the cliffs, boulders, and the outcrops known as 'Old Man's Hat', over two thousand rock carvings still adorn the physical environment of North Head, which at times must have been alive with the sound of rock being scratched, chipped, and carved. Far outnumbering literary records of quarantine, the carvings are a vast visual archive that reflects the changing role of the station. The earliest motifs date from 1813, before the cove officially became a quarantine station. By the early twentieth century, Asian writing covered the cliffs nearest the beach. From later still, etched graffiti and pencil-drawn maps depicting Fiji and Tonga decorate the painted walls inside the station's buildings. From the colonial government's earliest quarantines against British and Irish immigrants in the nineteenth century, to a strident defence of a nation defined by its sea borders and explicitly coded white in the twentieth century, the very fabric of the quarantine station charts Australia's changing global relationships in the modern era.[113]

Many of the etchings are in the form of initials, their creators unidentifiable. We cannot know who 'ECB' is, for example, or when he or she stayed at the station. Others inscribed surnames with dates or ships. One reads: 'G. Larnack, per William Rodger 1838'. Another records 'E. Medcalf Dec[r] 1839'; the date confirms that this was one of the emigrants of the *North Britain*. In 1995, Jean Foley recorded the existence of a much larger plaque, parts of which are now illegible, that reads:

> I Dawson landed here to perform quarantine
> on the 11th of September A.D. 1835 with his wife [Emily?]
> [with?] 3 sons 5 daughters from Lincolnshire
> on the ship Canton of London.
> In the reign of William IV
> Britain and Ireland.[114]

Dawson's record memorialised the arrival of a whole family in an unusually elaborate way. Many of the etchings, like Dawson's, are shallow and exposed, and some have disappeared. The most striking carvings are a series of large, formal plaques on the boulders set back from the quarantine landing beach. Each records the quarantine of a whole ship. One plaque memorialises the *Lady Elma Bruce*, from Liverpool in 1850 with 308 emigrants. Surgeon J.S. Hughes must have had mixed feelings as he watched Mr Marshall, the mason, carve a record of the *Neneveh*'s quarantine in 1875, next to the record of his earlier voyage with the *Annie Wilson* (Figure 6). Another plaque nearby records the arrival of the *Telegraph* from Liverpool with 370 emigrants in 1860 and reveals that Hughes in fact underwent three periods in quarantine.

The history of quarantine stations is a history of what it meant to make the transition from emigrant to immigrant, and it is never just about disease. In the middle of the nineteenth century Australian quarantine was all at once about the backgrounds from which British and Irish labouring people had come, the experience of voyaging, the problems of being at sea, and the wider moral and political concerns of rapidly expanding and changing colonies. In diaries, rock carvings, artistic impressions, maps, medical diagnoses, and the to and fro of newspaper debate, the primary function of quarantine – to confine people and things suspected of contagion – emerged in different ways, for different reasons, and with varying degrees of intensity for all the people involved.

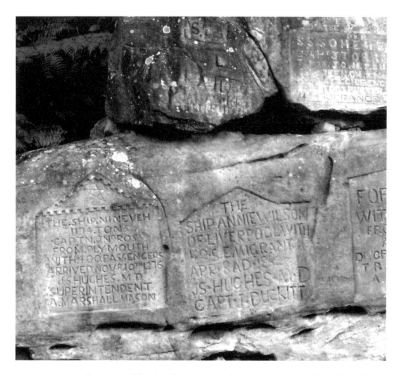

Figure 6   Surgeon Hughes' carvings, Quarantine Landing Beach,
Spring Cove, New South Wales.

For many of the early emigrants who spent days and weeks on the sheltered beach and cliffs of Spring Cove, the physical environment of the quarantine station (as opposed to its social implications) contained quite a positive meaning. The shoreline and beaches offered opportunities for exploration, a source of fresh food, and, for some, a chance to plan before embarking on a new life as colonists. Long after the vitriolic exchanges in the *Sydney Morning Herald* became yesterday's news, the presence of people who stayed at the quarantine ground has endured in the carvings that they left behind in this physical landscape. These fragments of individual and collective testimony are certainly suggestive of the limbo and tedium of quarantine, but they also reinforce in a very significant way the importance of travel that takes people from there to here, and changes them in the process.

Notes

1 TNA, ADM 101/7/10, Journal of surgeon William Evans on convict ship *Bencoolen* (1819), 25 August 1819.
2 Grace Karskens, *The Colony: A History of Early Sydney* (Sydney: Allen and Unwin, 2009), pp. 197–198.
3 ANMM, MS ALF, Anon, Diary on *Alfred* (1838–9), 16 January 1839.
4 TNA, ADM 101/1/10, Journal of surgeon John William Bowler on emigrant ship *Aliquis* (1838), General Remarks.
5 Governor Darling to W. Huskisson, 28 August 1828, *Historical Records of Australia* (Sydney: Library Committee of the Commonwealth Parliament, 1916), Series 1: Volume 14, pp. 347–348.
6 NMM, MS87/047, William Maybury, Convict's Log on the *Bussorah Merchant*, 27 March–26 July 1828, entry for '122nd day's sail'.
7 NMM, MS87/047, Maybury's Log, accompanying letter.
8 Milton J. Lewis, *The People's Health: Public Health in Australia 1788–1950* (Westport, CT: Greenwood, 2003), p. 29.
9 Viscount Goderich to Governor Bourke, 31 March 1832, *HRA* 1:16, pp. 583–586.
10 Viscount Goderich to Governor Bourke, 31 March 1832, *HRA* 1:16, pp. 583–586.
11 'Quarantine Proclamation', *New South Wales Government Gazette*, 27 February 1833, p. 1. For a history of the development of the quarantine station see Jean Duncan Foley, *In Quarantine: A History of Sydney's Quarantine Station 1824–1984* (Sydney: Kangaroo Press, 1995).
12 'Proclamation', *New South Wales Government Gazette*, 19 July 1837, p. 1.
13 For the dangers of the swamp in the nineteenth century see Conevery Bolton Valencius, *The Health of the Country: How American Settlers Understood Themselves and Their Land* (New York: Basic Books, 2004), pp. 145–152.
14 Foley, *In Quarantine*, p. 37–38; Jean Duncan Foley, 'Maritime Quarantine versus Commerce: The role of the Health Officer of Port Jackson in the nineteenth century', *Journal of the Royal Australian Historical Society* 90:2 (2004), pp. 152–174, p. 158.
15 Alison Bashford, 'Quarantine and the Imagining of the Australian Nation', *Health* 2 (1998), pp. 387–402.
16 TNA, ADM 101/12/8, Journal of surgeon Oliver Sproule on convict ship *Borneo* (1828); TNA, ADM 101/14/4, Journal of surgeon Robert Dunn on convict ship *Bussorah Merchant* (1828).
17 Foley, *In Quarantine*, p. 155.
18 Amy L. Fairchild, *Science at the Borders: Immigrant Medical Inspection and*

the Shaping of the Modern Industrial Labour Force (Baltimore and London: Johns Hopkins University Press, 2003), pp. 67–68.

19 Fairchild, *Science at the Borders*, p. 7.

20 Kirsten McKenzie, *Scandal in the Colonies* (Melbourne: Melbourne University Publishing, 2005), pp. 146–52; For contemporary debates see Elizabeth Elbourne, 'The Sin of the Settler: The 1835–36 Select Committee on aborigines and debate over virtue and conquest in the early nineteenth-century British white settler empire', *Journal of Colonialism and Colonial History* 4 (2004), http://muse.jhu.edu/journals/journal_of_colonialism_and_colonial_history/voo4/4. 3elbourne.html (accessed 22 September 2010); Anne O'Brien, 'Kitchen Fragments and Garden Stuff: Poor Law discourse and indigenous people in early colonial New South Wales', *Australian Historical Studies* 39 (2008), pp. 150–166.

21 See, for example, 'Emigration to New South Wales', *The Times*, 26 December 1834, p. 2; 'Female Emigration to New South Wales', *The Times*, 22 January 1838, p. 6. On the emigration of single women see A.J. Hammerton, '"Without Natural Protectors": Female Immigration to Australia, 1832–36', *Australian Historical Studies* 16:65 (1975), pp. 539–566.

22 Robin Haines, *Emigration and the Labouring Poor* (Basingstoke: Palgrave, 1997), pp. 261, 263–267.

23 David Neal, *The Rule of Law in a Penal Colony: Law and Power in Early Colonial New South Wales* (Cambridge: Cambridge University Press, 1991), p. 19.

24 TNA, CO 201/269, Report of Board: Emigrant Ship *Lady MacNaghten*, July 1837. Minutes of Evidence: Journal of surgeon Hawkins, pp. 111–184.

25 Foley, *In Quarantine*, p. 25.

26 United Kingdom, House of Commons, James Stuart, Minutes of Evidence, *Emigration* 1839 [536-I] [536-II], xxxix, p. 35.

27 'The Fever Ship', *Sydney Herald*, 27 February 1837, p. 3.

28 'The Female Emigrant Ship Lady McNaughton', *Sydney Monitor*, 27 February 1837, p. 2.

29 AONSW, 4/3892, Colonial Secretary's Papers: Copies of Letters sent re Quarantine, 26 February 1837–16 October 1838, Colonial Secretary to Military Secretary, 26 February 1837.

30 AONSW, 4/3892, E. Deas Thomson to Dr Inches, 28 February 1837.

31 'Quarantine', *New South Wales Government Gazette*, 1 March 1837, p. 1.

32 E.g. J. Booker, *Maritime Quarantine: The British Experience, c. 1650–1900* (Aldershot: Ashgate, 2007); Peter Baldwin, *Contagion and the State, 1830–1930* (Cambridge: Cambridge University Press, 1999). For an exception see Howard Markel, *Quarantine! East European Jewish Immigrants and the New York City Epidemics of 1892* (Baltimore and London: Johns Hopkins University Press, 1997), pp. 13–81.

33 Dale C. Smith, 'Medical Science, Medical Practice and the Emerging Concept of Typhus in Mid-eighteenth Century Britain', in W.F. Bynum and Vivien Nutton (eds), *Theories of Fever from Antiquity to the Enlightenment* (London: Wellcome Institute for the History of Medicine, 1981), pp. 121–134, p. 123; John Pickstone, 'Ferriar's Fever to Kay's Cholera: Disease and social structure in Cottonopolis', *History of Science* 22 (1984), pp. 401–419, p. 415.

34 David McConnell Reed, *Fever Physiologically Considered* (London: J. Churchill, 1846), p. 220.

35 Christopher Hamlin, *Public Health and Social Justice in the Age of Chadwick: Britain, 1800–1854* (Cambridge: Cambridge University Press, 1998), pp. 52–61.

36 O'Brien, 'Kitchen Fragments', p. 150.

37 TNA, ADM 105/36, Letters and Correspondence regarding sickness on convict and emigrant ships (1836–1851). Alexander Neill to the Physician General of the Admiralty regarding the safe arrival of the *Heber*, 28 October 1837.

38 TNA, ADM 105/36, Neill to the Physician General, 28 October 1837.

39 AONSW, 4/4821, Reports on Conditions of Immigrant Ships, July 1837– February 1840. Ship 'John Barry' from Dundee, dep. 25 March 1837, arr. 13 July 1837.

40 United Kingdom, House of Commons, James Stuart, Minutes of Evidence, *Emigration* 1839 [536-I] [536-II], xxxix, p. 36.

41 TNA, ADM 101/78/5, Journal of surgeon D.G. Miller on emigrant ship *North Britain*, Case 5: Laurence Rice; Case 14: William Fuller; Case 6: John Loyd; Case 10: Elizabeth Loyd.

42 TNA, ADM 101/78/5, Miller, Journal on *North Britain*, General Remarks.

43 United Kingdom, House of Commons, James Stuart, Minutes of Evidence, *Emigration* 1839 [536-I] [536-II], xxxix, p. 36.

44 TNA, ADM 101/78/5, Miller, Journal on *North Britain*, Cases 8, 9, 10, 13.

45 Foley, *In Quarantine*, pp. 34–39.

46 George Gipps to Lord Glenelg, 29 September 1838, *HRA* 1:19, pp. 598–599.

47 'Domestic Intelligence', *Sydney Gazette*, 11 October 1838, p. 2; George Gipps to Lord Glenelg, 22 Nov 1838, *HRA* 1:19, p. 683.

48 AONSW, 4/4836, John Reid, Report re immigrants on *William Roger* (1838).

49 AONSW, 4/4836, Reid, Report re *William Roger*.

50 TNA, ADM 101/79/6, Journal of surgeon James Lawrence on emigrant ship *Westminster* (1838), General Remarks.

51 George Gipps to Lord Glenelg, 20 January 1839, *HRA* 1:19, p. 767.

52 United Kingdom, House of Commons, *New South Wales. Correspondence between the Colonial Department and the Treasury* 1840 [509] xxxiii, p. 45.

53 TNA, ADM 101/78/1, Journal of surgeon Smith on emigrant ship *Maitland* (1838), General Remarks.

54 TNA, ADM 105/36, Report from John Smith re illness on board the *Maitland*, September 1838.

55 TNA, ADM 101/78/1, Smith, Journal on *Maitland*, General Remarks.

56 George Gipps to Lord Glenelg, 22 November 1838, *HRA*, 1:19, pp. 684–685.

57 'Domestic Intelligence', *Sydney Herald*, 3 July 1839, p. 2.

58 United Kingdom, House of Commons, *New South Wales. Correspondence*, p. 45.

59 George Gipps to Lord Glenelg, 22 November 1838, *HRA*, 1:19, p. 684.

60 George Gipps to Lord Glenelg, 20 January 1839, *HRA* 1:19, p. 767.

61 Booker, *Maritime Quarantine*, pp. 481–490.

62 Charles Nicolle discovered louse-borne typhus infection in 1909.

63 Baldwin, *Contagion*, pp. 123, 211.

64 For a critique of Baldwin with regard to Australia see Krista Maglen, 'A World Apart: Geography, Australian quarantine and the mother country', *Journal of the History of Medicine and the Allied Sciences* 60:2 (2005), pp. 196–217.

65 Alison Bashford, 'Smallpox: The spaces and subjects of public health', in *Imperial Hygiene* (Basingstoke: Routledge, 2004); Judith Walzer Leavitt, *Typhoid Mary: Captive to the Public's Health* (Boston: Beacon Press, 1996).

66 'The Fever Female Emigrant Ship', *Sydney Monitor*, 6 March 1837, p. 2.

67 'The Lady McNaughten', *Sydney Monitor*, 1 March 1837, p. 3.

68 'The Fever Female Emigrant Ship', *Sydney Herald*, 6 March 1837, p. 2.

69 'The Fever Ship', *Sydney Herald*, 9 March, 1837, p. 2.

70 'The Lady McNaghten', *Sydney Herald*, 20 April 1837, p. 2.

71 'The Lady McNaughten – The Sick Female Emigrant Ship', *Sydney Monitor*, 20 March 1837, p. 3.

72 TNA, CO 201/269, Report re *Lady MacNaghten*.

73 'The Late Emigration System', *Sydney Herald*, 14 August 1837, p. 2.

74 'Original Correspondence', *Sydney Herald*, 14 August 1837, p. 3.

75 'The John Barry', *Sydney Gazette*, 15 August 1837, p. 2.

76 'Original Correspondence', *Sydney Herald*, 21 August 1837, p. 3.

77 'To the Editor of the Sydney Gazette', *Sydney Gazette*, 5 September 1837, p. 3.

78 'Ship News' *Sydney Gazette*, 20 July 1837, p. 2.

79 'Original Correspondence', *Sydney Herald*, 21 August 1837, pp. 2–3.

80 'To the Editor of the Sydney Gazette', *Sydney Gazette*, 24 August 1837, p. 3.

81 ANMM, MS ALF, Anon, Diary on *Alfred* (1838–1839), 16 January 1839.

82 NLA, Ms 5071, John Whiting, Journal on emigrant ship *Lightning*, from Liverpool to Melbourne (1854), 28 May 1854.

83 TNA, ADM 101/ 76/10, Journal of surgeon I.J. Hampton on Emigrant Ship *Florist* (1839), General Remarks.

84 AONSW, 4/4821, *Florist* from Gravesend.

85 'Notice to Young Women', broadsheet of 1833, reproduced in Deborah Oxley, *Convict Maids: The Forced Migration of Women to Australia* (Cambridge: Cambridge University Press, 1996), p. 174.

86 On the weak Australian reaction to the Irish famine more broadly, see Patrick O'Farrell, 'Lost in Transit: Australian reaction to the Irish and Scots famines, 1845–50', in Patrick O'Sullivan (ed.) *The Meaning of the Famine: The Irish World Wide*, Vol. 6 (Leicester: Leicester University Press, 1997), pp. 126–139.

87 ML, Mss B1535 / CY 1024, Diary of Hugh May Wilson, 15th August 1849–9th December 1849 from Deptford and Plymouth on barque *Sarah*, 4 October 1849.

88 Louise Ann Meredith, *Notes and Sketches of New South Wales* (London: William Clowes and Sons, 1844), p. 34.

89 George French Angas, *Savage Life and Scenes in Australia and New Zealand*, Vol. 2 (London: Elder & Co., 1847), p. 200–201.

90 Angas, *Savage Life*, p. 201.

91 Two excellent recent histories have made a similar point about Sydney and Van Diemen's Land more generally. James Boyce has shown how convicts experienced Van Diemen's land as a place of refuge and freedom; James Boyce, *Van Diemen's Land* (Melbourne: Black Inc., 2010), p. 48. Grace Karskens has also argued that 'the horror of Botany Bay was not environmental at all, but social'; Karskens, *The Colony*, p. 323;

92 ML, Mss 599, Diary of Charles Scott on *Annie Wilson* (1859), 3–22 October 1859.

93 ML, Mss 599, Scott, Diary on *Annie Wilson*, 4 and 25 December 1859.

94 Foley, *In Quarantine*, pp. 156–157.

95 ML, Mss B784 / mfm CY 1117, Journal of William Usherwood, on *Beejapore*, Liverpool to Sydney (1852–3), 6 January 1853.

96 NLA, Ms 6118 / mfm G28208, Journal of surgeon Osborne Johnson on *Beejapore*, 1852–1853, 7 January 1853. For a more detailed discussion of the *Beejapore*'s quarantine see Robin Haines, *Doctors at Sea: Emigrant Voyages to Colonial Australia* (Basingstoke: Palgrave Macmillan 2005), pp. 1–6.

97 Karskens, *The Colony*, p. 158.

98 ML, Mss B784, William Usherwood's Journal on *Beejapore*, 20 December 1852.

99 'Letter to the Editor', *Sydney Morning Herald*, 19 January 1853, p. 2.

100 ML, Mss B784, Usherwood's Journal on *Beejapore*, 7 January 1853.

101 ML, Mss B1319, Charles Moore, Diary on emigrant ship *Constitution* (1855), 27 May 1855.

102 ML, Mss B1319, Moore's Diary on *Constitution*, 30 May 1855.

103 NLA, AJCP M2346, Journal of William Bray on *Great Britain*, Liverpool to Melbourne (1854), 14 and 19 August 1854.

104 In 1840, when the government emigrant ship *Glen Huntly* arrived in the fledgling colony with fever, La Trobe used Point Ormond, much closer to the town. A.G.L. Shaw, *A History of Port Phillip District: Victoria before Separation* (Melbourne: Melbourne University Press, 2003), pp. 145–147, 214.

105 A.G.L. Shaw, *Convicts and the Colonies* (London: Faber and Faber, 1966), p. 326.

106 Graeme Davison, 'Gold-rush Melbourne', in Iain McCalman, Alexander Cook and Andrew Reeves (eds) *Gold: Forgotten Histories and Lost Objects of Australia* (Cambridge: Cambridge University Press, 2001), pp. 52–66, p. 52.

107 Robin Haines, *Emigration and the Labouring Poor* (Basingstoke: Palgrave, 1997), p. 261.

108 NLA, AJCP M2346, Bray's diary on *SS Great Britain*, 19 August 1854, emphasis in original.

109 NLA, AJCP M2346, Bray's diary on *SS Great Britain*, 20 August 1854

110 NLA, AJCP M2346, Bray's diary on *SS Great Britain*, entries for '8th day' and '15th day'.

111 Alison Bashford, 'Foreign Bodies: Vaccination, contagion and colonialism in the nineteenth century', in Alison Bashford and Claire Hooker (eds), *Contagion: Historical and Cultural Studies* (London and New York: Routledge, 2001), pp. 39–60, p. 40.

112 Foley, *In Quarantine*, p. 155.

113 For more on the significance of quarantine etchings see Gareth Hoskins, 'A Place to Remember: Scaling the walls of Angel Island immigration station', *Journal of Historical Geography* 30 (2004), pp. 685–700; Bashford, 'Quarantine and the Imagining'.

114 J.D. Foley, 'Rock Carvings in the Area of Quarantine Beach' (unpublished manuscript, Quarantine Station, Manly, New South Wales: 1995).

Conclusion

Voyages did not just deliver people. Voyages helped to make colonists. At the same time, all emigrants and convicts brought something of their past lives with them, whether it was the effects of a night in drenching rain on a steamer in the Irish Channel, or of solitary confinement in a modern penitentiary. Over the time and space of a voyage south and then east through the oceans, new contexts for understanding health and illness modified the knowledge and histories people brought with them, and they gained a new understanding of their place in an expanding world. For most travellers, the physical results of being at sea caused nothing more than seasickness or a mild sunstroke. For others, the physical, mental, environmental, and social experiences of the voyage combined with the residue of their life histories to leave a more enduring mark.

If British convicts and emigrants came to understand something new about their place in the world through the process of travelling, they did so within the constraints imposed by the physical boundaries of the ship, and by the social, medical, political, and colonial contexts that shaped their voyages. Often, divisions of class, gender, and social status that had emphasised their low position in the social hierarchy of land were instantiated, rather than diminished, by the experience of being at sea. The tensions that emerge when we put medicine, environment, colonialism, and society together are important because they help us to understand why going to sea mattered. When we take voyages seriously as meaningful historical events, the boundaries of land and sea, metropolitan and colonial, diseased and healthy, 'above' and 'below', become blurred and unstable.

From convicts who concealed illness because a voyage was the only thing that might improve their failing health, to emigrants who objected to the post-mortem examination of a loved one, naval surgeons' journals are richly revealing of the variety of meanings that the subject of health encompassed at sea. Read against the grain, these official accounts reveal a great deal about the hopes and fears of convicts and emigrants, but they also show that surgeons were always interested in much more than the practicalities of preserving health on ships. Official journals served a particular purpose, whereby the surgeon had to ensure that he was paid. Often, surgeons' ideas and actions also reflected broader assumptions of class and gender, as well as an ethos of nineteenth-century naval medicine as it sought authority and status, particularly under the leadership of William Burnett at the Admiralty. Experiments with ventilation, therapeutics, and disinfection, as well as institutional backing for post-mortem examinations provided opportunities for surgeons to participate collectively in practices that increased their professional standing. On an individual level, these voyages were another stepping-stone through a career that might combine service in a British hospital, on a West African patrol, or in an Australian prison.

Placed side by side with a sailor's diary, emigrant's letter, or a passenger's diary, however, it is clear that these official medical accounts obscure as much as they reveal. The sailors' ceremonies at the equator, for example, are almost entirely absent from surgeons' official medical journals. These ceremonies turned medical authority on its head and mocked the surgeons' obsession with dryness on such a vast expanse of water. Surgeons' collective silence suggests that they remained deeply troubled by such acute ridicule of the medical principles they held so dear. So too, Henry Kelsall made no mention of the nightly scenes of sailors carrying women through the hatches of the *Andromeda* as they fainted in the heat of the tropics. When he wrote for the eyes of the colonial governor George Gipps, Obadiah Pineo urged all surgeons to call at the Cape of Good Hope if they would prevent scurvy. In a letter to William Burnett, however, Pineo expressed the contrary belief, that such measures would only 'save appearances'. At the same time as Pineo struggled with colonial scrutiny of his conduct, surgeons of emigrant ships were constructing their own vigorous defences as their ships arrived with typhus. Examining surgeons' journals in the broader contexts that surround them reveals chinks in their authoritative armour. Contemporary medical debates, professional tensions, political arguments, and colonial priorities shaped what surgeons wrote and how they explained their decisions. The myriad events that they left out of their journals, if only we could see most of them, would be just as significant as the carefully worded detail that went in.

Most importantly, going to sea was an environmental experience shaped by the geography, character, and colonial associations of the maritime regions through which people sailed. In 1841, as the emigrant ship *Lord Auckland* sailed east through the southern oceans en route to

New Zealand, Mrs Green died on the day after 'the most severe storm [the captain] was ever out in'. In his diary, Alfred Fell wrote that she had been 'very delicate ever since we came on board'. The storm had certainly accelerated the woman's demise, but Fell also believed that it was 'impossible for her to live long'. Mrs Green had been 'a tall, delicate, & very strange looking young woman about 23 years of age, seriously inclined and always kept herself very quiet'. She was 'not at all calculated for the wear and tear, the wife of a first settler will have to endure'.[1]

Throughout the preceding chapters, we have moved far beyond the idea that convicts and emigrants were a silent cargo who arrived safely in Australia because their surgeons, endowed with growing authority, heroically enforced sanitary measures that reduced mortality. Instead, we see that medical knowledge and authority was never a given, and convicts and emigrants actively invested in and shaped the meanings and outcomes of voyages. These observations have real implications for our understanding of how convicts, emigrants, and surgeons participated in the country that Australia became.

The career trajectories of men like Obadiah Pineo and John Hampton show how investing heavily in the practicalities of convict transportation reaped colonial rewards (and not a little controversy) for surgeons. Pineo, the surgeon so frustrated by scurvy, and investigated twice by the Medical Board in Sydney when he sent over a hundred convicts to the colonial hospital at the end of the *Lord Lyndoch*'s disastrous voyage, went on to become the superintendent of Deloraine probation station.[2] In 1856, John Hampton would become comptroller of convicts for Van Diemen's Land.[3] It is relatively easy to see how we might critically place naval surgeons in Australian colonial history, but we need to go further than this. As this book has tried to show, the experiences that emigrants, convicts, and surgeons had were always implicated in, and woven through, a much bigger colonial story. To conclude, I want to give a final example that emphasises how the interconnectedness that has been at the heart of the voyages in this book continued to matter far beyond the time that people spent at sea.

In August 1832 assistant surgeon George Imlay sailed to Dublin with the *Roslin Castle*, where the cholera was 'still raging'. After 152 convicts and eight free settlers had embarked, the *Roslin Castle* 'put to sea immediately to prevent communication between the prisoners and their friends, thinking by so doing to lessen the chances of infection'. Between Dublin and Cork most of the convicts suffered from diarrhoea, and 'seven who had neglected to apply for advice, when suffering from looseness, were served with cholera'. Imlay gave his opinion on the nature of the illness. 'The germs of the disease must, in all probability, have been in the constitution previous to their leaving the hulk and the debility incident to sea-sickness rendered their systems susceptible of its baleful influence.' Imlay took 'every precaution' to prevent infection. He ensured that clothing and bedding were boiled in water, and then immersed in chloride of lime. He destroyed every article of bedding and clothing used by the patients, and washed the hospital and its utensils with soap, hot water, and solution of chloride of lime.[4]

Imlay's journal is neat, his case notes mercifully legible, compared to some of his colleagues'. Nevertheless, his single page of general remarks bears little of the political or theoretical engagement that concerned many of his contemporaries or, indeed, of the prolonged explanations that betrayed the surgeon's constant need to justify his actions. Had he wished, Imlay could certainly have involved himself in the debate about whether or not cholera was contagious, as other naval surgeons were doing at that time. Imlay's fastidious attention to clothing and bedding is evidence that he believed cholera to be contagious, an opinion with which most of his naval colleagues would have disagreed. Neither did Imlay make any mention of the state in which he received prisoners from Dublin's *Essex* hulk. Nine months later, Andrew Henderson would argue bitterly with Dr Edward Trevor, the Inspector General for Irish Prisons, about whether or not the men from the *Essex* were fit to undertake, or even likely to survive, the Australian voyage.

As the sparse detail of his journal suggests, Imlay was not by nature the kind of career naval surgeon who complained about convicts who were unfit to become colonists; he was a colonist himself. When he arrived in Sydney with the *Roslin Castle* in February 1833, his two brothers, Alexander and Peter, had already established themselves in the colony. Alexander had used service as an army surgeon to pay his way to New South Wales. He arrived in 1829. His other brother, Peter, also a naval surgeon, had arrived on the *Greenock* in 1830.[5] By the time George arrived, Governor Bourke had granted the men over a thousand hectares of New South Wales land. They soon extended their holdings to South Australia and Van Diemen's Land as well.

In early 1847, colonial newspapers reported that George Imlay had shot himself dead in the bush near his hut.[6] He never met Henry Wellings, the young father from north-west England who wrote his emigrant's diary and drew his map of the world over a decade later on the *David McIvor* in 1858. After their arrival, the Wellings family lived in Sydney, where Wellings worked as a painter and builder and was one of the founding members of the Balmain Working Men's Institute. Later the family moved to Eden, the town now associated with the

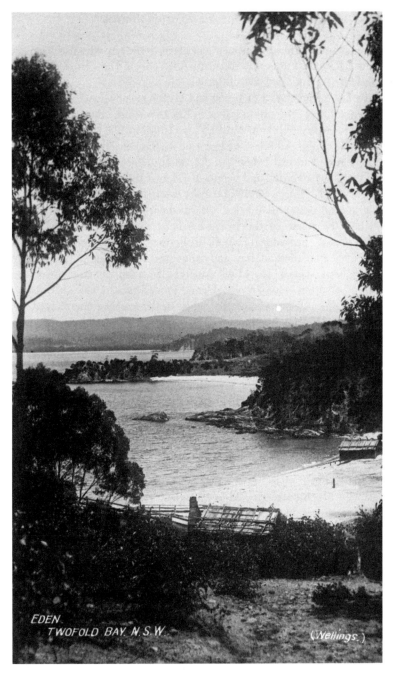

Figure 7 Charles Eden Wellings, 'View of Twofold Bay from Cattle Bay, Eden; Mount Imlay in Background' (c. 1910–12).

name of Imlay. There, Wellings' son Harry – the boy who had been six years old when the family sailed to Australia on the *David McIvor* – would marry and have five children.

In Eden, the stories of Imlay and Wellings converged. In no small part, the Imlay brothers' presence in Eden's modern cultural memory is due to the oldest of Harry Wellings' two children: Charles and (another) Henry Wellings. Charles became a photographer. His collection, now held in the National Library of Australia, depict the beaches, creeks, buildings, whaleboats, and people of Eden at the turn of the twentieth century. In *Looking for Blackfella's Point* (2002), Mark McKenna observes that around present-day Eden, a rural town in south-east New South Wales, 'the spirit' of the Imlay brothers, the 'first 'pioneers' of the Eden area … pervades the area'.[7] In Figure 7, Mount Imlay overlooks the town and Twofold Bay and fades into the background of many of Wellings' scenes. The Hotel Australasia on Imlay Street forms the subject of other photographs. Henry P. Wellings, Charles's brother, became a local historian and journalist. In the 1930s he interviewed the old men of Eden who remembered Tongihi, the 'last of the Monaro blacks'. One man, 'Old Bill' told Henry that 'every member of Tongihi's tribe had been shot by settlers'. Wellings told also of tribal warfare, and felt keenly that 'the Aboriginal population of Australia has little to thank European invasion for'.[8] In Henry's writings, the Imlays drove cattle and sheep 'unwittingly' through the 'wild and undeveloped' New South Wales terrain, but they were also apparently regarded as 'safe' by the Aboriginal people.[9] In 1967, Henry P. Wellings wrote the Imlays' entry for the *Australian Dictionary of National Biography*, an entry that still stands.

The histories of these two families – and their role in Australian history – became intertwined in ways that no one could have imagined as George and Henry sailed from England a decade apart and on different ships, with new lives ahead of them. I want to argue that these confluences must have been repeated thousands and thousands of times around Australia through the nineteenth and twentieth centuries. Individual Australian voyages – such as George Imlay's on the *Roslin Castle* in 1832–33 and Henry Wellings' on the *David McIvor* in 1858 – are worthy of study in their own right, but they also linked together land and land, people and people, across time and space. Travelling from Britain through the tropics and southern oceans to Australia, a powerful sense of continuity emerges. George Imlay, Henry Wellings, Eliza Baldwinson, Mrs Bateup, Alexander Bryson, William Dooly, Charles Picknell, and Fanny Davis, to name only a few of the varied cast of characters we have met along the way, all experienced their voyages in very different ways. Each voyage also contributes something new to our understanding not just of colonial travel, but of what was at stake when individuals went to Australia.

Delving into the history of voyaging and bringing emigrants, wealthy passengers, convicts, surgeons, and ships together affords important insights about the hardships and power relationships that occurred at sea. If it has also become clear that these nineteenth-century voyages were not just the 'floating vision[s] of hell' that we often assume they must have been, neither should revising these assumptions be an occasion to rejuvenate a triumphant narrative of British naval mastery, medical progress, and colonial expansion.[10] By using health as a lens through which to look at what going to sea meant, and seeing voyages as events that connected rather than separated much more of Britain and Australia than their ports, we must also acknowledge in all its messy, often uncomfortable reality that these voyages helped to make colonialism. Precisely because Australian voyages were complex social and environmental events, they help to illuminate the world-view that colonists of all kinds brought to the process of Australian colonialism in the nineteenth century, the consequences of this colonialism for the people who already lived on the land, and the social and political legacy of settlement and dispossession for all the generations who have followed.

Notes

1 NMM, MRF/151, Journal of Alfred Fell, Diary on board the emigrant ship *Lord Auckland*, 1841–1842, 2 January 1842.

2 Tom Dunning and Hamish Maxwell-Stewart, 'Mutiny at Deloraine: Ganging and convict resistance in 1840s Van Diemen's Land', *Labour History* 82 (2002), pp. 35–47, p. 41.

3 A.G.L. Shaw, *Convicts and the Colonies* (London: Faber and Faber, 1966), p. 356.

4 TNA, ADM 101/64/6, Journal of surgeon George Imlay on convict ship *Roslin Castle* (1832–3), General Remarks.

5 H.P. Wellings, 'Imlay, George (1794?–1846)', *Australian Dictionary of Biography*, Volume 2 (Melbourne: Melbourne University Press, 1967), pp. 2–3.

6 'Family Notices', *The Colonial Times* (Hobart), 22 January 1847, p. 2.

7 Mark McKenna, *Looking for Blackfella's Point: An Australian History of Place* (Sydney: University of New South Wales Press, 2005), pp. 42, 71.

8 Henry Wellings, writing in *Eden Magnet*, 1 and 8 August, 1931, cited in McKenna, *Looking for Blackfella's Point*, p. 76.

9 McKenna, *Looking for Blackfella's Point*, p. 40.

10 Ironically, the digitisation of The National Archives' collections of naval surgeons' journals has tended so far to reinforce rather than dispel this narrative. For the 'floating' vision quote see 'Doctors at sea – but little to laugh about', *Navy News*, December 2010, p. 22.

Bibliography

Archives

Australian National Maritime Museum (Sydney)
Manuscript Collections

Bristol Record Office

Kings College London
Foreign and Commonwealth Office Collection

The National Archives (London, Great Britain)
Admiralty Records
Colonial Office Records
Home Office Records
Prison Commission Records

National Archives of Ireland (Dublin)
Chief Secretary's Office Papers
Convict Office Correspondence

National Library of Australia (Canberra)
Manuscript Collections

National Maritime Museum (London)
Manuscripts

Public Records Office of Northern Ireland (Belfast)
Manuscripts

State Archives of New South Wales (Sydney)
Immigration Reports

State Archives of Tasmania (Hobart)
Convict Records

State Library of New South Wales (Sydney)
Dixson Library
Mitchell Library

Warwickshire County Record Office

Newspapers and periodicals

The Argus (Melbourne)
British Medical Journal
Colonial Times (Hobart)
The Lancet
Liverpool Mail
Liverpool Standard and Commercial Advertiser
London Medical Gazette
The Maitland Mercury and Hunter River General Advertiser
Medical Times
Sydney Gazette and New South Wales Advertiser
Sydney Herald
Sydney Monitor
The Times

Official sources

Historical Records of Australia Series 1 (Sydney: Library Committee of the Commonwealth Parliament, 1916).
New South Wales Government Gazette.
United Kingdom, House of Commons. *Report from the Select Committee on Transportation* 1812 [341] ii.
United Kingdom, House of Commons. *Report of the Commissioner of Enquiry into the state of the colony of New South Wales* 1822 [448] xx.
United Kingdom, House of Commons. *Gaols* 1825 [5] xxiii.
United Kingdom House of Commons. *Report and Evidence of the Select Committee on Anatomy* 1828 [568] vii.
United Kingdom, House of Commons. *Report from the Select Committee on Transportation* 1837 [518].
United Kingdom, House of Commons. *Emigration* 1839 [536–1] [536 II] xxxix.
United Kingdom, House of Commons. *New South Wales. Correspondence between the Colonial Department and the Treasury* 1840 [509] xxxiii.
United Kingdom House of Commons, *Two Reports from John Henry Capper* 1842 [122] xxxii.
United Kingdom House of Commons, *Convicts, Two Reports of John Henry Capper* 1843 [113] xlii.

United Kingdom, House of Commons, General Board of Health, *Report on Quarantine* 1849 [1070] xxiv.

United Kingdom. *Report of the General Board of Health on the Epidemic Cholera of 1848 & 1849* 1850 [1273–5] xxi.

United Kingdom, House of Commons. *Report from the Select Committee on the Passengers' Act; with the Proceedings of the Committee, Minutes of Evidence, Appendix and Index* 1851 [632] xix.

United Kingdom, House of Commons. *Reports Relating to the Mortality on Board Certain Ships* 1852–3 [205].

United Kingdom, House of Commons. *Emigrant Ship 'Dirigo'* 1854 [492] xlvi.

United Kingdom, House of Commons. *Papers Relative to Emigration to Australian Colonies* 1857 [144], x.

Unpublished manuscript

Foley, Jean Duncan. 'Rock Carvings in the Area of Quarantine Beach' (unpublished manuscript, Quarantine Station, Manly, New South Wales: 1995).

Published sources

Admiralty. *Instructions for the Royal Naval Hospitals at Haslar and Plymouth* (London: William Clowes, 1834).

Admiralty. *Instructions for Surgeons-Superintendents on Board Convict Ships* (London: William Clowes, 1838).

Anderson, Clare. '"The Ferringees are Flying – the Ship is ours!": the Convict Middle Passage in Colonial South and Southeast Asia, 1790–1860', *Indian Economic and Social History Review* 41:3 (2005), pp. 143–186.

Anderson, Clare. *The Indian Uprising of 1857–8: Prisons, Prisoners and Rebellion* (London and New York: Anthem Press, 2007).

Anderson, Warwick. *The Cultivation of Whiteness: Science, Health and Racial Destiny in Australia* (New York: Basic Books, 2003).

Anderson, Warwick. *Colonial Pathologies: American Tropical Medicine, Race, and Hygiene in the Philippines* (Durham and London: Duke University Press, 2006).

Angas, George French. *Savage Life and Scenes in Australia and New Zealand*, Vol. 2 (London: Elder & Co., 1847).

Anon. *The Kains: Female Convict Vessel* (Adelaide: Sullivan's Cove, 1989).

Archer, Thomas. *The Pauper, the Thief and the Convict* (London: Groombridge and Sons 1865).

Arnold, David. *Colonising the Body* (London, Berkeley and Los Angeles: University of California Press, 1993).

Arnold, David. *The Tropics and the Traveling Gaze: India, Landscape and Science, 1800–1856* (Seattle and London: University of Washington Press, 2006).

Arnott, Neil. *On Warming and Ventilating; with Directions for making and using the Thermometer Stove, or Self-Regulating Fire, and other new apparatus* (London: Longman, Orme, Brown, Green, and Longmans, 1838).

Baldwin, Peter. *Contagion and the State, 1830–1930* (Cambridge: Cambridge University Press, 1999).

Bashford, Alison. 'Quarantine and the Imagining of the Australian Nation', *Health* 2 (1998), pp. 387–402.

Bashford, Alison. 'Foreign Bodies: Vaccination, contagion and colonialism in the nineteenth century', in Alison Bashford and Claire Hooker (eds) *Contagion: Historical and Cultural Studies* (London and New York: Routledge, 2001), pp. 39–60.

Bashford, Alison. *Imperial Hygiene. A Critical History of Colonialism, Nationalism and Public Health* (Basingstoke: Palgrave, 2004).

Bateson, Charles. *The Convict Ships, 1787–1868* (Glasgow: Brown, Son & Ferguson, 1985), pp. 48–49, 382–3.

Bayliss, Robert A. and C. William Ellis. 'Neil Arnott, F.R.S. Reformer, Innovator and Popularizer of Science', *Notes and Records of the Royal Society of London* 36:1 (1981), pp. 103–123.

Beddoes, Thomas. *Observations on Calculus, Sea Scurvy, Consumption, Catarrh, and Fever* (Philadelphia: T. Dobson, 1797).

Bennett, Michael J. 'Smallpox and Cowpox under the Southern Cross: The smallpox epidemic of 1789 and the advent of vaccination in colonial Australia', *Bulletin of the History of Medicine* 83:1 (2009), pp. 37–62.

Bentley, Jerry H. 'Sea and Ocean Basins as Frameworks of Historical Analysis', *Geographical Review* 89:2 (1999), pp. 215–224.

Bentley, Jerry H., Renate Bridenthal and Karen Wigen (eds) *Seascapes: Maritime Histories, Littoral Cultures and Transoceanic Exchanges* (Honolulu: University of Hawaii Press, 2007).

Bird, Samuel Dougan. *On Australasian Climates and their Influence in the Prevention and Arrest of Pulmonary Consumption* (London: Longman, 1863).

Blane, Gilbert. *Select Dissertations on Several Subjects of Medical Science* (London: T. & G. Underwood, 1822).

Bolton Valencius, Conevery. *The Health of the Country: How American Settlers Understood Themselves and Their Land* (New York: Basic Books, 2002).

Booker, J. *Maritime Quarantine: The British Experience, c. 1650–1900* (Aldershot: Ashgate, 2007).

Boyce, James. *Van Diemen's Land* (Melbourne: Black Inc., 2008).

Braudel, Fernand. *The Mediterranean and the Mediterranean World in the Age of Philip II*, 2 vols, trans. S. Reynolds (New York: Harper and Row, 1972).

Brooke, Alan and David Brandon, *Bound for Botany Bay: British Convict Voyages to Australia* (London: The National Archives, 2005).

Brown, Michael. 'From Foetid Air to Filth: The cultural transformation of British epidemiological thought, c. 1780–1848', *Bulletin of the History of Medicine* 82 (2008), pp. 515–544.

Bryder, Linda. '"A Health Resort for Consumptives": Tuberculosis and Immigration to New Zealand, 1880–1914', *Medical History* 40:4 (1996), pp. 453–471.

Burrell, Sean and Geoffrey Gill. 'The Liverpool Cholera Epidemic of 1832 and Anatomical Dissection – Medical Mistrust and Civil Unrest', *Journal of the History of Medicine and Allied Sciences* 60:4 (2005), pp. 478–498.

Burton, Antoinette. 'Archive Stories: gender in the making of imperial and colonial histories', in Philippa Levine (ed.) *Gender and Empire* (Oxford: Oxford University Press, 2004), pp. 281–293.

Butlin, Noel George. *Forming a Colonial Economy: Australia 1810–1850* (Cambridge: Cambridge University Press, 1994).

Campbell, Judy. *Invisible Invaders: Smallpox and Other Disease in Aboriginal Australia, 1780–1880* (Melbourne: Melbourne University Press, 2002).

Cannadine, David (ed.) *Empire, the Sea and Global History: Britain's Maritime World, c. 1760–1840* (Basingstoke: Palgrave Macmillan, 2007).

Carpenter, Kenneth J. *The History of Scurvy and Vitamin C* (Cambridge: Cambridge University Press, 1986).

Carter, Paul. *The Road to Botany Bay: An Essay in Spatial History* (London and Boston: Faber and Faber, 1987).

Cartwright, Frederick F. and Michael Biddiss. *Disease and History*, 2nd edn (Stroud: Sutton, 2000).

Casella, Eleanor Conlin. 'Prisoner of His Majesty: Postcoloniality and the archaeology of British penal transportation', *World Archaeology* 37:3 (2005), pp. 453–467.

Charters, Erica. '"The Intention is Certainly Noble": The Western Squadron, Medical Trials and the Sick and Hurt Board during the Seven Years War', in David Boyd Haycock and Sally Archer (eds) *Health and Medicine at Sea, 1700–1900* (Woodbridge: Boydell Press, 2009), pp. 19–37.

Christopher, Emma. 'Steal a Handkerchief, See the World: The transoceanic voyaging of Thomas Limpus', in Ann Curthoys and Marilyn Lake (eds), *Connected Worlds: History in Transnational Perspective* (Canberra: ANU Press, 2005), pp. 77–88.

Christopher, Emma. *Slave Ship Sailors and their Captive Cargoes* (Cambridge: Cambridge University Press, 2006).

Christopher, Emma, Marcus Rediker and Cassandra Pybus (eds) *Many Middle Passages: Forced Migration and the Making of the Modern World* (Los Angeles and London: University of California Press, 2007).

Clark, James. *A Treatise on Pulmonary Consumption Comprehending an Enquiry into the Causes Nature Prevention and Treatment of Tuberculous and Scrofulous Diseases in General* (London: Sherwood, Gilbert and Piper, 1835).

Coleborne, Catharine. *Madness in the Family: Insanity and Institutions in the Australasian Colonial World, 1860–1914* (Basingstoke: Palgrave Macmillan, 2010).

Collier, Stephen J. and Aihwa Ong. *Global Assemblages: Technology, Politics and Ethics as Anthropological Problems* (Oxford: Blackwell, 2005).

Colley, Linda. *Captives* (London: Pimlico, 2002).

Corbin, Alain. *The Lure of the Sea: The Discovery of the Seaside in the Western World, 1750–1840* (Cambridge: Polity Press, 1994).

Corbin, Alain. *The Foul and the Fragrant: Odour and the Social Imagination* (London: Papermac, 1996).

Cosgrove, Denis. 'Tropic and Tropicality', in Felix Driver and Luciana Martins (eds) *Tropical Visions in an Age of Empire* (Chicago and London: Chicago University Press, 2005), pp. 197–216.

Creighton, Margaret S. *Rites and Passages: The Experience of American Whaling, 1830–1870* (Cambridge: Cambridge University Press, 1995).

Crosby, Alfred. *Ecological Imperialism: The Biological Expansion of Europe* (Cambridge: Cambridge University Press, 1986).

Cullen, William. *First Lines of the Practice of Physic, with Practical and Explanatory Notes*, 4 vols (Edinburgh: C. Elliott, 1788).

Cumpston, J.H.L. *The History of Smallpox in Australia, 1788–1908* (Melbourne: Commonwealth of Australia Quarantine Service, 1914).

Cunningham, Peter. *Two Years Experience in New South Wales* (London: Henry Colburn, 1827).

Curtin, Phillip D. *The Image of Africa: British Ideas and Action, 1780–1850* (Madison: University of Wisconsin Press, 1964).

Damousi, Joy. *Depraved and Disorderly: Female Convicts, Sexuality and Gender in Colonial Australia* (Cambridge: Cambridge University Press, 1997).

Dana, Richard Henry. *Two Years before the Mast: A Personal Narrative of Life at Sea* (New York: Harper and Brothers, 1842).

Deacon, Harriet. 'The Politics of Medical Topography: Seeking healthiness at the Cape during the nineteenth century', in Richard Wrigley and George Revill (eds), *Pathologies of Travel* (Atlanta: Rodopi, 2000), pp. 279–297.

Dening, Greg. *Mr Bligh's Bad Language: Passion, Power and Theatre on the Bounty* (Cambridge: Cambridge University Press, 1992).

Dixon, Thomas. 'Patients and Passions: Languages of medicine and emotion, 1789–1850', in Fay Bound Alberti (ed.) *Medicine, Emotion and Disease, 1700–1950* (Basingstoke: Palgrave Macmillan, 2006).

Drayton, Richard. 'Maritime Networks and the Making of Knowledge', in David Cannadine (ed.), *Empire, the Sea and Global History: Britain's Maritime World, c. 1763–c. 1840* (Basingstoke: Palgrave Macmillan, 2007), pp. 72–82.

Driver, Felix. 'Moral Geographies: Social science and the urban environment in mid-nineteenth century England', *Transactions of the Institute of British Geographers* 13:3 (1988), pp. 275–287.

Driver, Felix and Luciana Martins (eds) *Tropical Visions in an Age of Empire*, (Chicago and London: Chicago University Press, 2005).

Duffield, Ian and James Bradley (eds) *Representing Convicts: New Perspectives on Convict Forced Labour Migration* (Leicester: Leicester University Press, 1997).

Duncan M.D., William Henry. *On the Physical Causes of the High Rate of Mortality in Liverpool* (Liverpool: J. Walmsley, 1843).

Dunkley, Peter. 'Emigration and the State, 1803–1842: The nineteenth-century revolution in government reconsidered', *Historical Journal* 23:2 (1980), pp. 353–380.

Dunning, Tom and Hamish Maxwell-Stewart. 'Mutiny at Deloraine: Ganging and convict resistance in 1840s Van Diemen's Land', *Labour History* 82 (2002), pp. 35–47.

Durbach, Nadja. 'They Might as Well Brand Us: Working class resistance to compulsory vaccination in Victorian England', *Social History of Medicine* 13:1 (2000), pp. 45–62.

Elbourne, Elizabeth. 'The Sin of the Settler: The 1835–36 Select Committee on Aborigines and Debate over virtue and conquest in the early nineteenth-century British white settler empire', *Journal of Colonialism and Colonial History* 4 (2004). Online, http://muse.jhu.edu/journals/journal_of_colonialism_and_colonial_history/v004/4.3elbourne.html.

Equiano, Olaudah. *The Interesting Narrative and Other Writings*, first publ. 1789 (London: Penguin, 2003).

Erickson, Charlotte. *Leaving England: Essays on British Emigration in the Nineteenth Century* (Ithaca, NY: Cornell University Press, 1994).

Errington, Elizabeth Jane. *Emigrant Worlds and Transatlantic Communities: Migration to Upper Canada in the First Half of the Nineteenth Century* (Montreal and Kingston: McGill-Queen's University Press, 2007).

Evans, Robin. *The Fabrication of Virtue: English Prison Architecture, 1750–1840* (Cambridge: Cambridge University Press, 1982).

Ewell, James. *The Medical Companion*, 3rd edn (Philadelphia: printed for the author, 1819).

Fairchild, Amy L. *Science at the Borders: Immigrant Medical Inspection and the Shaping of the Modern Industrial Labour Force* (Baltimore and London: Johns Hopkins University Press, 2003).

Few, Martha. 'Circulating Smallpox Knowledge: Guatemalan doctors, Mayan Indians and designing Spain's smallpox vaccination expedition', *British Journal for the History of Science* 43 (2010), pp. 1–19.

Finer, Samuel E. *The Life and Times of Edwin Chadwick* (London: Methuen, 1980).

Finlayson, M.D., Robert. 'An Essay Addressed to Captains of the Royal Navy, and those of the Merchant's Service; On the Means of Preserving the Health of their Crews: With Directions for the Prevention of Dry Rot in Ships', *Pamphleteer* 26:51 (1825).

Fitzpatrick, David. '"A Peculiar Tramping People": the Irish in Britain, 1801–1870', in W.E. Vaughan (ed.), *A New History of Ireland*, Vol. 5: *Ireland under the Union, 1801–1870* (Oxford: Oxford University Press, 1989), pp. 623–657.

Foley, Jean Duncan. *In Quarantine: A History of Sydney's Quarantine Station 1824–1984* (Sydney: Kangaroo Press, 1995).

Foley, Jean Duncan. 'Maritime Quarantine versus Commerce: the role of the Health Officer of Port Jackson in the nineteenth century', *Journal of the Royal Australian Historical Society* 90:2 (2004), pp. 152–174.

Foster, R.F. *Modern Ireland, 1600–1972* (London: Penguin, 1989).

Frost, Lucy and Hamish Maxwell-Stewart. 'Introduction', in *Chain Letters: Narrating Convict Lives* (Carlton, Victoria: Melbourne University Press, 2001).

Gallman, J. Matthew. *Receiving Erin's Children* (Chapel Hill and London: University of North Carolina Press, 2000).

Garland, Chris and Herbert S. Klein. 'The Allotment of Space for Slaves aboard Eighteenth-century British Slave Ships', *The William and Mary Quarterly* 42:2 (1985), pp. 238–248.

Gascoigne, John. *The Enlightenment and the Origins of European Australia* (Cambridge: Cambridge University Press, 2002).

Gilchrist, Ebenezer. *The Use of Sea Voyages in Medicine, and particularly in a Consumption: with Observations on that Disease*, new edition (London: T. Cadell, 1771).

Gilroy, Paul. *The Black Atlantic* (Cambridge, MA: Harvard University Press, 1993).

Gómez, Nicolas Wey. *The Tropics of Empire: Why Columbus Sailed South to the Indies* (Cambridge, MA: MIT Press, 2008).

Green, Toby. *The Rise of the Trans-Atlantic Slave Trade in Western Africa, 1300–1589* (Cambridge: Cambridge University Press, 2011).

Griffiths, Arthur. *Memorials of Millbank* (London: Chapman and Hall, 1884).

Guy, William A. 'On Sufficient and Insufficient Dietaries, with Special Reference to the Dietaries of Prisoners, *Journal of the Statistical Society of London*, 26:3 (1863).

Haines, Robin. *Emigration and the Labouring Poor* (Basingstoke: Palgrave, 1997).

Haines, Robin. 'Medical Superintendence and Child Health on Government-assisted Voyages to South Australia in the Nineteenth Century', *Health and History* 3:2 (2001), pp. 1–29.

Haines, Robin. *Doctors at Sea: Emigrant Voyages to Colonial Australia* (Basingstoke: Palgrave Macmillan, 2005).

Haines, Robin and Ralph Shlomowitz. 'Explaining the Modern Mortality Decline: What can we learn from sea voyages?' *Social History of Medicine* 11:1 (1998), pp. 15–48.

Hales, Stephen. *A Description of Ventilators whereby Great Quantities of Fresh Air May with Ease Be Conveyed into Mines, Gaols, Hospitals, Work-Houses and Ships* (London: W. Innys, 1743).

Hamlin, Christopher. *Public Health and Social Justice in the Age of Chadwick: Britain, 1800–1854* (Cambridge: Cambridge University Press, 1998).

Hammerton, A.J. '"Without Natural Protectors": Female immigration to Australia, 1832–36', *Australian Historical Studies* 16:65 (1975), pp. 539–566.

Harms, Robert W. *The Diligent: A Voyage through the Worlds of the Slave Trade* (New York: Basic Books, 2002).

Harper, Marjory and Stephen Constantine. *Migration and Empire* (Oxford: Oxford University Press, 2010).

Harrison, Mark. *Medicine in an Age of Commerce and Empire* (Oxford: Oxford University Press, 2010).

Harrison, Mark. 'Tropical Medicine in Nineteenth-century India', *British Journal for the History of Science* 25:3 (1992), pp. 299–318.

Harrison, Mark. 'From Medical Astronomy to Medical Astrology: Sol-lunar and planetary theories of disease in British medicine, c. 1700–1850', *British Journal for the History of Science* 33 (2000), pp. 25–48.

Harrison, Mark. *Climates and Constitutions: Health, Race, Environment and British Imperialism in India, 1600–1850* (New Delhi and Oxford: Oxford University Press, 2002).

Harrison, Mark. '"An Important and Truly National Subject": The West Africa service and the health of the Royal Navy in the mid nineteenth century', in David Boyd Haycock and Sally Archer (eds) *Health and Medicine at Sea, 1700 –1900* (Woodbridge: Boydell Press, 2009), pp. 108–127.

Hassam, Andrew. *Sailing to Australia: Shipboard Diaries by Nineteenth-century British Emigrants* (Manchester: Manchester University Press, 1994).

Hassam, Andrew. *No Privacy for Writing: Shipboard Diaries 1852–1879* (Melbourne: Melbourne University Press, 1995).

Hathaway, Jane (ed.) *Rebellion, Repression, Reinvention: Mutiny in Comparative Perspective* (Westport, CT: Praeger, 2001).

Haycock, David Boyd and Sally Archer (eds) *Health and Medicine at Sea 1700–1900* (Woodbridge: Boydell Press, 2009).

Henningsen, Henning. *Crossing the Equator: Sailor's Baptisms and Other Initiation Rites* (Copenhagen: Munksgaarde, 1961).

Henry, William. *The Elements of Experimental Chemistry* (London: Baldwin, Cradock and Joy, 1826).

Hitchins, Fred H. *The Colonial Land and Emigration Commission* (Philadelphia: University of Philadelphia Press, 1931).

Hood, John. *Australia and the East* (London: John Murray, 1843).

Hoskins, Gareth. 'A Place to Remember: Scaling the walls of Angel Island immigration station', *Journal of Historical Geography* 30 (2004), pp. 685–700.

Howard, John. *The State of the Prisons in England and Wales with Preliminary Observations, and An Account of Some Foreign Prisons* (Warrington: Cadell, 1777).

Howell, Raymond. *The Royal Navy and the Slave Trade* (London: Croom Helm, 1987).

Humphery, Kim. 'A New Era of Existence: Convict transportation and the authority of the surgeon in colonial Australia', *Labour History* (Australia) 59 (1990), pp. 59–72.

Ignatieff, Michael. *A Just Measure of Pain* (New York: Pantheon, 1978).

Jacoby, Karl. *Crimes against Nature: Squatters, Poachers, Thieves and the Hidden History of American Conservation* (Berkeley and Los Angeles: University of California Press, 2003).

Jalland, Pat. *Australian Ways of Death: A Social and Cultural History 1840–1918* (Oxford: Oxford University Press, 2002).

Jankovic, Vladimir. 'The Last Resort: A British perspective on the medical south', *Journal of Intercultural Studies* 27:3 (2006), pp. 271–298.

Jennings, Eric T. *Curing the Colonizers: Hydrotherapy, Climatology and French Colonial Spas* (Durham and London: Duke University Press, 2006).

Johnson, James. *The Influence of Tropical Climates on European Constitutions*, 6th edn (London: James Ranald Martin, 1841).

Jukes, J.B. *Narrative of the Surveying Voyage of H.M.S. Fly* (London: T. & W. Boone, 1847).

Karskens, Grace. *The Colony: A History of Early Sydney* (Sydney: Allen and Unwin, 2009).

Kearns, Gerry. 'Town Hall and Whitehall: Sanitary intelligence in Liverpool, 1840–1863', in Sally Sheard and Helen Power (eds) *Body and City: Histories of Urban Public Health* (Aldershot: Ashgate, 2000), pp. 89–108.

Kennedy, Dane. 'The Perils of the Midday Sun: Climatic anxieties in the colonial tropics', in J.M. Mackenzie (ed.) *Imperialism and the Natural World* (Manchester: Manchester University Press, 1990).

Kisacky, Jeanne, 'Restructuring Isolation: Hospital architecture, medicine and disease prevention', *Bulletin of the History of Medicine* 79:1 (2005), pp. 1–49.

Kraut, Alan M. *Silent Traveler: Germs, Genes and the Immigrant Menace* (Baltimore and London: Johns Hopkins University Press, 1994).

Kruithof, Mary. *Fever Beach: The Story of the Migrant Clipper 'Ticonderoga' and its Ill-fated Voyage and Historical Impact* (Mount Waverly, Victoria: QI Publishing, 2002).

Kudlick, Catherine J. *Cholera in Post-revolutionary Paris: A Cultural History* (Berkeley: University of California Press, 1996).

Kupperman, Karen Ordahl. 'Fear of Hot Climates in the Anglo-American Colonial Experience', *William and Mary Quarterly* 3rd series 41:2 (1984), pp. 213–240.

Lamb, Jonathan. *Preserving the Self in the South Seas, 1680–1840* (Chicago: University of Chicago Press, 2001).

Land, I. (ed.) 'New Approaches to the Founding of the Sierra Leone Colony, 1786–1808', Special Issue of *Journal of Colonialism and Colonial History* 9:3 (2008).

Lawlor, Clark and Akihito Suzuki. 'The Disease of the Self: Representing consumption, 1700–1830', *Bulletin of the History of Medicine* 74 (2000), pp. 459–494.

Lawrence, Christopher. 'Disciplining Disease: Scurvy, the navy, and imperial expansion, 1750–1825', in David Philip Miller and Peter Hans Reill (eds), *Visions of Empire: Voyages, Botany and Representations of Nature* (Cambridge: Cambridge University Press, 1996), pp. 80–106.

Leavitt, Judith Walzer. *Typhoid Mary: Captive to the Public's Health* (Boston: Beacon Press, 1996).

Levere, Trevor H. 'Dr Thomas Beddoes (1750–1808): Science and medicine in politics and society', *British Journal of the History of Science* 17:2 (1984), pp. 187–204.

Levine, Philippa. *Prostitution, Race and Politics: Policing Venereal Disease in the British Empire* (New York and London: Routledge, 2003).

Lewis, Milton J. *The People's Health: Public Health in Australia 1788–1950* (Westport, CT: Greenwood, 2003).

Lind, James. *An Essay on the Most Effectual Means of Preserving the Health of Seamen, in the Royal Navy*, 2nd edn (London: D. Wilson, 1762).

Livingstone, David. 'Tropical Hermeneutics: Fragments for a Historical Narrative, An Afterword', *Singapore Journal of Tropical Geography* 21:1 (2000), pp. 92–98.

Lloyd, C.C. 'The Conquest of Scurvy', *British Journal for the History of Science*, 1 (1962–63), pp. 357–363.

Lloyd, Frank. *The Navy and the Slave Trade* (London: Frank Cass and Co., 1968).

McCalman, Iain, Alexander Cook and Andrew Reeves (eds) *Gold: Forgotten Histories and Lost Objects of Australia* (Cambridge: Cambridge University Press, 2001).

McConnell Reed, David. *Fever Physiologically Considered* (London: J. Churchill, 1846).

McConville, Sean. *A History of English Prison Administration*, 2 vols (London: Routledge, 1981).

MacCormac, Henry. *On the Nature, Treatment and Prevention of Pulmonary Consumption* (London: Longman, Brown Green and Longmans & J. Churchill, 1855).

MacDonald, Helen. *Human Remains: Dissection and Its Histories* (New Haven and London: Yale University Press, 2006).

McDonald, John and Ralph Shlomowitz. 'Mortality on Convict Voyages to Australia, 1788–1868', *Social Science History* 13:3 (1989), pp. 285–313.

McKenna, Mark. *Looking for Blackfella's Point: An Australian History of Place* (Sydney: University of New South Wales Press, 2005).

McKenzie, Kirsten. *Scandal in the Colonies* (Melbourne: Melbourne University Press, 2005).

MacLaren, A.C. 'On the Origin and Spread of Cholera in the 8th District of Plympton St. Mary, Devonshire', *Journal of the Statistical Society of London* 13:2 (1850), pp. 103–134.

McLean, David. 'Protecting Wood and Killing Germs: "Burnett's Liquid" and the origins of the preservative and disinfectant industries in early Victorian Britain', *Business History* 52:2 (2010), pp. 285–305.

McLean, David. *Surgeons of the Fleet: The Royal Navy and its Medics from Trafalgar to Jutland* (London and New York: I.B. Tauris, 2010).

McWilliam, J.O. *Medical History of the Expedition to the Niger during the years 1841–2: comprising an account of the fever which led to its abrupt termination* (London: John Churchill, 1843).

Maglen, Krista. 'A World Apart: Geography, Australian quarantine and the mother country', *Journal of the History of Medicine and the Allied Sciences* 60:2 (2005), pp. 196–217.

Markel, Howard. *Quarantine! East European Jewish Immigrants and the New*

York City Epidemics of 1892 (Baltimore and London: Johns Hopkins University Press, 1997).

Marland, Hilary. *Medicine and Society in Wakefield and Huddersfield, 1780–1870* (Cambridge: Cambridge University Press, 1987).

Marsden, Ben and Crosbie Smith. *Engineering Empires: A Cultural History of Technology in Nineteenth-Century Britain* (New York: Palgrave Macmillan, 2005).

Martins, Luciana. 'Navigating in Tropical Waters: British maritime views of Rio de Janeiro', *Imago Mundi* 50 (1998), pp. 141–155.

Maury, Matthew F. *Physical Geography of the Sea* (New York: Harper and Brothers, 1855).

Melville, Henry. *Redburn: His First Voyage* (New York: Harper and Brothers, 1850).

Meredith, Louise Ann. *Notes and Sketches of New South Wales* (London: William Clowes and Sons, 1844).

Milman, Francis. *An Enquiry into the source from whence the symptoms of the scurvy and of putrid fevers arise* (London: J. Dodsley, 1782).

Milne, Graeme J. *Trade and Traders in Mid-Victorian Liverpool* (Liverpool: Liverpool University Press, 2000).

Murphy, Michelle. *Sick Building Syndrome and the Problem of Uncertainty* (Durham, NC: Duke University Press, 2006).

Nadel, George. *Australia's Colonial Culture* (Cambridge, MA: Harvard University Press, 1957).

Neal, David. *The Rule of Law in a Penal Colony: Law and Power in Early Colonial New South Wales* (Cambridge: Cambridge University Press, 1991).

Neal, Frank. 'Liverpool, the Irish Steam Ship Companies and the Famine Irish', *Immigrants and Minorities* (1986), pp. 28–61.

Nicholas, Stephen (ed.) *Convict Workers, Reinterpreting Australia's Past* (Cambridge: Cambridge University Press, 1988).

O'Brien, Anne. 'Kitchen Fragments and Garden Stuff: Poor Law discourse and indigenous people in early colonial New South Wales', *Australian Historical Studies* 39 (2008), pp. 150–66.

O'Brien, Gerard, 'The New Poor Law in Pre-famine Ireland', *Irish Economic and Social History* 12 (1985), pp. 33–48.

O'Connor, Erin. *Raw Material: Producing Pathology in Victorian Culture* (Durham and London: Duke University Press, 2003).

O'Farrell, Patrick. 'Lost in Transit: Australian reaction to the Irish and Scots famines, 1845–50', in Patrick O'Sullivan (ed.) *The Meaning of the Famine: The Irish World Wide*, Vol. 6 (Leicester: Leicester University Press, 1997), pp. 126–139.

Ó Gráda, Cormac. *Black '47 and Beyond: The Great Irish Famine in History, Economy and Memory* (Princeton: Princeton University Press, 2000).

Oxley, Deborah. *Convict Maids: The Forced Migration of Women to Australia* (Cambridge: Cambridge University Press, 1996).

Paterson, D. *A Treatise on the Scurvy, Containing a New and Effectual Method of Curing That Disease; and the Cause and Indications of Cure, Deduced from Practice; And Observations Connected with the subject* (Edinburgh: Manners & Miller, 1795).

Paul, G.O. *Observations on the Alarming Progress of the Gaol or Typhus Fever* (Gloucester: D. Walker and Sons, 1817).

Pickford, James H. *Hygiene, or, Health as Depending upon the Conditions of the Atmosphere, Foods and Drinks, Motion and Rest, Sleep and Wakefulness, Secretions, Excretions and Retentions, Mental Emotions, Clothing, Bathing, &c.* (London: Churchill, 1858).

Pickstone, John. 'Ferriar's Fever to Kay's Cholera: Disease and social structure in Cottonopolis', *History of Science* 22 (1984), pp. 401–419.

Poovey, Mary. *Making a Social Body: British Cultural Transformation, 1830–1864* (Chicago and London: University of Chicago Press, 1995).

Porter, Dorothy and Roy Porter. 'The Politics of Prevention: Anti-vaccinationism and public health in nineteenth-century England', *Medical History* 32 (1988), pp. 231–252.

Powell, J.M. 'Medical Promotion and the Consumptive Immigrant to Australia', *Geographical Review* 63:4 (1973), pp. 449–476.

Pringle, John. *Observations on the Nature and Cure of Hospital and Jayl-Fevers* (London: A. Millar & D. Wilson, 1750).

Rediker, Marcus. *Between the Devil and the Deep Blue Sea* (Cambridge: Cambridge University Press, 1989).

Rediker, Marcus and Peter Linebaugh. *The Many-headed Hydra: The Hidden History of the Revolutionary Atlantic* (Boston: Beacon Press, 2000).

Rees, Sian. *The Floating Brothel: the Extraordinary True Story of an Eighteenth-century Ship and its Cargo of Female Convicts* (New York: Hyperion, 2002).

Reid, Kirsty. *Gender, Crime and Empire: Convicts, Settlers and the State in Early Colonial Australia* (Manchester: Manchester University Press, 2007).

Reverby, Susan M. '"Normal exposure" and Inoculation Syphilis: a PHS "Tuskegee" doctor in Guatemala, 1946–1948', *Journal of Policy History* 23 (2011), pp. 6–28.

Reynolds, Henry. *An Indelible Stain?* (Ringwood, Victoria: Viking, 2001).

Richards, Eric. 'How Did Poor People Emigrate from the British Isles to Australia in the Nineteenth Century?', *Journal of British Studies* 32:3 (1993), pp. 250–279.

Richardson, Ruth. *Death, Dissection and the Destitute* (London: Penguin Books, 1989).

Riehl, H. *Tropical Meteorology* (London: McGraw Hill, 1954).

Risse, Guenter. '"Typhus Fever" in Eighteenth Century Hospitals: New approaches to medical treatment', *Bulletin of the History of Medicine* 59:2 (1985), pp. 176–195.

Risse, Guenter. 'Britannia Rules the Seas: The health of seamen, Edinburgh, 1791–1800', *Journal of the History of Medicine and Allied Sciences* 43 (1988), pp. 426–446.

Ritchie, John. 'Towards Ending an Unclean Thing: The Molesworth Committee and the abolition of transportation to New South Wales, 1837–1840', *Historical Studies (Melbourne)* 17:3 (1976), pp. 144–164.

Roe, Michael. *An Imperial Disaster: The Wreck of the George III* (Hobart: Blubberhead Press, 2006).

Rosenberg, Charles E. *The Cholera Years: The United States in 1832, 1849 and 1866* (Chicago: University of Chicago Press, 1962).

Rosenberg, Charles. 'The Therapeutic Revolution: Medicine, meaning and social change in nineteenth-century America', in Morris Vogel and Charles Rosenberg (eds) *The Therapeutic Revolution: Essays in the Social History of American Medicine* (Philadelphia: University of Pennsylvania Press, 1979), pp. 3–25.

Rousseau, George S. and David Boyd Haycock. 'Coleridge's Choleras: Cholera morbus, Asiatic cholera and dysentery in early nineteenth-century England', *Bulletin of the History of Medicine* 77:2 (2003), pp. 298–331.

Royal Jennerian Society. *Yearly Report* (London: John Westley and Co., 1830).

Sankey, Francis F. *Familiar Instructions in Medicine and Surgery, with Observations on the Means of Maintaining the Health of Men on Ship Board, or when Employed in Unhealthy Localities* (London: Parker, Furnivall, and Parker, 1846).

Scally, Robert. 'Liverpool Ships and Irish Emigrants in the Age of Sail', *Journal of Social History* 17:1 (1983), pp. 5–30.

Shaw, A.G.L. *Convicts and the Colonies* (London: Faber and Faber, 1966).

Shaw, A.G.L. *A History of Port Phillip District: Victoria before Separation* (Melbourne: Melbourne University Press, 2003).

Smith, A.E. *Colonists in Bondage: White Servitude and Convict Labour in America, 1607–1776* (Gloucester, MA: Peter Smith, 1965).

Smith, Babette. *Cargo of Women* (Kensington, NSW: New South Wales University Press, 1992).

Smith, Dale C. 'Medical Science, Medical Practice and the Emerging Concept of Typhus in Mid-eighteenth Century Britain', in W.F. Bynum and Vivien Nutton (eds), *Theories of Fever from Antiquity to the Enlightenment* (London: Wellcome Institute for the History of Medicine, 1981), pp. 121–134.

Stoler, Ann Laura and Frank Cooper. 'Between Metropole and Colony:

Rethinking a research agenda', in *Tensions of Empire: Colonial Cultures in a Bourgeois World* (Berkeley and Los Angeles: University of California Press, 1997), pp. 1–56.

Sutton, Samuel. *An Historical Account of a New Method for Extracting the Foul Air out of Ships &c* (London: J. Brindley, 1745).

Sweetser, William. *A Treatise on Consumption; Embracing an Inquiry into the Influence Exerted upon it by Journeys, Voyages and Changes of Climate* (Boston: T.H. Carter, 1836).

Thackrah, Charles Turner. *The Effects of Arts, Trades and Professions … On Health and Longevity: With Suggestions for the removal of many of the Agents which produce disease and shorten the duration of life … Second Edition, Greatly Enlarged* (London: Longman, Rees, Orme, Brown, Green, & Longman, 1832).

Thomas, E.G. 'The Old Poor Law and Medicine', *Medical History* 24 (1980), pp. 1–19.

Thomson, Frederick. *An Essay on the Scurvy: Shewing Effectual and Practicable Means for its Prevention at Sea. With some observations on Fevers, and proposals for the More Effectual Preservation of the Health of Seamen* (London: G.G.J. & J. Robinson, 1790).

Thomson, T.R.H. 'On The Value of Quinine in African Remittent Fever', *The Lancet* (28 February 1846), pp. 244–245.

Trotter, Thomas. *Observations on the Scurvy* (London: J.S. Jordan, 1795).

Trotter, Thomas. *Medicina Nautica*, 3 vols (London: Longman, Hurst, Rees, and Orme, 1797–1804).

Trotter, Thomas. *A View of the Nervous Temperament* (London: Wright, Goodenow, & Stockwell, 1808).

Tuckey, James Hingston. *An Account of a Voyage to Establish a Colony at Port Philip in Bass Strait* (London: Longman, Hurst, Rees, and Orme, 1805).

Turnbull, William. *The Naval Surgeon; Comprising the Entire Duties of Professional Men at Sea* (London: R. Phillips, 1806).

Ulrich, Laurel Thatcher. *A Midwife's Tale: The Life of Martha Ballard, Based on Her Diary, 1785–1812* (New York: Vintage Books, 1991).

van Vugt, William E. *Britain to America: Mid-nineteenth-century Immigration to the United States* (Urbana: University of Illinois Press, 1999).

Vickery, Amanda. 'An Englishman's Home Is His Castle? Thresholds, boundaries and privacies in the eighteenth-century London house', *Past and Present* 199 (May 2008), pp. 147–173.

Vink, Marcus. 'Indian Ocean Studies and the "New Thalassology"', *Journal of Global History* 2:1 (2007), pp. 41–62.

Wallace, Alfred Russel. *The Wonderful Century: Its Successes and Failures* (Toronto: George N. Morang, 1898).

Walton, John K. *The English Seaside Resort: A Social History, 1750–1914* (Leicester: Leicester University Press, 1983).

Ward, Kerry. *Networks of Empire: Forced Migration in the Dutch East India Company* (Cambridge and New York: Cambridge University Press, 2009).

Waugh, David Lindsay. *Three Years Practical Experience of a Settler in New South Wales; being extracts from letters to his friends in Edinburgh, from 1834–1837*, 8th edn, with a map (Edinburgh: John Johnstone, 1838).

Wellings, Henry P. 'Imlay, George (1794? –1846)', *Australian Dictionary of Biography*, Volume 2, (Melbourne: Melbourne University Press, 1967), pp. 2–3.

Willmer, George. *The Draper in Australia* (London: Freeman, 1856).

Wilson, William S. *The Ocean as a Health Resort* (London: J. & A. Churchill, 1880).

Worboys, Michael. 'Germs, Malaria and the Invention of Mansonian Tropical Medicine: From "diseases in the tropics" to "tropical diseases"', in David Arnold, *Warm Climates and Western Medicine'* (Amsterdam: Rodopi, 1996) pp. 181–207.

Zoli, Corri. 'Black Holes of Calcutta and London: Internal colonies in Vanity Fair', *Victorian Literature and Culture* 35 (2007), pp. 417–449.

Zuckerman, Arnold. 'Scurvy and the Ventilation of Ships in the Royal Navy: Samuel Sutton's contribution', *Eighteenth Century Studies* 10:2 (1976–77), pp. 222–234.

Index